IMMUNOLOGIC PHYLOGENY

ADVANCES IN EXPERIMENTAL MEDICINE AND BIOLOGY

IMMUNOLOGIC PHYLOGENY

Edited by

W. H. Hildemann

Hilo College
University of Hawaii
Hilo, Hawaii

and

A. A. Benedict

University of Hawaii at Manoa
Honolulu, Hawaii

SPRINGER SCIENCE+BUSINESS MEDIA, LLC

Library of Congress Cataloging in Publication Data

International Conference on Immunologic Phylogeny, University of Hawaii, 1975.
Immunologic phylogeny.

(Advances in experimental medicine and biology; v. 64)
Includes bibliographical references and index.
1. Immunotaxonomy—Congresses. 2. Immunology, Comparative—Congresses. I.
Hildemann, W. H., 1927-   II. Benedict, Albert Alfred, 1921-   III. Hawaii.
University. IV. Title. V. Series.
QR183.8.I57 1975   591.2'9   75-35524

Proceedings of the International Conference on Immunologic Phylogeny
held at the University of Hawaii, Manoa and Hilo campuses, June 11-14, 1975

© 1975 Springer Science+Business Media New York
Originally Published by Plenum Press, New York in 1975
Softcover reprint of the hardcover 1st edition 1975

Preface

There are two now classic reasons for the widespread and continuing interest in the phylogeny of immune reactivities and structure. First is the fundamental concern of biologists with the evolution of defense mechanisms. We are eager to discover origins, mechanisms, and adaptive specializations of immunocompetence because the very existence of individuals and entire species is involved in a most essential way. Second is the strong biomedical interest in adaptive immune mechanisms to increase understanding of health and disease in man. If man and placental mammals represent the quintessence of immunoresponsiveness with complex interdependent pathways, the less elaborate but fully functional systems of immunity in "lower" animals proffer insights applicable to immediate concerns in medicine. Recent approaches to organ transplantation, immunotherapy of cancer and repair of immunodeficiency diseases, to name just a few areas, have depended greatly on phylogenetic perspectives. In a larger sense, intelligent wildlife conservation, utilization of food resources, and adequate environmental protection all hinge on knowing how diverse species survive or otherwise succumb to insults, injuries, and disease.

The phylogenetic immunologist also seeks detailed information on the structure of the immunoglobulins which relates directly to the evolutionary history of living animals. Perhaps genetic mechanisms responsible for the evolution of these proteins may be revealed as spin-off information. The vast number of immunoglobulin specificities and effector structures, coupled with the remarkable phylogenetic conservation of certain polypeptide regions, makes these molecules especially useful to protein chemists as well as immunologists.

Although many still talk glibly about higher and lower animals as if a hierarchy of superior versus relatively inferior functions were being classified, the immunologic phylogeneticist already knows better. The lower animals, including invertebrates of course, have a much longer history of coping successfully with a myriad of potentially infectious and pathogenic agents in every conceivable habitat.

Several major new insights are emerging from studies presented at this conference on Immunologic Phylogeny. Different levels of recognition and reaction to foreign agents are now discernible in phylogenetic progression all the way from coelenterates to mammals. The immune systems of advanced vertebrates may represent highly specialized versions of more general systems of receptors and mediators. Recent findings summarized in this monograph indicate that immunologic specificity and memory may both be viewed as adaptively evolving characteristics.

Cell-mediated immunity associated with so-called T-cell functions is evident in advanced invertebrates and surely precedes in phylogeny the B-cell immunoglobulin production first detectable in primitive fishes. Integrated cellular and humoral antibody immunity as shown by helper T-lymphocyte and B-lymphocyte cooperation is demonstrable in advanced bony fishes. At this level, two distinct molecular classes of immunoglobulins are also first discernible. Much still remains to be discovered about the structure and functions of vertebrate antibodies. At the level of primitive fishes (i.e., cyclostomes or agnathans), even the essential polypeptide composition of the apparently singular immunoglobulin remains in doubt. Indeed, the homology of non-mammalian immunoglobulins to those of mammals cannot be made until covalent structures are revealed.

Complex immunoregulation now being extensively studied in certain birds and mammals appears to depend upon selective synthesis of multiple molecular classes and subclasses of immunoglobulins. Parallel specialization of T-cell functions may also be characteristic of these advanced vertebrates. However, earlier manifestations of immunoreactivity (e.g., mitogen and allogeneic responsiveness, transplantation immunity, tumor immunity) seem to have been retained during progressive evolution and diversification of immunocyte functions. Although the generalization that invertebrates lack specific immunologic capability must now be rejected, assumption of a continuous phylogenetic progression in immune mechanisms extending from primitive invertebrates to advanced vertebrates is surely debatable. Many information gaps remain at all levels of phylogeny!

The immunologic phylogenist or phylogenetic immunologist in 1975 retains two unusual joys as a biological scientist. First is the realization that many orders, classes, and even whole phyla of animals have yet to be studied in any detail by anyone. In other words, it is not too late to become a "founding father" - to put forward and test quite new hypotheses. Second is the realization that with so few workers studying the immunocompetence of any unusual species or group, one can truly enjoy his research with little worry of someone else publishing first on the same topic.

Maybe this is why participants at this conference have been so friendly and communicative. For many of us, this realm of experimental biology is still more pleasure than work.

Finally, the international flavor of the University of Hawaii/ East-West Center surrounded by an ocean rich with "lower" animals was a most appropriate setting for this conference. We are grateful to the East-West Center for use of their fine facilities and to the University of Hawaii Graduate Division for the generous support given to the conference.

A. A. Benedict
University of Hawaii at Manoa

W. H. Hildemann
University of Hawaii at Hilo

June, 1975

Contents

Immunodiscrimination and Integrity of Metazoans

Allogeneic Incompatibility and Transplantation Immunity

Primordial Cell-Mediated Immunity and Memory

VERTEBRATE IMMUNOLOGY

Structure and Functions of Antibodies

Evolution of Lymphoid and Immunocyte Systems

Mitogen Responsiveness, MLC Reactions, and Lymphocyte Heterogeneity

Maturation and Modulation of Immune Functions

Specific Immunoregulation and Histocompatibility Systems

INVERTEBRATE IMMUNOLOGY

Heterophile Precipitins, Protectins, and Agglutinins

TRIDACNIN, A POTENT ANTI-GALACTAN PRECIPITIN FROM THE HEMOLYMPH OF TRIDACNA MAXIMA (RÖDING)

B. A. Baldo and G. Uhlenbruck
Clinical Immunology Unit, Children's Medical Research Fdn.
Princess Margaret Hospital, Subiaco, Western Australia, 6008
and Medical University Clinic, Dept. Immunobiology
Cologne, W. -Germany

INTRODUCTION

In discussing the evolution of the immune process, Burnet (1) stated that invertebrate hemocytes possess at least a limited capacity to recognise foreignness and that agglutinins from body fluids demonstrate pseudo-immunological capacities. This, he concluded, provided the basis from which the more sophisticated antibody system of vertebrates could be developed given strong enough evolutionary forces. Many invertebrate species have been shown to be capable of phagocytosing pathogens and other materials (2) and, although a degree of specificity has been observed in the agglutinins present in the hemolymph of some invertebrates (3), phagocytosis may be the most important defense against infection in the organisms. As pointed out by Hildemann(4), invertebrates have obviously resisted infection for many millions of years without the aid of the more sophisticated adaptive immune mechanisms found in vertebrates. The ability to recognise and distinguish self from foreignness is a characteristic of all animal species and this capacity is well developed in invertebrates (4). Two good examples of this capacity amongst the invertebrates are the aggregation of sponge cells (5) and the species specificity demonstrated by fusing tunicate colonies (6). Specific interactions such as these appear to be due to glycoproteins on the cell surfaces (7, 8) and, as suggested by Marchalonis and Cone (9), vertebrate immunological mechanisms may have evolved from such invertebrate recognition phenomena.

We have approached the problem of recognition in immunology by examining some of the highly active agglutinins which can be extracted from

3

a number of invertebrates including clams, snails and sponges. Just as a knowledge of the specificities of antibodies is often necessary for an understanding of the specific functions of the vertebrate immune mechanisms, it also seems important to become thoroughly familiar with the specificities of the invertebrate agglutinins if their biological role is to be elucidated. Various suggestions have been made as to the function of these agglutinins including their participation in immune-like defense mechanisms, symbiotic relationships, cell-cell recognition in fertilization and embryogenesis and the trapping of nutritional components (10) but, the question must be considered to be still open to speculation.

We now present some of our preliminary studies on tridacnin (11), a potent anti-galactan precipitin found in the hemolymph of the elongate clam, Tridacna maxima (Röding) (12). In this report, emphasis has been placed on the purification and specificity data obtained so far.

REACTION OF T. MAXIMA HEMOLYMPH WITH PREPARATIONS OF
DIFFERENT ORIGIN

T. maxima hemolymph contains a potent natural agglutinin which, in the presence of Ca^{++}, possesses both hemagglutinating (HA) and precipitating activities. The agglutinin, which we have termed tridacnin (11), agglutinates erythrocytes and other cells from a variety of animal species and precipitates with a number of glycopeptides, galactans and other polysaccharides. Using inhibition of tridacnin-induced HA of human erythrocytes, gel diffusion and quantitative precipitin methods, we have found that tridacnin reacts with a wide range of preparations from vertebrates, invertebrates, plants and microorganisms (13, Baldo and Uhlenbruck, unpublished). Figs. 1 and 2 clearly demonstrate the potency of the precipitin reactions which are observed between T. maxima hemolymph and some polysaccharide-containing solutions. For example, T. maxima hemolymph containing only 9.6 μgN precipitates approximately 7 μgN when mixed with 20 μg of larch galactan (Fig. 2). Other preparations which react with T. maxima hemolymph include bovine erythrocyte and pig amnion mucoids, human serum, human milk and saliva (Fig. 1a), a number of invertebrate preparations including polysaccharide extracts from Lymnaea stagnalis (Fig. 1b), Ascaris lumbricoides, Lumbricus terrestris and house dust mites, plant arabinogalactans, pneumococcus type XIV polysaccharide (Fig. 1b) and a purified polysaccharide from the yeast Torulopsis groppengresseri. A number of preparations which react with tridacnin contain terminal 0-ß-D-Galp-(1-6)-D-Gal structures (13-16) and in this respect, tridacnin resembles certain mouse myeloma proteins (15, 16).

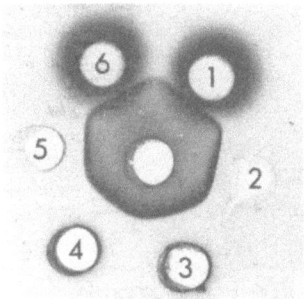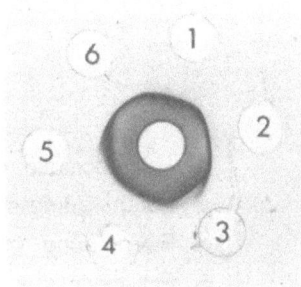

Fig. 1. Agar gel diffusion patterns formed from the reaction of
Tridacna maxima hemolymph extract with some polysaccharides, glycopeptides and human saliva and milk. Center wells: T. maxima extract
202 μg N/ml. Peripheral wells: a. 1 and 6. Human group A_1 secretor
milk. 2. Hog H blood group substance 0.8 mg/ml. 3 and 4. Human
group 0 secretor saliva. 5. Human H blood group substance 0.9 mg/ml.
b. 1 and 4. Pomacea urceus galactan 1.8 mg/ml. 2. Helix pomatia
galactan 1 mg/ml. 3. Pneumococcus type XIV polysaccharide 1.1 mg/ml.
5. Bovine lung galactan 1 mg/ml. 6. Lymnaea stagnalis galactan
1 mg/ml.

PURIFICATION OF TRIDACNIN

Experiments have shown that tridacnin can be isolated in high yield
from the hemolymph by a number of simple affinity chromatography techniques. Experiments with Sepharose 2B, 4B and 6B (Pharmacia, Uppsala)
and acid-treated Sepharose 2B, 4B and 6B, have demonstrated that the
degree of cross-linkage on these polymers is important in the ability of
tridacnin to react with these insoluble supports. In the presence of Ca^{++},
some purified agglutinin can be isolated from Sepharose 2B but little or
no reaction occurs with Sepharose 4B and Sepharose 6B (Baldo and Uhlenbruck, unpublished). Acid treatment of the polymers, however, (17) gives
a product which readily reacts with the agglutinin. Fig. 3 shows the result
of a typical experiment in which tridacnin was isolated from whole hemolymph on a column of acid-treated Sepharose 6B. This increased reactivity after acid treatment of the cross-linked gel presumably results from
an increased number of end groups being exposed and thus becoming available for reaction with the agglutinin. Adsorbed agglutinin is easily eluted
from the columns by the addition of N-acetyl-D-galactosamine (0.025 M)
or lactose (0.1 M) giving yields of at least 20% purified agglutinin from
whole hemolymph. Tridacnin can also be isolated in high yield from columns of the product formed from the copolymerization of larch arabino-
galactan with the N-carboxyanhydride of L-leucine (11).

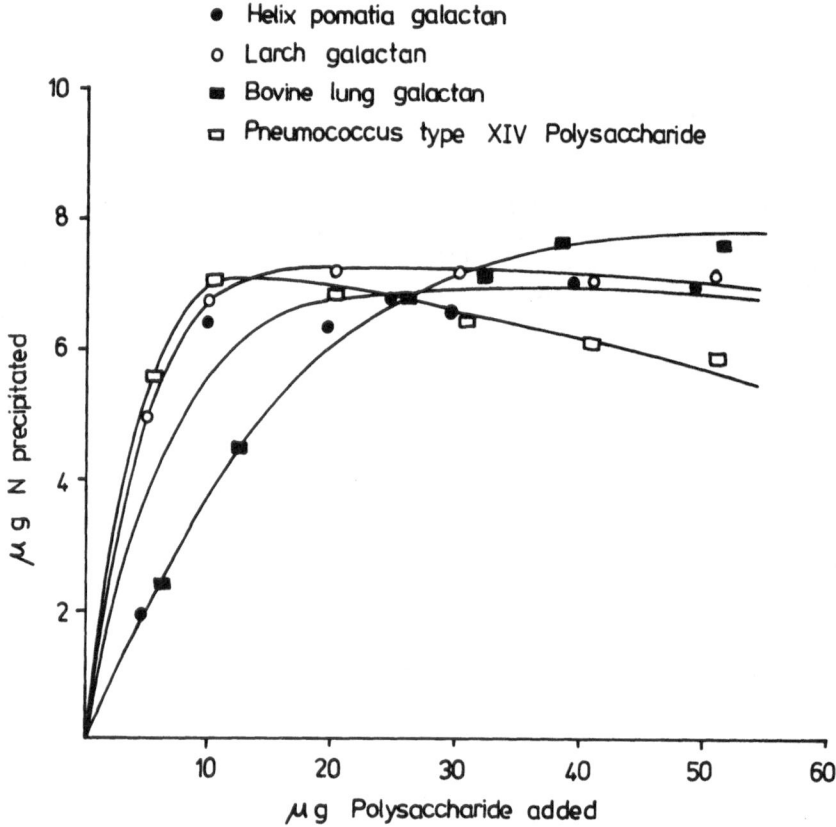

Fig. 2. Precipitation of some galactans and purified pneumococcus
type XIV polysaccharide by <u>Tridacna</u> <u>maxima</u> hemolymph extract: 25 μl,
9.6 μg N was added to tubes containing increasing amounts of the
following preparations: <u>Helix</u> <u>pomatia</u> galactan (●), larch galactan
(o), bovine lung galactan (▬), pneumococcus type XIV polysaccharide
(▭). Total volume 135 μl.

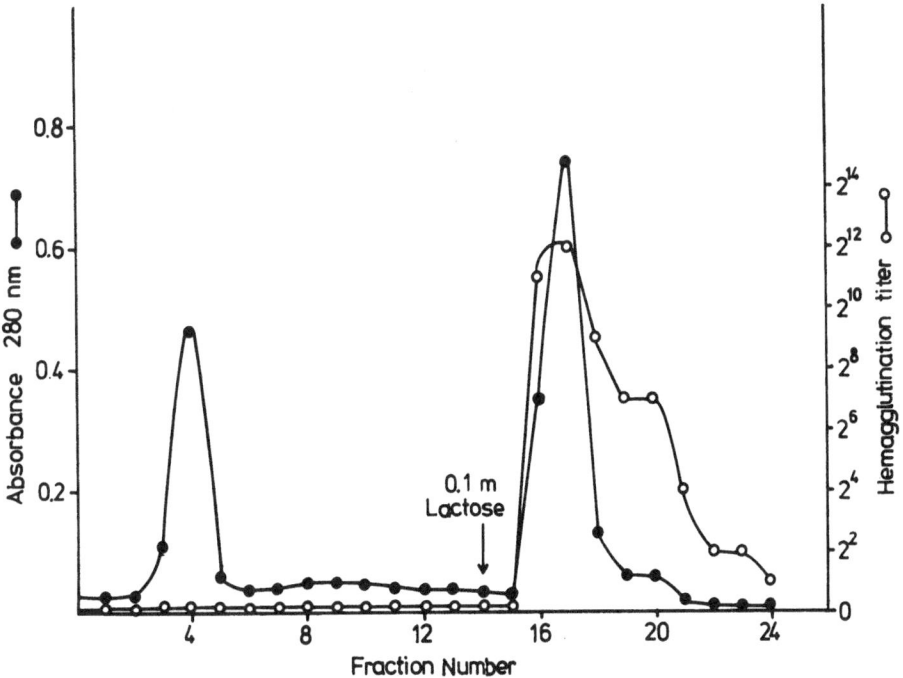

Fig. 3. Isolation of tridacnin from an acid-treated Sepharose 6B
column (1 x 26 cm). Lyophilized Tridacna maxima hemolymph (10 mg
in 1 ml) was applied to a column of Sepharose 6B which had previously
been treated with 0.2 M HCl for 2 hours at 50°C. Column washed with
saline containing 0.01 M Ca^{++} and then eluted (tube 15) with 0.1 M
lactose. Each fraction was examined for protein (•) by measuring
the absorbance at 280 nm and for its (o) HA activity against human
group 0 erythrocytes. Yield purified agglutinin, 2.1 mg.

SPECIFICITY STUDIES

Of the sugars tested so far, N-acetyl-D-galactosamine has been found
to be the best inhibitor of tridacnin in both hemagglutination inhibition and
quantitative precipitin inhibition experiments (18, Baldo and Uhlenbruck,
in preparation). Inhibition was also observed with some other sugars but
in all cases good inhibitors were found to have a D-galacto configuration
(Table 1). p-Nitrophenyl-ß-D-galactoside was a better inhibitor than
p-nitrophenyl-α-D-galactoside and lactose proved a more potent inhibitor
than melibiose, raffinose and stachyose, each of which contain α-linked
D-galactose. On a molar basis, lactose was approximately nine times as
effective an inhibitor as melibiose and raffinose and approximately twenty
times as effective as stachyose. These results indicate that the Tridacna
lectin shows a preference for ß-anomeric linkages.

B. A. BALDO AND G. UHLENBRUCK

Table 1. Inhibition of T. maxima Extract-Induced Hemagglutination and Precipitation by D-Galactose and some Derivatives of D-Galactose.

Test Substance	Result using		
	Hemagglutination Inhibition [a]		Quantitative Precipitin Inhibition [b]
	mg/ml	μmole/ml	μmoles
D-galactose	5.0	27.7	0.52
D-galactosamine HCl	5.0	23.2	0.27
Lactose	2.5	7.3	0.36
N-acetyl-D-galactosamine	0.3	1.4	0.017
p-Nitrophenyl ß-D-galactopyranoside	2.5	8.3	0.15
p-Nitrophenyl ∝-D-galactopyranoside	13.0	43.1	1.9
p-Nitrophenyl 2-acetamido-2-deoxy-ß-D-galactopyranoside	0.4-0.8	1.2-2.4	N.T.

[a] Minimum concentration completely inhibiting the agglutination of human group 0 erythrocytes by 8 HA doses of T. maxima extract.

[b] Amount of inhibitor needed for 50 per cent inhibition of the precipitation between T. maxima and pneumococcus type XIV polysaccharide.

N. T. = Not tested.

PROPERTIES OF TRIDACNIN

Isoelectric focusing in gel (Fig. 4) and disc gel electrophoresis at
pH 8.9 showed that more than one component was present in the immuno-
adsorbent-purified tridacnin. This result is similar to findings with the
agglutinin isolated from the mollusc Helix pomatia (19). On Sephadex
G-200 gel filtration, whole T. maxima hemolymph shows only 2 peaks
one of which elutes at the void volume of the column. HA activity occurs
throughout the gel profile. This result, and the finding of heavily stained
material at the top of 5 per cent and 7 per cent polyacrylamide disc gels
indicates that at least some of the purified agglutinin consists of high MW
material. Studies of the structure of tridacnin are now in progress and
preliminary results have shown that mercaptoethanol treatment produces
subunits which migrate freely into 7 per cent acrylamide gels (Baldo and
Uhlenbruck, unpublished).

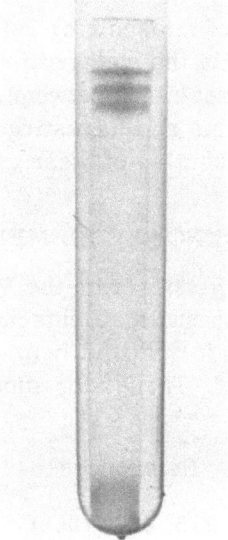

Fig. 4. Gel isoelectric focusing pattern obtained with immuno-
adsorbent-purified tridacnin. Tridacnin, 25 μg used with gel
consisting of 4.6 per cent acrylamide and 3 per cent ampholytes
pH 3-10. The 3 bands focused in the pH range 3.9-4.3. Gel stained
with Coumassie blue.

FUTURE WORK

Further work is needed to more fully characterize the potent precipitating anti-galactan found in T. maxima hemolymph but the data already obtained may even now help in studies designed to investigate the biological role of the agglutinin. The anti-galactan properties of tridacnin may, for example, play a part in the symbiotic relationship between Tridacna and Gymnodinium microadriaticum algae or in the utilization of plankton. In this connection it may be worth mentioning that most of these organisms contain galactans or arabinogalactans within their cell walls as an integrated constituent. For instance we have found in collaboration with the Max Planck Institute for Plant Breeding in Cologne-Vogelsang, that chloroplsts or certain subcellular particles from plant sources (thylacoids) can be agglutinated or precipitated by tridacnin. Thus, tridacnin may provide a valuable tool not only for studying and influencing metabolic processes in plants, but also, after appropriate labelling, for investigating the localization of galactans within the membrane mosaic structure. Furthermore, the injection of galactans from different origin, which are very easily available, into the hemolymph or organs of tridacnids should provide us with an experimental model for elucidating the biological role of this precipitin. In addition, we intend to investigate several other tridacnids for the occurrence of tridacnin or related agglutinins or precipitins and to compare them with the composition of the respective photosynthetic algae. Also crossreactions between different tridacnins - "isotridacnins" - may then become an interesting research project, which can show us the way to the function of these antibody-like substances.

ACKNOWLEDGEMENTS

This study was aided by grants from the Princess Margaret Children´s Medical Research Foundation and the Deutsche Forschungsgemeinschaft. We thank Gisela Steinhausen for skillful help, Jill Butler for expert technical assistance and Dr. K.J. Turner for support.

References

1. Burnet, F.M., Nature, 218: 426 (1968)
2. Grey, H.M., Adv. Immunol., 10: 51 (1969)
3. McKay, D. and Jenkin, C.R., Aust. J. Exp. Biol. Med. Sci., 48: 139 (1970)
4. Hildemann,W.H., Life Sciences, 14: 605 (1974)
5. Humphreys, T.D., Transplant. Proc., 2: 194 (1970)
6. Oka, H. and Watanabe, H., Bull. Biol. Asamushi, 10: 153 (1960)

7. Margoliash, E. , Schenck, J. R. , Hargie, M. P. , Burokas, S. , Richter, W. R. , Barlow, G. H. and Moscona, A. A. , Biochem. Biophys. Res. Commun. , 20: 383 (1965)

8. Henkart, P. , Humphreys, S. and Humphreys, T. , Biochemistry, 12: 3045 (1973)

9. Marchalonis, J. J. and Cone, R. E. , Aust. J. Exp. Biol. Med. Sci. , 51: 461 (1973)

10. Uhlenbruck, G. , Dahr, W. , Rothe, A. and Baldo, B. A. , Forschungsberichte NRW, No. 2475, Westdeutscher Verlag, Opladen, FRG, (1974)

11. Baldo, B. A. and Uhlenbruck, G. , FEBS Letters, in press (1975)

12. Rosewater, J. , The Indo-Pacific Mollusca, 1: 347 (1965)

13. Uhlenbruck, G. , Baldo, B. A. and Steinhausen, G. , Z. Immunforsch. , in press (1975)

14. Baldo, B. A. and Uhlenbruck, G. , Immunology, in press (1975)

15. Eichmann, K. , Uhlenbruck, G. and Baldo, B. A. , Immunochemistry, submitted for publication (1975)

16. Glaudemans, C. P. J. , Jolley, M. E. and Potter, M. , Carbohydr. Res. , 30: 409 (1973)

17. Ersson, B. , Aspberg, K. and Porath, J. , Biochim. Biophys. Acta, 310: 446 (1973)

18. Baldo, B. A. and Uhlenbruck, G. , Carbohydr. Res. , 40: 143 (1975)

19. Hammarström, S. and Kabat, E. A. , Biochemistry 8: 2696 (1969)

ANTI-GALACTAN PRECIPITINS IN THE HEMOLYMPH OF TRIDACNA MAXIMA AND LIMULUS POLYPHEMUS

E. Cohen, B.A. Baldo and G. Uhlenbruck

Roswell Park Memorial Institute, Buffalo, NY, USA
PMH, The University of Western Australia, Subiaco, W.A. 6008
Medical University Clinic, Cologne, W. Germany

In the course of our investigations on the anti-neuraminyl-specificity of the hemagglutinin from the hemolymph of the horseshoe crab Limulus polyphemus (Cohen et al., 1972; Cohen, 1968), we included the hemolymph of this living fossil also in our experiments, dealing with the occurrence and distribution of blood group A like active structures in nature as detected by the heterophile anti-N-acetyl-D-galactosamine agglutinin/precipitin from the albumin gland of the snail Helix pomatia (see Prokop et al., 1974).

In this case we found, using the agargel diffusion technique, a strong precipitin reaction between the Limulus hemolymph on the one side, and the snail albumin gland extract on the other side. However, it soon turned out, quite unexpectedly and very surprising to us, that this precipitin reaction was not due to the presence of blood group A like structures in the hemolymph of Limulus polyphemus, but has to be considered as a reaction between a precipitin in the hemolymph of the horseshoe crab and a component in the albumin gland of the snail. This component subsequently could be identified and characterized by us as galactan (Voigtmann, Salfner and Uhlenbruck, 1971). So for the first time an anti-galactan reagent has been described.

Independently, in 1972, another group of anti-galactans has been found by Potter and his associates, the specificity of which was thought to be directed towards the O-ß-D-galactopyranosido-(1-6)-D-galactose configuration of the bovine lung galactan. This group of anti-galactans was represented by certain mouse myeloma IgA proteins.

The next step was again done by our team in so far as we discovered
that certain heterophile antibody-like proteins from plant and other sources, showing anti-"H"-like blood group specificity, strongly reacted with
certain galactans, obviously this could be attributed to the terminal, non-
reducing bound ß-L-galactosido and L-fucopyranosido structures. Interesting also was the reaction of catfish "anti-H" and the crossreaction of
Pneumococcus Type XIV antiserum (anti-S-XIV) from horse with snail
and pneumogalactan. Remarkable in this connection, too, is the other
crossreaction between Mycoplasma galactan and pneumogalactan (see also Table 1).

In our search for additional anti-galactans in the world of invertebrates, in order to elucidate their physiological function or to find an explanation for their biological role (symbiosis with algae?, defense mechanisms?), we discovered a most potent anti-galactan in the hemolymph of
the clam Tridacna maxima Röding (for references see Table 1). It reacted very strongly with quite a number of different galactans and agglutinated a number of red cells, bacteria, microorganisms, lymphocytes, sper-
matozoa, and plant particles. In fact, when taking all results together, a
new field in the "Immunochemistry" of polysaccharides - anti-polysaccha-
rides has been opened and recently summarized in form of a monography
(Uhlenbruck, Steinhausen and Baldo, 1975). Bretting and Renwrantz, in
collaborating with us, found another, very similar anti-galactan in the
more primitive Axinella sponge (see Table 1).

By a newly developed comparatative and competitive precipitation method, we were then able to demonstrate that obviously the combining specificities of mouse myeloma IgA, Tridacnin and the Axinella precipitin
were nearly identical, in so far as they all precipitated with substances
containing the same immunodeterminant structure, namely the terminal
Digalactobiose O-ß-D-galactopyranosido-(1-6)-D-galactosido residue.
For this disaccharide, which we have also isolated from vertebrate
sources (bovine red cell mucoid, Uhlenbruck 1964), we propose the name
Digalactobiose I. According to all our experiments (Eichmann, Uhlenbruck and Baldo, 1975), this anti-digalactobiose I specificity of the Tri-
dacnin/Axinella/Myelom Type seems now to be confirmed and established.

The reaction of eel serum is understandable on the basis of the occurrence of L-fucose and L-galactose in the respective galactans (see
Table 1). The same holds for the other heterophile antibodies (Table 1,
II, 3) and the lectins listed under III in Table 1. It is noteworthy that also some immune antibodies do react with the galactofuranosyl structure
which plays a role in some galactans or galactomannans in microorga-
nism (for review see Uhlenbruck, Steinhausen and Baldo, 1975).

Table 1. Anti-Galactans and Galactans from Different Sources:
Suggested Mode of Interaction

Classification of Anti-Galactans	Proposed Combining Specificities	MG	SG	PG	AG	Refer.
I. Invertebrates						
1. Tridacna clam	ß-D-galp(1-6)-D-galp	0	++	++	++	1-6
2. Axinella sponge	ß-D-galp(1-6)-D-galp	0	++	++	++	3, 7
3. Horseshoe crab	ß-D-galp(1-3)-D-galp	0	++	-	-	8, 9
II. Vertebrates						
1. eel serum	∝, ß-L-fucp, ß-L-galp	0	++	-	-	10,11
2. mouse myeloma	ß-D-galp(1-6)-D-galp	0	++	++	++	4,12,13
3. Immune antibodies						
a. camel	ß-D-galf(1-6)-D-galp	++	0	++	0	15
b. sheep	ß-D-galf(1-2)-D-manp	++	0	0	0	16,17
c. catfish	∝, ß-L-fucp-, ß-L-galp	0	++	0	0	10
d. anti-S-XIV	ß-D-galp-D-galp	0	++	++	-	5,13
III. Plant Lectins						
1. non-group-specific (Ricinus, Abrus)	ß-D-galp→	+	(++)+	-	-	10,11,18
2. "Anti-H" (Evonymus, Cytisus)	ß-L-galp; ∝, ß-L-fucp	0	+	-	-	10,11

Legends:

0	=	not yet tested
-	=	no reaction
+	=	hemagglutination and hemagglutination inhibition
++	=	visible precipitin reaction
( )	=	very weak reaction
galp	=	galactopyranosido structure
galf	=	galactofuranosido structure
fucp	=	fucopyranosido structure
manp	=	mannopyranosido structure
G	=	galactan
MG	=	microorganism-G (Mycoplasma, Dermatophytes)
SG	=	snail-G (Invertebrate-G)
PG	=	Pneumo-G (Vertebrate-G)
AG	=	Arabino-G (Plant-G)

References to Table 1:   ( ) indicates running number under "References"

 1 = Baldo and Uhlenbruck, 1975   (11)
 2 = Uhlenbruck, Dahr, Rothe and Baldo, 1974   (12)
 3 = Eichmann, Uhlenbruck and Baldo, 1975   (9)
 4 = Uhlenbruck, Steinhausen, Baldo and Kareem, 1975   (13)
 5 = Uhlenbruck, Steinhausen and Baldo, 1975   (6)
 6 = Uhlenbruck, Steinhausen, Gauwerky, Baldo and Renwrantz, 1975 (14)
 7 = Bretting and Renwrantz, 1974   (7)
 8 = Voigtmann, Salfner and Uhlenbruck, 1971   (4)
 9 = this paper here first report
10 = Baldo and Uhlenbruck, 1973   (15)
11 = Baldo, Uhlenbruck and Salfner, 1974   (16)
12 = Potter, Mushinski and Glaudemans, 1972   (5)
13 = Glaudemans, Jolley and Potter, 1973   (17)
14 = Glaudemans, Zissis and Jolley, 1975   (18)
15 = Kakoma and Kinyanjui, 1974   (19)
16 = Grappel, Blank and Bishop, 1968; 1969   (20)
17 = Shifrine and Gourlay, 1965   (21)
18 = Schiefer, Gerhardt, Brunner and Krüpe, 1974   (22)

Although the specificity of the anti-galactan from Tridacna hemolymph, called Tridacnin, clearly seems to be   an anti-digalactobiose I precipitin – with the exception that not all hemagglutination and hemagglutination inhibition study have fully confirmed the combining specificity of this antibody-like substance –, we have some difficulties in giving a correct interpretation for the specificity of the Limulus polyphemus anti-galactan.

From the data we have, however, we may conclude that this precipitin is directed towards another digalactobiose which occurs in some galactans of snail origin and which has the structure of an O-ß-D-galactopyranosido-(1-3)-D-galactose. We suggest to call this second disaccharide Digalactobiose II. The evidence that the Limulus polyphemus precipitin does detect and recognize this structure can be deduced from the following experimental results:

1)   It does not react with structures carrying the Digalactobiose I type. (see Table 1) (For instance AG or PG)

2)   We found that it precipitates only with snail galactans having also the Digalactobiose II structure: Helix pomatia galactan and the one from Lymnaea stagnalis.

3)   It is in its serological behaviour not identical with the heterophile agglutinins and precipitins from eel serum and anti-S-XIV horse serum:
     a)   because of non-identity reaction in agargel diffusion, where nonidentity with Tridacnin also can be observed (Uhlenbruck, Stein-

hausen and Baldo, 1975);

b) because of its quite different erythro-agglutination behaviour (see also next point), preliminary results have indicated that it is not related to the so-called Limulin (anti-neuraminyl-specificity).

4) The same holds for distinguishing it from plant lectins listed in Table 1. Here especially is to note that all these react enhanced with different red blood cells after neuraminidase treatment, whereas total Limulus hemolymph, on the contrary (containing Limulin and this anti-galactan) does not react at all after neuraminidase treatment with erythrocytes from different sources (Cohen et al., 1972) and the original agglutination is completely abolished, as we found. This was actually the first clue to the anti-neuraminyl-specificity of Limulin (Cohen, 1968).

5) It does not react with the T antigen on red cells (O-ß-D-galactosido-(1-3)-N-acetyl-D-galactosamine).

Accordingly, we are left with the conclusion that most probably the precipitin with anti-galactan specificity from the horseshoe crab is also, like the one from Tridacna hemolymph, directed towards a disaccharide structure in the galactan, namely Digalactobiose II, as no other partner seems to be present in the reactive snail galactans and terminal monosaccharides must be excluded as reactants. Is it pure speculation to predict, that in future also a myeloma protein with this same anti-Digalactobiose II specificity will be described?

In conclusion, we may summarize, that in the hemolymph of Tridacna and in the one of Limulus certain precipitins do naturally occur, which are directed against Digalactobiose units of galactans: While Tridacnin may be complementary to Digalactobiose I, the other anti-galactan from Limulus may detect Digalactobiose II. Although these anti-galactans being no immunoglobulins, this combining specificity resembles very closely the one of certain mouse myeloma IgA, which however, as we have observed, do not show any red cell agglutinating properties, even after neuraminidase and protease-treatment this could not be achieved using several sorts of erythrocytes. Therefore one may assume, that the combining sites of both types - myeloma and invertebrate origin - may be very similar but not identical. Probably they may even show crossreactivity with respect to antibodies to their combining sites. These and other questions still await further experimental research (Eichmann et al., to be published; Uhlenbruck, Steinhausen and Baldo, see monography 1975).

This work has been supported by Deutsche Forschungsgemeinschaft.

References:

1. Cohen, E. , Roberts, S.C. , Nordling, S. and Uhlenbruck, G.. Vox. Sang. 23, 300-307 (1972)

2. Cohen, E. Trans. N.Y. Acad. Sci. 30, 427-443 (1968)

3. Prokop, O. , Uhlenbruck, G. , Rothe, A. and Cohen, E. Ann. N.Y. Acad. Sci. 234, 228-231 (1974)

4. Voigtmann, R. , Salfner, B. and Uhlenbruck, G. Z. Immun.-Forsch. 141, 488 (1971)

5. Potter, M.E. , Mushinski, E. and Glaudemans, C.P.J. J. Immunol. 108, 295 (1972)

6. Uhlenbruck, G. , Steinhausen, G. and Baldo, B.A. "Galactane und Anti-Galactane", Verlag Josef Stippak, Aachen, (1975)

7. Bretting, H. and Renwrantz, L. Z. Immun.-Forsch. 147, 250 (1974)

8. Uhlenbruck, G. Z. Immun.-Forsch. 127, 9 (1964)

9. Eichmann, K. , Uhlenbruck, G. and Baldo, B.A. Immunochemistry, in press

10. Eichmann, K. , Uhlenbruck, G. and Baldo, B.A. to be published

11. Baldo, B.A. and Uhlenbruck, G. Carbohydrate Res. 40, 143 (1975)

12. Uhlenbruck, G. , Dahr, W. , Rothe, A. and Baldo, B.A. Forschungsber. NRW, 2475 (1974). Westdeutscher Verlag, Opladen

13. Uhlenbruck, G. , Steinhausen, G. , Baldo, B.A. and Kareem, H.A. Naturwiss., in press

14. Uhlenbruck, G. , Steinhausen, G. , Gauwerky, Ch. , Baldo, B.A. and Renwrantz, L. Biol. Zentralbl. 94, 205 (1975)

15. Baldo, B.A. and Uhlenbruck, G. Immunology 25, 649 (1973)

16. Baldo, B.A. , Uhlenbruck, G. and Salfner, B. Z. Immun.-Forsch. 148, 330 (1975)

17. Glaudemans, C.P.J. , Jolley, M.E. and Potter, M. Carbohydrate Res. 30, 409 (1973)

18. Glaudemans, C.P.J. , Zissis, E. and Jolley, M.E. Carbohydrate Res. 40, 129 (1974)

19. Kakoma, I. and Kinyanjui, Res. vet. Sci. 17, 397 (1974)

20. Grappel, S.F. , Blank, F. and Bishop, T.C. Bacteriol. 95, 1238 (1968)

21. Shifrine, M. and Gourlay, R.N. Nature 208, 498 (1965)

22. Schiefer, M. , Gerhardt, U. , Brunner, H. and Krüpe, M. J. Bacteriol. 120, 1 (1974)

PROTECTINS IN ARGENTINE MOLLUSKS:

IMMUNOLOGICAL AND IMMUNOCHEMICAL ASPECTS

M. Palatnik, G. R. Vasta, N. E. Fink and M. E. Chiesa

Facultad de Ciencias Exactas, Universidad Nacional de

La Plata, 47 y 115, La Plata, Argentina

The agglutinating activities of the organs, fluids and spawn from snails and slugs toward various human blood groups has now been examined in detail. The effect of calcium salts and aspects of the variation of agglutinins and hemolysins between individuals of a single species or between species are described in the present paper. Two families of the order Stylommatophora, Vaginulidae and Strophocheilidae, as well as a family of subclass Prosobranchia, order Mesogastropoda, Ampullariidae, represent very primitive groups of the class Gastropoda native to Argentina. O. lactea and H. aspersa are introduced species well known with respect to their serological behaviour. They were studied for possible populational or geographic differences in reactivities. V. solea is a slug of not yet clear taxonomical classification. To some authors it belongs to a new order Systellommatophora which is different from Stylommatophora and Basommatophora (1). Borus, which is of a large size, has a number of morphological features that assign it to Strophocheilidae group A, the most primitive of the family (2).

The family Ampullariidae constitutes a group exhibiting primitive features of Prosobranchia with adaptations related to its ecology (3). The great rivers are the habitat of A. insularum d'Orbigny, while A. canaliculata Lamarck (A. australis d'Orbigny) prefers the still sun-warmed waters of small lakes, ponds, pools, ditches and other reservoirs that collect rain water or water from seasonal river overflow. Both species are very widespread in our region and exhibit variability as to characteristics of the shell (3). A. canaliculata, known under the name of "La Plata apple snail" was gathered from three artificial lakes from public parks in the city and from the flats of a stream distant 25 km from La Plata.

MATERIAL AND METHODS

The specimens were gathered over the summer months and kept in the laboratory either in a terrarium or in running water tanks, with proper feed. Spawn was preserved prior to usage at $-28^{\circ}C$, after washing several times in isotonic sodium chloride solution. Methods for obtaining organs and fluids, the preparation of extracts, enzyme treatment and calcium medium utilization have been described elsewhere (4). D-galactose and L-fucose were prepared in 0.2 M solutions in 0.85% sodium chloride solution; N-acetyl-D-galactosamine was prepared at 0.1 M concentration. The agglutination inhibition method followed was that of Bathia et al. (5). The same method was applied for saliva against A_1-ficinated red cells. The reading and scoring methods have already been described (4) and hemolysins were read by direct observation.

RESULTS

V. solea shows weak activity of hepatopancreas and of hemolymph; the latter, absorbed with O erythrocytes provides a presumptive anti-A,B (Table I).

The Borus albumen gland is inactive for normal erythrocytes but exhibits activity for bromelinized red cells in calcium medium. Eggs have higher titers, also in calcium medium (Table I). Of the two introduced species with their usual high anti-A scores, the zoning phenomena detected in H. aspersa should be noted (Tables I, II).

Ampullaria has variable reactivity to ABO erythrocytes related to organ, fluid, animal development, geographic place of origin, species and specimen. With only one exception, the specimens lacked hepatopancreas activity (Table III); in one case there was a weak activity with ficin. The uterus has a high titer, both in A. insularum and in Zoo A. canaliculata and, irrespective of the enzyme employed, activity is similar for all erythrocytes. In the other animals the titer for this organ ranges from low to medium; in one juvenile form and in an adult with a hypotrophic gland, the uteri have no activity. In another juvenile form of the "El Pescado" stream the titer is 16-32. Hemolymph has titration scores that tend to correlate negatively with those of the uterus. Hemolysins are found in the uteri of A. insularum and in one specimen from the "Bosque Lake". Hemolysins are never found in the hemolymph. The extrapalleal fluid is also devoid of agglutinins. Spawn exhibits optimum agglutinating activity with bromelin in calcium medium. Some samples are inactive against normal erythrocytes with Ca^{++} ion. There are also hemolysins more active against bromelin-treated red cells (Table IV). There are no differences between fresh and frozen samples. Manifest individual variability is found in Ampullaria and there is apparently less variability in spawn than in uteri titers.

Table 1. - Agglutinins in terrestrial gastropods

	A_1	A_2	B	A_1B	A_2B	O
Family Vaginulidae						
1. Vaginula soleiformis Orbigny* (Vaginula solea Hylton Scott); "Parque Saavedra", La Plata						
Hemolymph: N;	4	2	1	2	2	1
Hemolymph(absorbed with O):N;	2	1	1	1	1	0
Hepatopancreas: N;	1	1	1	1	1	0
Family Strophocheilidae						
2. Strophocheilus(Megalobulimus) oblongus lorentzianus(Doering);** Tucumán						
Albumen gland: B;***	1	1	4	2	4	1
Eggs: N; ****	4	4	16	8	16	4
Family Odontostomidae						
3. Plagiodontes daedalus(Deshayes); "Villa del Dique", Río Tercero, Córdoba						
Albumen gland: N;	32	16	16	32	16	16
F;	8	2	0	4	0	0
Family Helicidae						
4. Otala lactea (Müller); Mar del Plata						
Albumen gland: N;	1024	256	0	512	0	2
T;	8192	2048	4	4096	4	64
5. Helix(Cryptomphalus)aspersa Figueiras(Helix aspersa Müller); Mar del Plata						
Albumen gland: F;	32768	65536	32	32768	2048	16
T;	32768	32768	16	32768	1024	0

N=normal red cells; F=ficin; T=trypsin; B=bromelin. * Albumen gland and spawn yielded negative results against normal, ficinized, papainized and trypsinized ABO cells at 20ºC and 37ºC. ** Hepatopancreas at 20ºC and 37ºC gave negative reactions with A, B, O, A^p and O^p normal cells; hemolymph at 20ºC gave negative results with ABO normal cells. *** 2% red cell suspension in 1 M $CaCl_2$ solution. **** 2% red cell suspension in 0.7 M $CaCl_2$ solution. The specimens belong to class Gastropoda, subclass Pulmonata, order Stylommatophora. Following the name of each species, the geographical location of samples are given. 1, 2 and 3 are autochthonous species; 4 and 5 are introduced species. Figures are given as end-point titers.

Table II. – Prozones in titrations of Helix aspersa

Erythrocytes & treatment	2^0	2^1	2^2	2^3	2^4	2^5	2^6	2^7	2^8	2^9	2^{10}	2^{11}	2^{12}	2^{13}
Ficin														
A_2B	½	½	1	0	4	2	2	4	2	2	1	½	0	0
0	0	½	0	0	0	2	0	0	0	0	0			
B	0	0	0	0	4	3	0	0	0	0				
Trypsin														
A_2B	½	1	3	3	4	4	4	4	3	1	1	0	0	0
B	½	0	0	½	4	0	0	0	0	0				
O^p	0	1	1	4	4	2	0	0	0	0				

Table III. – Agglutinins and hemolysins in Ampullaria

	A_1	A_2	B	A_1B	A_2B	O
1. A. insularum, d'Orbigny; "Arroyo Miguelín", Punta Lara						
Uterus: T;	256	256	512	256	512	512
T;	(8)	(8)	(8)	(8)	(8)	(8)
F;	256	256	512	256	1024	256
F;	(16)	(16)	(16)	(16)	(16)	(16)
Hemolymph: T;	8	8	8	4	8	8
F;	8	8	4	8	4	4
2. A. canaliculata Lamarck (A. australis d'Orbigny); La Plata						
(a) "Arroyo El Pescado" *, ***						
Uterus: T;	16	16	32	32	32	16
F;	32	4	32	16	32	16
Hemolymph: T;	32	16	32	32	16	8
F;	16	8	8	16	8	8
(b) "Lago del Bosque" Individual A						
Uterus: T;	4	4	2	4	2	4
T;	(4)	(4)	(2)	(4)	(2)	(4)
F;	8	4	4	4	4	8
F;	(4)	(4)	(4)	(4)	(4)	(4)
Hemolymph: T;	16	16	16	16	16	16
F;	32	32	32	16	32	16
Hepatopancreas: T;	0	0	0	0	0	0
F;	2	0	0	1	2	0

Table III (Continued). - Agglutinins and hemolysins in <u>Ampullaria</u>

(continued)	A_1	A_2	B	A_1B	A_2B	O
2. <u>A</u>. <u>canaliculata</u> Lamarck						
(<u>A</u>. <u>australis</u> d'Orbigny);						
La Plata						
(b) "Lago del Bosque"						
Individual B**						
Uterus: T;	0	0	0	0	0	0
F;	4	2	1	1	2	1
Hemolymph: T;	0	2	2	1	2	2
F;	8	4	8	8	8	8
Hepatopancreas: T;	1	1	1	1	1	1
F;	4	2	1	1	1	1
(c) "Parque Saavedra" *						
Uterus: T;	0	0	0	0	0	0
F;	0	0	0	0	0	0
Hemolymph: T;	2	1	1	2	4	4
F;	4	2	1	2	1	2
(d) Zoological Garden						
Individual A						
Uterus: T;	256	256	256	256	256	256
F;	512	256	512	512	512	256
Hemolymph: T;	16	16	8	4	8	16
F;	16	16	16	16	16	16
Individual B						
Uterus: T;	4	4	4	4	8	4
F;	8	4	8	8	8	4
Hemolymph: T;	4	4	2	1	4	4
F;	4	4	2	2	2	2

T=trypsin; F=ficin. * Juvenile forms. ** Adult with a small uterus.
*** 25 km from La Plata. All the animals are of female sex. The
specimens belong to class <u>Gastropoda</u>, subclass <u>Prosobranchia</u>, order
<u>Mesogastropoda</u>, family <u>Ampullariidae</u>. Hepatopancreas from
individuals 1, 2a, 2c, 2dA, 2dB showed no reactivity against
trypsin and ficin treated cells. The extrapalleal fluid from
all the listed individuals was serologically negative. Figures are
given as end-point titers; figures in parentheses are hemolysin
end-point titers.

Table IV. – Agglutinins and hemolysins in spawn from
Ampullaria canaliculata

		A_1	A_2	B	A_1B	A_2B	O
(a) "Arroyo El Pescado"							
Specimen A*:	N;	16	32	2	16	0	0
	F;	0	0	0	0	0	0
	B;	2	2	2	32	2	4
Specimen B*:	N; F;	0	0	0	0	0	0
	B;	1	2	1	2	8	4
(b) "Lago del Bosque"							
Specimen A*:	N; F;	0	0	0	0	0	0
	B;	4	4	0	4	32	0
Specimen B**:	N;	0	0	0	0	0	0
	F;	16	8	8	8	8	8
	F;	(4)	(4)	(4)	(4)	(4)	(4)
	B;	32	16	8	8	16	32
	B;	(2)	(2)	(2)	(4)	(2)	(2)
(c) "Parque Saavedra"							
Specimen A*:	N;	16	8	16	16	32	16
	F;	16	8	32	16	16	16
	B;	64	64	64	64	64	64
	B;	(32)	(32)	(32)	(4)	(1)	(32)
(d) Zoological Garden							
Specimen A**:	N; F;	0	0	0	0	0	0
	B;	32	32	16	32	32	32
Specimen B*:	N;	32	64	16	16	64	64
	N;	(1)	(1)	(2)	(1)	(0)	(2)
	F;	64	16	64	32	64	32
	F;	(1)	(1)	(0)	(0)	(0)	(0)
	B;	32	32	64	32	64	32
	B;	(1)	(32)	(4)	(32)	(8)	(32)

N=normal red cells; F=ficin; B=bromelin.
* Frozen samples.
** Fresh samples.
2% suspensions of normal cells in 0.7 M $CaCl_2$ of bromelinized cells
in 1 M $CaCl_2$; of ficinized cells in 0.85% NaCl.
Figures are given as end-point titers; figures in parentheses are
hemolysin end-point titers.

Table V. - Inhibitions with sugars and saliva

Extract	Minimal dosage for total inhibition (moles)			
	N-acetyl-D-galactosamine	L-fucose	D-galactose	Red cells
O. lactea				
Albumen gland *	0.025			A_1
	0.0125			A_2
		0.0125		O tryp.
H. aspersa				
Albumen gland **	0.025			A_1tryp.
	0.0125			A_2tryp.
A. canaliculata				
Uterus ***	No inh.		No inh.	A_1tryp.
	No inh.		No inh.	B tryp.
Spawn ***	No inh.	No inh.	No inh.	A_1 ⎫ in
	No inh.	No inh.	No inh.	B ⎬ 0.7 M
	No inh.	No inh.	No inh.	O ⎭ $CaCl_2$
V. solea				
Hemolymph ***	No inh.	No inh.	No inh.	A_2
		No inh.	No inh.	B
		No inh.		O
P. daedalus				
Albumen gland ***	Total inhibition with A_1 secretor saliva			A_1 fic.

* Dilution of the extract, 1/8;

** 8 agglutinating doses;

*** 2-4 agglutinating doses.

V. solea and A. canaliculata extracts are not inhibited by sugars.
P. daedalus is inhibited with group A_1 secretor saliva (Table V).

DISCUSSION

Comparison of our O. lactea protectins with those described in
the literature reveals very similar activities to those reported by
Bathia et al. (5). However, in the case of the former, a weak anti-H
activity with normal erythrocytes is detected, while protectins from
North American specimens are only active with enzyme-treated cells.
Though detection methods are not strictly comparable, H. aspersa
immunological behaviour is closer to that of Spanish origin than
to that of French origin (6).

Some features of enzyme action should be noted. On the one
hand, ficin exposes an A receptor detected by P. daedalus extracts;
on the other hand, bromelin is the only enzyme that activates an
agglutinin from albumen gland and eggs of Borus in Ca^{++} ion containing
medium. Bromelin is a selective enzyme for complete and cold human
antibodies such as anti-A and anti-H (7). Its peculiar activity with
respect to Ampullaria spawn and Borus extracts mentioned above may be
accounted for by the effect of enzyme potentiating activity inherent
in the extracts, as proposed for bromelin in human serum (8,9). The
prozone observed in H. aspersa titrations against human and pig red
cells may be due to an incomplete agglutinin that reacts faster or
to an excess of antibody-like substance (10); it may also be due to
extract viscosity, as is the case described for human antibodies in
20% bovine albumin medium (11). The prozone phenomenon shows another
difference in enzyme activity between protectins and immunoglobulins:
though trypsination eliminates the prozone of anti-Rh antibodies (11),
it does not cancel that of a protectin.

In view of their Ca-dependence, these agglutinins (12) can be
said to have a primitive behaviour by comparison to vertebrate
immunoglobulins and to suggest a conglutinin-like activity. In
man and in higher vertebrates, certain types of antibodies such as
saliva conglutinins and immunoconglutinins are active only in the
presence of Ca^{++} ion (13). The conglutinin is involved in a number
of non-specific immunity processes in bacterial infections, is
closely linked to the mechanism of immune hemolysis and is heat
stable (14).

We do not know whether protectins are under close genetic
regulation but even if their variation is non-genetic in origin we
should bear in mind that non-genetic variation is usually adaptive
and controlled by natural selection (15). The relation between
protectins and Ca^{++} ion on the other provide for speculation along
two lines in connection with their evolution, their variability and

biological role. Hermaphrodites have protectins in their female reproductive organs, but in dioic species such as Ampullaria, males are practically devoid of those substances (16). Consequently, if they actually do condition their protection, one sex would appear to be exposed to a greater selective pressure. This sexual difference, in some species, in resistance to pathogens in the environment would be a primitive form of the immune system. The evolution of higher vertebrates towards "sex-independent" immunocompetence may have represented a radical change in the phylogeny of immunity.

Just as the reproductive-linked protectin is of unquestionable significance to the adaptability of the population, the Ca^{++} ion, linked to the protection of the embryo and of the adult, must also have implications for embryonic viability or for pre-reproductive and adult mortality. As protectin is apparently linked to Ca^{++} and this ion is subject to selective pressure, the lack of calcium coverings prevents the survival of the embryo and of the developing animal. It follows then that an immune system of this kind is not optimum and the independence from Ca^{++} for the activity of vertebrate immunoglobulins is another transcending evolutionary step.

Hepatopancreas and extrapalleal fluid are both involved in shell regeneration (17) and as was seen in Ampullaria are both devoid of agglutinins. The extrapalleal fluid is not very different from hemolymph in chemical composition and gives rise to shell-forming deposits (18). The absence of antibody-like substances in both tissues is noteworthy. This could be interpreted to mean that either they are not active in the hepatopancreas-extrapalleal fluid-shell pathway, or that being active, they undergo a process of denaturation.

SUMMARY

Protectins and agglutinins in several organs, fluids and spawn from Argentine terrestrial and fresh-water gastropod species were examined. Differences or analogies with vertebrate immunoglobulin serological behaviour are summarized. Individual or group variability and the evolutionary meaning of the reproductive system-linked and the Ca^{++} ion-linked protectins are discussed.

ACKNOWLEDGMENTS

To Dr. Zulma J. A. de Castellanos for her help with gastropod classification. This work received partial financial support from Consejo Nacional de Investigaciones Científicas y Técnicas, and a Travel Grant from Fundación de Genética Humana.

REFERENCES

1. Grassé, P. P., Traité de Zoologie, 5(3), 1083 pp. (Masson, Paris, 1968).

2. Moreira Leme, J. L., Arq. Zool. São Paulo, 23: 295 (1973).

3. Hylton Scott, M. I., Rev. Museo Arg. Cienc. Nat., 3: 233 (1957).

4. Vasta, G. R., Ciesa, M. E. and Palatnik, M., Submitted for publication (1975).

5. Bathia, H. M., Boyd, W. C. and Brown, R., Transfusion, 7: 53 (1967).

6. Uhlenbruck, G. and Weis, A., Z. Immunitaetsforsch., 145: 356 (1973).

7. Dybkjaer, E., Proc. 10th Congr. Int. Soc. Blood Transf., Stockholm 1964; p. 1030 (Karger, Basel/New York, 1965).

8. Pirofsky, B., Vox Sang., 5: 442 (1960).

9. Cawley, L. P., Schneider, D. and Eberhardt, L., Vox Sang., 11: 81 (1966).

10. Dunsford, I. and Bowley, C. C., Techniques in Blood Grouping, two vol. (Oliver and Boyd, Edinburgh, 1967).

11. Wheeler, W. E., Luhby, A. L. and Scholl, M. L. L., J. Immunol., 65: 39 (1950).

12. Grey, H. M., in Advances Immun., 10: 51 (Academic Press, New York, 1969).

13. Mollison, P. L., Blood Transfusion in Clinical Medicine, 5th ed., 830 pp. (Blackwell, Oxford, 1972).

14. Coombs, R. R. A., Coombs, A. and Ingram, D. G., The Serology of Conglutination and its Relation to Disease, 210 pp. (Blackwell, Oxford, 1961).

15. Mayr, E., Animal Species and Evolution, 792 pp. (Belknap Press, Cambridge, Massachusetts, 1969).

16. Kothbauer, H. and Schenkel-Brunner, H., Z. Naturfursch. (B), 26: 1082 (1971).

17. Abolins-Krogis, A., Symp. Zool. Soc. Lond., 22: 75 (1968).

18. Digby, P. S. B., Symp. Zool. Soc. Lond., 22: 93 (1968).

IMMUNOLOGIC SIGNIFICANCE OF SPECIFICITIES OF CELLULAR AGGLUTININS

OF LIMULUS POLYPHEMUS

Elias Cohen

Dept. Lab. Med., Roswell Park Memorial Institute and

Dept. Microb., SUNYAB, 666 Elm Street, Buffalo NY 14263

From the earliest investigations of blood group antigens, plant extracts (lectins) were found with hemagglutinating ability. The hemolymph of selected invertebrate animal species were found to contain agglutinins for a variety of animal cells and specificity for human erythrocyte blood groups.

Similarities in specificity and serologic activity between lectins of plant origin and certain agglutinins of invertebrate origins have been described by a number of investigators in a recent international conference, subsequently published (18). Although some workers use the designation "lectin" for agglutinins of both plant and animal origin, the original designation by Boyd (19) was applicable to plant seed protein agglutinins. In this author's opinion, for historical reasons, the term "lectin" should be restricted to an agglutinin of plant origin. My presentation is concerned with agglutinins of invertebrate origins.

Noguchi, in 1903 (1), first reported cellular agglutinins in the serum of Limulus polyphemus, the Horseshoe crab. Marchalonis (2) and Cohen, Rowe and Wissler (3) independently described and investigated Limulus agglutinins. However, Drs. Ralph J. DeFalco, Alan A. and Mabel Boyden of Rutgers University had routinely utilized Limulus hemagglutinins for graduate study serological demonstrations during the 1950's. First isolation of the agglutinin by Marchelonis and Edelman (4) and first description of the N-acetyl neuraminic acid (NANA) specificity by Cohen (5) with collaboration of Dr. Stig Nordling, stimulated a host of investigations. Uhlenbruck (6), with Pardoe and Birch (7) included the cell receptor site for Limulus agglutinin as an integral part of the topographic concept of cell membranes. Cohen et al (8) utilized anti-NANA$_{LP}$

29

(Limulus) agglutinins to demonstrate a common N-acetyl-neuraminyl
receptor for both M and N human blood group determinants.

"Natural" agglutinins of marine invertebrates, crustaceans
and mollusks are speculated to be of some selective advantage due
to their ability to immobilize or opsonize bacteria or foreign particles. However, Marchalonis and Edelman (4), on basis of their work
concluded that Limulus agglutinin and mammalian immunoglobulin are
not related evolutionary developments. Tripp (8)(9) has studied
molluscan immunity and Pauley (10) investigated the natural agglutinins of the Blue Crab, as well as extensively reviewing the work
of many investigators on the immune advantage of the presence of
hemolymph agglutinins.

In view of absence of agglutinins in young moulting land crabs
(Birgus latro), it was speculated (11)(12) that agglutinins of
Birgus (possibly Limulus) may be part of a saccharide transport or
storage mechanism of the shell formation of those invertebrates.
Shell of both species is chitin (polysaccharide) impregnated with
calcium carbonate (particular Birgus). Primitive origins of protective function (immune response) may have arisen from natural
selective advantage of manifold functions of Limulus-like hemolymph
agglutinins. For example, Limulus has been a most successful
arachnoid-like living fossil.

Anti-galactan precipitins discovered and reported at this conference by Uhlenbruck and Baldo (13) present a new serologic and
immunochemical dimension -- with specificity as an anti-N-acetyl-
D galactosamine. Invertebrates as Tridacna (clam), Axinella (sponge)
and Limulus (horseshoe crab) have a common anti-galactan similar
to mouse myeloma IgA proteins, although the invertebrate ones are
not immunoglobulins per se.

At present, it is only speculative, as to how Limulus-like
agglutinins fit into the phylogeny of the immune response. Nevertheless, agglutinating ability of a humoral substance directed
against an ubiquitous N-acetyl neuraminyl cellular receptor would
be an effective defensive shield against invasive foreign organisms.

Purification procedures for agglutinins have been reported by
Finstad et al (14) and others (19)(20) for Limulus and Hall and
Rowland (15)(16) for the lobster (Homarus). Pauley (17) has purified agglutinins of the Blue Crab (Callinectes) and other marine
invertebrates.

It is hoped that isolation and purification procedures will
facilitate appropriate labelling experiments that may help to explain (a) the diverse physiologic functions of invertebrate agglutinins and (b) their interrelationship to the phylogeny of the
immune response.

References

1. Noguchi, H., Zentr. Bakt. Abt. I. Orig. 34:286 (1903).

2. Marchalonis, J.J., Feder. Proc. 23:1468 (1964).

3. Cohen, E., Rowe, A.W. and Wissler, F.C., Life Sciences 4:2009, (1965).

4. Marchalonis, J.J. and Edelman, G.M., J. Molec. Biol. 32:453, (1968).

5. Cohen, E., Trans. N.Y. Acad. Sci. 20:427 (1968)

6. Uhlenbruck, G., Vox Sang. 16:200 (1968)

7. Pardoe, G.I. Uhlenbruck, G., and Bird. G.W.G., Immunology 18: 73 (1970).

8. Tripp, M.R.,Annals, N.Y. Acad. Sci. 234:18 (1974).

9. Tripp, M.R.,Annals, N.Y. Acad. Sci. 234:23 (1974).

10. Pauley, G.B., Contemporary Topics in Immunobiol. 4:241 (1973).

11. Cohen, E., in Protein Metabolism and Biological Function, 87, Rutgers Univ. Press. N. Brunswick, N.J. (1970).

12. Cohen, E., Rozenberg, M. and Massaro, E.J., Annals N.Y. Acad. Sci., 234:28 (1974).

13. Baldo, B.A., Uhlenbruck, G. and Cohen, E., Advances in Exper. Med. and Biol. (In press) 1975.

14. Finstad, C.L., Good, R.A. and Litman, G.W., Annals N.Y. Acad. Sci. 234:170 (1974).

15. Hall, J.L. and Rowlands, D.T., Jr., Biochem. 13:821 (1974).

16. Hall, J.L. and Rowlands, D.T., Jr., Biochem. 13:828 (1974).

17. Pauley, G.B., Annals N.Y. Acad. Sci. 234:145 (1974).

18. Cohen, E., (Editor) Annals, N.Y. Acad. Sci. 234:1-412 Publ. N.Y. Acad. Sci., New York, N.Y. (1974).

19. Boyd, W., Introduction to immunochemical specificity, Interscience Publ. Inc., New York, New York (1962).

Supported by the Juliette and Israel Cohen Memorial Research Fund.

INVERTEBRATE IMMUNOLOGY

Cell Surface Receptors
and Recognition Factors

SOME SPECIFIC ASPECTS OF CELL-SURFACE RECOGNITION

BY SIPUNCULID COELOMOCYTES

John E. Cushing
Biological Sciences, University of California
Santa Barbara, California 93106

David K. Boraker
Medical Microbiology, College of Medicine
University of Vermont
Burlington, Vermont 05401

INTRODUCTION

Sipunculid worms have been the subject of research on the phylogeny of immune responses since the investigations of Canta-cuzene (1). These marine worms comprise a distinctive group that inhabit intertidal areas scattered over the world. While a variety of discoveries has been made in sipunculids that are of immunological interest, emphasis is made that no specific molecular or cellular reactions have been found in this phylum that are comparable to those of vertebrate adaptive immunity. The discoveries that have been made include the phagocytic and encapsulation reactions common to invertebrates, the occurrence in some species of specialized free-swimming phagocytic structures in coelomic fluid termed "urns" (1), an inducible lysin for a protozoan (2), inducible and noninducible bactericidins (3,4,5), a capacity to hemolize (6,7) and agglutinate vertebrate erythrocytes (8), an agent capable of immobilizing dinoflagellates (6), substances with specificities related to vertebrate blood groups (9) and an inhibitory effect on phagocytosis by bovine serum (10).

The continually accelerating increase in research related to to the phylogeny of the immune response, as exemplified by the

numerous references in such publications as 11, 12, 13, 14, 15,
16, and 17, as well, of course, as this symposium, would seem to
make this a particularly favorable place to present a combined
"big-picture" look at a series of researches concerned, over a
number of years in our laboratory, with the encapsulation responses
of male sipunculid worms (Dendrostomum zostericolum Chamberlain)
to homologous eggs placed in their coelom. This work is based on
earlier observations which showed that severed homologous tentacles
placed in sipunculid coelomic cavities, while remaining viable for
long periods of time, were efficiently encapsulated (8). Three
related areas of investigation will be reported. The first established the methods and fundamental nature of the reactions
involved (18), the other two are summaries of further investigations
currently available as masters theses (19,20).

MATERIALS AND METHODS

Dendrostomum individuals exist as separate sexes and retain
their respective gametes within their coelomic cavities for long
periods of time. Here they are associated with hemerythrocytes
containing the respiratory pigment hemerythrin, and various cells
(here termed coelomocytes and not yet readily distinguished from
each other) that act in phagocytosis and encapsulation. Mature
gametes in the coelom are eventually released and react through
fertilization in the surrounding sea water. These circumstances
made it possible to inject eggs (using 24 or 26 gauge needles),
either normal or manipulated, into the coelomic cavities of males
or other females and subsequently (usually at 24 and/or 48 hours)
to withdraw samples of coelomic fluids and make microscopic examination and counts of the relative numbers of encapsulated and unencapsulated eggs. Sterile precautions were taken throughout the
experiments and initial usage of sterile sea water was supplanted
by the use of artificial sea water (21) without effect on the results. The numbers of eggs injected were quantitatively controlled,
10 to 30 thousand being injected, from an initial suspension containing approximately 150,000 eggs per ml., in proportion to the
total sea water displacement volume of the worm receiving them.
Encapsulation counts were made using a Spencer Bright-Line Hemo-
cytometer. Degree of encapsulation was assessed for individual
eggs on a scale ranging from four plus for complete encapsulation
through zero for no encapsulation. Eggs scoring one or higher
were counted as positive in the tabulations presented. Eggs
were stained using a combination of glycerol fixative and Sudan
IV, a method giving a pink color and specific for lipids in the
yolk (22). Eggs so treated and washed by two centrifugations and
resuspensions in sea water free from reagents were very stable for
long periods.

RESULTS

Capsule Formation

Like other sipunculids, Dendrostromum has two separate circulatory systems, one in the tentacles and the long hollow tubes
termed compensatory sacs, the other in the coelom (23). Capsule
formation by circulatory amoebocytes occurs in both systems. As
the present paper is concerned only with those found in the coelomic
fluid, the amoebocytes involved are termed coelomocytes. Most
worms are relatively free of capsules, some have many small capsules plus larger aggregates of these and others a few larger aggregates. The impression is that the smaller masses normally tend
to aggregate into larger ones. This is known to be true in the
case of capsules around injected materials discussed below. The
fate of the coelomocytic masses is unknown, but some homeostatic
mechanism must keep the blood relatively clear. Observations on
injected eggs showed that at least autodisintegration occurred,
and made it improbable that, unlike gametes, the aggregates passed
out through nephridial pores. As the data given below shows, it
was relatively easy to distinguish encapsulated from unencapsulated
eggs, provided account was taken of the fact that the process involved is a dynamic one.

Normal Encapsulation

Series of female worms were examined over the course of the
experiments to determine the extent to which encapsulated eggs
appear in normal coelomic fluid. The following ratios of encapsulated to unencapsulated eggs from three series of several worms
each were typical: series one, 3 to 3225; series two, 1 to 3575;
series three, 3 to 5366. One other series showing 15 to 1264 was
unique in having the greatest amount of capsule formation of
normal eggs observed in females. The number of encapsulations did
not increase in worms kept one or more days in running sea water
following an initial "bleeding" or injection of sterile sea water.
Together these observations showed that autoencapsulation was not a
significant factor.

Reaction to Heterospecific Eggs

Eggs from the sea urchin Strongylocentrolus purpuratus and
from the sipunculid Golfingia gouldii were essentially totally
encapsulated by male coelomocytes within 24 hours, while accompanying normal Dendrostomum eggs were not. These observations show the
extremes and selectivity of the encapsulation response. Note is
made that the failure of male coelomocytes to encapsulate homologous
eggs,even though these do not normally occur in their coelomic

cavities, is paralleled by similar reactions of earthworms noted briefly by Cameron (24). This failure to recognize eggs as "not self" is the response that forms the basis for further research to be reported.

Reactions to Injections of Whole Blood

A series of worms was injected with whole blood according to the following scheme. One ml. of blood was taken from each of two female partners. One half ml. of blood from one of the females was injected into the other, and the other half ml. into a male from which one half ml. had just been withdrawn and discarded. Counts of encapsulated and unencapsulated eggs were made on each of three succeeding days, coelomocytic masses being looked for on the last day. The percentage of encapsulated eggs in the females at the start of the experiment was found to be below one percent as in the other normal counts reported above. Injected bloods contained totals of between 7,000 and 18,500 eggs. Table I shows that

Table I. Encapsulation of Eggs Following Exchanges of Whole Blood. Counts were made of eggs observed in drops of blood taken at 24, 48, and 62 hours. The combined totals of these counts for each worm given above show that no enhanced encapsulation occurred as the result of transfusions of whole blood.

| | Females | | | Males | |
worm	# eggs counted	# capsules	worm	# eggs counted	# capsules
1	7442	2	1	603	1
2	2958	2	2	502	1
3	6152	0	3	1279	0
4	5429	3	4	759	0
5	3780	0	5	1002	2
6	5921	1	6	461	0

capsule formation was not increased in the adulterated blood of females, and that males also did not encapsulate untreated eggs. No reactions were observed that might have been attributed to the injection of other components of blood. An experiment in which the blood was diluted with an equal volume of artificial sea water just prior to injection did not bring about any increased response.

These experiments support the view that males and females do not recognize normal allogeneic (homologous) eggs as "not self."

Reactions to Eggs Washed in Sterile Sea Water

Table II shows the responses of males and females to stained
and normal eggs previously washed in sterile sea water and that
the coelomocytes readily discriminated between stained and unstained
eggs. Five experiments like the one reported showed degrees of
discrimination similar in magnitude.

Table II.   Encapsulation of Stained and Normal Eggs Washed
            in Sterile Sea Water. This table shows the relative
            numbers of encapsulated (+) and uncapsulated (-)
            eggs in a series of worms observed over a three
            day period after injection. The figures given are
            the totals of eggs found in drops of coelomic fluid
            taken from series of ten male and ten female worms
            respectively.

	\multicolumn{3}{c}{Stained}	\multicolumn{3}{c}{Normal}
	+	-	(%+)	+	-	(%+)
\multicolumn{7}{c}{24 hrs.}
Males (10)	73	24	(75.2)	5	88	(5.4)
Females (10)	88	8	(91.7)	7	4610	(.15)
\multicolumn{7}{c}{48 hrs.}
Males (10)	92	14	(86.8)	6	112	(5.1)
Females (10)	57	23	(71.3)	2	4499	(.05)
\multicolumn{7}{c}{66 hrs.}
Males (10)	63	5	(92.7)	4	67	(5.6)
Females (10)	53	8	(86.8)	1	4645	(.02)

Variations in the percentage of capsule formation around
normal eggs by males ranged from the neighborhood of eight percent
to occasional individuals that formed no capsules. The female
response was relatively difficult to determine because of the large
numbers of eggs normally present in the coelom. Estimates were
made based upon the expected number of injected normal eggs
that should have been seen during the scoring of stained eggs.
While rough, these estimates suggest that the degree of capsule
formation about injected normal eggs is similar in both sexes.
Consideration of the male response alone with relation to the preceding sections shows that while washing has some effect on encapsulation of normal eggs this is slight compared to that of staining.

Additional Observations

Eggs heated in artificial sea water for 10 minutes at 30° and 50° C did not show any visible damage. At 70° C eggs still retained their structure, but appeared to suffer some damage to external membranes and formed into large aggregates. An experiment with male worms showed that enhanced capsule formation did not take place at 30° C but was markedly enhanced at the higher temperatures. In contrast, eggs frozen and thawed at -5° C for 24 hrs. were not encapsulated. These preliminary experiments were considerably extended by the work of Hand as summarized in the following sections.

The effect of extended washing of eggs was studied. The variability between parts of the repeated portions of the experiment showed that better control will be needed to obtain accurate quantitative data. However, while extensive washing seemed to increase encapsulation somewhat, the effect was never nearly as marked as with the case of staining.

Filter paper discs 0.6 cm. in diameter were soaked in a mixture of serum from a male and female sipunculid for thirty minutes. Each of four worms received two of these discs through a slit in the body wall. This was prepared by squeezing the blood anteriorly and clamping off a portion of the posterior end. The slit was subsequently sealed with Eastman 910 monomer tissue glue. Four other worms received similar discs soaked in sterile sea water. Two from each group were opened at four hours, and all were found to have initiated capsule formation. The remaining worms all had heavily encapsulated the discs at twenty-one hours, showing that no transfer of self-markers had been effected through serum treatment.

Contrasting results were obtained when nephridia were transplanted. Each of three males received an intercoelomic transplant of a whole nephridium from a female. Reciprocal transplants were also made into three females. Sixty-two hours later the coelmocytes of all worms were found to have ignored these transplants excepting for heavily encapsulation of the small bits of skin around the external openings of the nephridia. Intrusions of catalyzed Eastman 910 monomer tissue glue were also covered. The cilia of all nephridia were functioning and the organ itself retained its motility. Transplanted bits of retractor muscle and intestine were also ignored. It was also observed that coelomocytes collected at places where breaks in the muscle layers of worms exposed the inner surface of the integument to the coelomic cavity.

Experiments have shown that it is possible to establish parabiosis by joining the posterior ends of worms together using

Eastman 910 monomer and pieces of capillary tubing. An exchange
of circulation was established and two pairs of worms lived in
good health for several weeks. Worms drained of most of their
blood with a syringe were observed to regenerate the elements of
the coelomic fluid in a few days. These observations offer promise
for experimentation with the establishment of tolerance, the mani-
pulation of sex cells, and the localization of formation of coelomic components etc.

RELATIONSHIPS OF VITAL STAINS TO TREATMENT AND ENCAPSULATION

This section summarizes the work of Hand (19) concerning the
reactions with vital stains of eggs treated in various ways, and
the relation of encapsulation responses to these reactions. The
stains used were as follows: tetrazolium (25,26) an indicator
of functioning respiratory enzymes that causes the normally grey-
ish eggs to turn red if undamaged; trypan blue which stains damaged
eggs blue, leaving normal ones uncolored; and eosin which stains
eggs pink and again leaves normal eggs unchanged (27). Artificial
sea water was used throughout. Several series of experiments determined the optimal usage of stains with the realization that
"death" of a cell should be considered arbitrarily as a progression of events resulting in irreversible damage. Quantitative
methods were used that were similar to those already described.

Experimental groups consisted of four male worms, two of
which received untreated eggs and two of which received eggs subjected to different treatments. These were studied in order to
determine optimal conditions of minimal treatment to achieve
maximum damage. The results of heat (50° C for ten minutes),
freezing (-5° C for 24 hrs.) and sonification (MSE Sonicator
for 20 seconds) with respect to staining and encapsulation reactions
are summarized in Table III (next page).

The outstanding result is the demonstration that, while all
treatments badly damaged eggs even though leaving them structurally
intact, eggs that were heated and sonicated were heavily encapsulated while those that were frozen were not. In other words,
frozen eggs that reacted to vital stains as though dead still
retained the "self" recognition signal of normal eggs.

THE ANTIGENIC SPECIFICITIES OF SIPUNCULID GAMETES

Brown (20) has made an extensive study of the antigenic
specificities of sipunculid eggs, sperm, and coelomic fluid. He
utilized rabbit antiserums and the agar-gel double diffusion
technique to investigate soluble substances diffusing from these
materials. This work demonstrated that eggs and sperm had at

Table III.   Comparative Results of the Effects of Different Treatments and the Encapsulation Response. Each percentage is based on a count of approximately 500 eggs following treatments as referred to in the text above.

Test	Heat	Percentage of eggs damaged by: Freezing	Sonication
Tetrazolium	100%	100%	100%
	100%	99.4%	96%
	100%		
Eosin	97.2%	96.3%	91.5%
	61.5%	100%	99.0%
	57.5%	97.0%	94.3%
	88.7%		85.8%
			98.2%
Trypan Blue	70.0%	90.9%	91.0%
	96.6%		

	Worm Encapsulation		
	87.1%	2.4%	96.5%
	85.0%	0.3%	96.0%
	83.6%	2.4%	96.9%

least two antigenic components in common and also that it was possible to obtain antibodies specific for at least three antigens on eggs which could not be demonstrated on sipunculid sperm and hemerythrocytes or in male coelomic fluid. Experiments indicated that two of the antigens involved survived freezing well, but that one at least was damaged by heat treatment, a result compatible with Hand's observations.

DISCUSSION AND SUMMARY

The research reported showed that the encapsulation response of male sipunculid coelomocytes to injected homologous eggs provides a useful system for the study of "self" vs. "not self" recognition signals detected by coelomocytes. The basis of this system is the failure of male coelomocytes to encapsulate untreated homologous eggs injected into their coelom, even though such eggs normally never occur there. In contrast, homologous eggs that have been altered by staining, heating, and sonication are readily recognized as "not self" and rapidly encapsulated. The possibility of "dissecting" the "self" vs. "not self" relationships was shown by the discovery that frozen eggs, while apparently dead as determined by their reactions with vital stains, were not encapsulated. Of additional potential interest was the demonstration that eggs possessed some antigens which also occurred on sperm, and others which were unique to themselves.

The conclusion seems valid that normal egg viability _per se_ is not necessary to self-recognition. Therefore, the distinction between "self" and "not self" being made by coelomocytes would appear to involve some sort of precise molecular basis. That this involves a "self" tolerance is obvious in that coelomocytes do not phagocytize or encapsulate the normal constituents of their environment, nor as noted above, transplanted nephridia beyond their damaged portions (the contrasting encapsulation of homologous tentacle transplants (8) is most probably due to extraneous microorganisms and other foreign adherents). While the degree of specificity of the "not self" aspects of encapsulation remains to be elucidated it appears that this will prove to be complex. Reasons for concluding this include the demonstration that eggs not only share soluble antigens with sperm, but apparently have unique ones of their own not found on sperm or coelomic fluid. Speculation is premature, but the well studied properties of fertilizen and antifertilizen (28,29) make it reasonable to believe that at least some unique egg antigens are not shared with other sipunculid tissues accessible to coelomocytes. It is apparent that further investigations also will have to bring into account recent researches relevant to the initial observations of Tripp (30). These show that at least some invertebrate agglutinins can enhance phagocytosis. Additionally, attention could be directed to the possible interactions of specific molecular forces with relatively nonspecific ones such as the Zeta potential that acts in hemagglutination. Finally, potentially relevant to this paper is the demonstration (10) that bovine serum markedly inhibits the phagocytosis of yeast by sipunculid coelomocytes (without damaging them), that this inhibition can be reversed by sipunculid coelomic fluid, and that coelomocytes can apparently be made "tolerant" to the inhibition.

REFERENCES

1. Bang, F.B., Fedn. Proc., 26: no. 6, 1664 (1967).
2. Bang, F.B., J. Immunol., 96: 960 (1966).
3. Krassner, S.M., Biol. Bull., 125: 382 (1963).
4. Rabin, H. and Bang, F.B., Biol. Bull., 125: 388 (1963).
5. Evans, E.E., Cushing, J.E. and Evans, M.L., Infect. Immunol., 8: 355 (1973).
6. Cushing, J.E., McNeely and Tripp, M.R., J. Invert. Pathol., 14: no. 1, 4 (1969).
7. Weinheimer, P.F., Acton, R.T., Cushing, J.E. and Evans, E.E., Life Sciences, 9 part II: 145 (1970).
8. Triplett, E.L., Cushing, J.E., and Durall, G.E., Amer. Naturalist 92: 287 (1958).

9. Cushing, J.E., Calaprice, N.L. and Trump, G., Biol. Bull.
    125: 69 (1963).
10. Cushing, J.E., Tripp, M.R. and Fuzessery, S. (abst.) Federn.
    Proc. 29 no. 2 Mar.-Apr. (1970).
11. Bang, F.B., Biosci., 23 no. 10, 584 (1973).
12. Cushing, J.E., Immunochemistry 12: in proof (1975).
13. Cooper, E.L., Non-Specific Factors Influencing Host Resistance
    (Braun, W. and Ungar, J. ed) p. 11, Karger, Basel (1973).
14. Cooper, E.L., Contemporary Topics in Immunobiology, vol. 4,
    Invertebrate Immunology, 299 pp. (Plenum, New York, 1974).
15. Hildemann, W.H., Chpt. 1 pp. 3-73 (in Transplantation Anti-
    gens, Kahan, B.D. and Reisfeld, R.A., Academic Press, New
    York, 1972).
16. Hildemann, W.H., Nature, 250 no. 5462: 116 (1974).
17. Wright, R.K. and Cooper, E.L., Amer. Zool., 15: 21 (1975).
18. Cushing, J.E., Boraker, D. and Keough, E., Fedn. Proc.
    (abst.), 24 No. 2: 504 (1965).
19. Hand, J.H., Reactions of Sipunculid Eggs to Vital Stains as
    related to the Encapsulation Response, M.A. Thesis Univ.
    of Calif., Santa Barbara (1966).
20. Brown, S.J., The Relation of Antigenic Specificities to
    Sipunculid Egg Allografts, M.A. Thesis Univ. of Calif.,
    Santa Barbara (1970).
21. Tyler, A., Biol. Bull., 104: 224 (1953).
22. Humason, G.L., Animal Tissue Techniques, 468 pp. (W.H. Free-
    man, San Francisco, 1962).
23. Manwell, C., Science, 139: 755 (1963).
24. Cameron, G.R., J. Path. and Bacteriol., 35: 933 (1932).
25. Smith, F.E., Science, 113: 751 (1951).
26. Jensen, L., Pierpoint, M. and Hayes, P., Proc. of Assoc.
    Official Seed Analysts, 47: 141 (1957).
27. Tennant, J.R., Transplantation, 2: 685 (1964).
28. Tyler, A., Amer. Naturalist, 99:309-334
    (1965).
29. Vacquier, V.D., Tegner, M. and Epel, D., Exp. Cell Research,
    80: 111 (1973).
30. Tripp, M.R., J. Invert. Pathol., 8: 478 (1966).

The authors acknowledge the technical assistance of Elizabeth
Keough and Nancy Williams in the first part of this study. Partial
support was received from the U.S. Office of Naval Research, the
U.S. Public Health Service and the Faculty Research Committee,
University of California, Santa Barbara.

RESPONSE OF EARTHWORM LEUKOCYTES TO CONCANAVALIN A

AND TRANSPLANTATION ANTIGENS

ROCH, Ph., VALEMBOIS, P. and DU PASQUIER, L.

Laboratoire de Zoologie A de l'Université de Bordeaux 1
et Centre de Morphologie Expérimentale du CNRS,
Avenue des Facultés, 33405 TALENCE (France);
Basel Institute for Immunology, Grenzacherstrasse 487,
CH 4058 BASEL (Switzerland)

INTRODUCTION

There are several reasons to believe that rejection of both
allogenic and xenogenic tissues by earthworms is due to an active
immune response: a second graft from a same donor to a same receptor
is more actively rejected (1); graft immunity can be transfered by
coelomic cells from a sensitized animal to a non sensitized one (2).
Coelomic cells, which are the free cells of the coelomic cavity,
mainly consist in leukocyte-like cells. The leukocytes undoubtly
play a prominent role in graft rejection in earthworms: it seems
that they recognize the immunogenic stimulus and then proliferate
and differentiate into cells that attack the grafted tissues (3).
In vertebrates, specific recognition is achieved by a special group
of leukocytes, the lymphocytes (4), that generally proliferate after
antigenic stimulation. The leukocytes can also exibit an increase of
DNA synthesis after a wound. But, in vertebrates, stimulated cells
involved in inflammation are different from lymphocytes. In order to
check whether graft reaction in earthworms was different from inflammatory process, we have compared the leukocyte stimulation induced
by wound with that occuring after graft. The quantitative aspects
of the stimulation have been investigated as well as the nature of
the stimulated cells.

In vertebrates, a variety of extracts from plant or bacterial
origin, which are called mitogens, can induce lymphocyte proliferation (5-6-7-8). Mitogenic stimulations follow the binding of mitogen
molecules with specific saccharide-containing-receptors of the cell
membrane. It has been showed that cells responding to different
mitogens belonged to separate populations of lymphocytes: for

instance, lymphocytes activated by phytohemagglutinin (PHA) or by soluble concanavalin A (Con A) are involved in cellular immunity (T cells); those responding to lipopolysaccharide of E. coli (LPS) are associated with humoral immunity (B cells). The following studies on the reactivity of invertebrate leukocytes to Con A were undertaken to ascertain the phylogenetic relations between invertebrate leukocytes and vertebrate lymphocytes.

MATERIAL and METHODS

Animals

The worms used for these experiments belonged to two genera, Eisenia foetida and Allolobophora caliginosa (Lumbricidae family). Wounds, grafts and Con A assays are made on Eisenia. Allolobophora was the donor of xenografts.

A first series of experiments consisted in wounds of about 1 mm performed in the dorsal body-wall. The wounds were then stitched with silver wire (9).

In grafted animals a piece of body-wall of about 1 mm^2 was transplanted in the coelomic cavity through an incised wound.

Second grafts were studied on animals which were transplanted one week after the first implantation with a fragment of body-wall from a donor of the same species than the first one. Such grafts can be considered as second set grafts for the species specific antigens.

Operated animals were always compared with control animals which had undergone no surgical treatment.

Cells donors for Con A assays had undergone no preliminary treatment.

Culture Methods

When excited by a current of low voltage (6v) earthworms throw through their dorsal pores the greater part of their coelomic cells (10). Suchatreatment which does not affect the viability of the cells was used to harvest leukocytes. A slight electric discharge, performed 24 hours before harvesting, eliminated the greater part of the chloragocytes. The harvesting was performed on pools of at least 10 animals. The coelomic liquid was collected in tubes containing the culture medium and centrifuged 5 mn at 250 g. Leukocytes were then recovered from the supernatant, whashed twice in culture medium and brought to the final concentration of 1.6 10^6 cells per ml. Culture medium contained 60 % L-15 medium (DIFCO),15 % fetal calf serum (DIFCO), 25 % bidistilled water, 100 U/ml penicillin and 50 µg/ml streptomycin and EGTA at final concentration of 0.005 M to prevent rapid aggregation of the cells. This medium was different from those previously used for earthworms (11-12-13) by the high concentration of amino-acids. The medium was buffered at pH 7.2 with HEPES (Microbiological Associates Inc.) at the concentration of 0.033 M. Finally, aliquots of 200 µl (3.2 10^5 cells) were put

in culture in Microtest Plates 220 AR (Falcon Plastics). All cultures
were set up in triplicates.

Con A Assays

20 µl of soluble Con A (Miles Yeda Ltd, Rehovot) purified by
Dr J. ANDERSSON following a method described by AGRAWAL and GOLDSTEIN
(14) was added at various dilutions (see Fig. 4) immediately after
washing. Fluorescent studies were made with tetramethyl-rhodamine-
labelled-Con A (kindly provided by Dr F. LOOR).

Labelling of Cells with Tritiated Thymidine

DNA synthesis was determined by incorporation of tritiated thymidine (CEA, Saclay) added 16 hours before termination of cultures.
Each 200 µl culture was pulsed with 1 µCi ^{3}H-thymidine (specific
activity 25 Ci/mM). At the end of the pulse, the cells from the
cultures were collected with a semi automatic apparatus (MIGGIANO
and WYSS unpublished) on glass fiber filters (Whatman) and washed
in 0.65 % NaCl. The acid insoluble material was precipitated by 5 %
TCA. The filters were then treated with 0.5 ml Protosol (Nuclear
Chicago) and processed for liquid scintillation counting after addition of 10 ml PPO–POPOP toluene solution.

Autoradiographs

For optical observations: smears were air dried 5 mn and then
fixed (3 hours) in glutaraldehyde vapour. Autoradiographs were done
using stripping film technic (Kodak AR 10 film, 18 days of exposure).
After development, slides were stained with May–Grunwald Giemsa and
a differential count was performed on at least 500 labelled cells
per experiment.

For high resolution: the cells deposited on Millipore 0.22 µ
filters were fixed in 2 % glutaraldehyde cacodylate 0.1 M buffered,
postfixed in 1 % buffered osmium tetroxyde and embedded in Epon 812.
Sections were stained with uranyl acetate and lead citrate. A monolayer of Ilford L 4 emulsion was applied to sections which were
exposed for 5–6 weeks in a dry atmosphere at 4 °C. The sensitivity
of the developer (Elon 0.045 %, ascorbic acid 0.3 %) was increased
by gold latensification (15–16). Grids were studied with Philips
201 electron microscope.

RESULTS

It has been previously proposed (3) that earthworm leukocytes
involved in inflammatory process were different from those initia-
ting reactions of specific rejection. To delineate the characters
of each of these reactions and to understand the modalities of mitogenic stimulation in earthworm leukocytes, we have studied in vitro
DNA synthesis of leukocytes removed from animals stimulated in
various ways. Xenograft stimulation (by comparison with wound action)
allograft stimulation and Con A action on cultured cells have been
successively studied.

Graft Stimulation

In a first series of experiments the amount of tritiated thymidine incorporated in vitro by leukocytes of operated animals was measured by standard scintillation technique. At various intervals after wound or graft application leukocytes were withdrawn from the animals and pulsed in vitro with tritiated thymidine for 16 hours. Several pools (usually 5) were set up for each stage. Results are summarized in Fig. 1 and Fig. 2. A first graft (xenograft as well as allograft) showed a slightly higher peak than a wound. In a same way the stimulation induced by a second graft (xenograft or allograft) was slightly higher than the one given with second wound. Only mild differences were noticed when comparing first and second grafts.

We have then studied the morphological features of the stimulated cells by the mean of autoradiography. Both autoradiographies on cells smeared on slides and in high resolution have shown that labelled cells could be arranged in two size categories: leukocytes with a diameter below 10 μm and leukocytes above 10 μm in diameter. Cells of the first group had a large nucleous and many free ribosomes in most of the available cytoplasm. Cells of the second group were irregular in shape and had a well developed cytoplasm with an abundant vesicular component. As shown in Fig. 3, percentage of labelled cells in different size categories, was affected by the modalities of the stimulation. The proportion of stimulated small cells reached a higher value after a graft stimulation than after a wound stimulation. This trend was more marked after a second set response.

Phytomitogen Stimulation

In a first series of experiments we have studied the effect of various concentrations of soluble Con A on tritiated thymidine incorporation. For each concentration the stimulation was studied as a function of the time of contact between mitogen and cells. The results are given in Fig. 4. It was possible to get a stimulation of DNA synthesis for Con A doses between 0.5 and 5 μg/ml. Con A doses higher than 10 μg/ml had no effect. Whatever the active concentrations no stimulation was noticed before 3 days. A peak of incorporation occurred at 5 days. Several experiments have been performed to see whether methyl-α-D-mannopyranoside (α-MM) abolishes the effect of Con A in earthworms like in vertebrates (17). The inhibitory effect of various concentrations of α-MM on DNA synthesis has been tested (Table 1). Control assays with D-galactose have shown no inhibitory effect of this sugar on the Con A activity. Similar results with α-MM were obtained in another experiment where the specificity of D-galactose was not tested. An autoradiographic study of Con A stimulated cells has shown that only a slight population of leukocytes was concerned with ^{3}H-thymidine incorporation. Less than 1 % of the cells were labelled at the time when the scintillation measurement showed peaked activity. An attempt has been made to label the leukocyte binding sites for Con A with

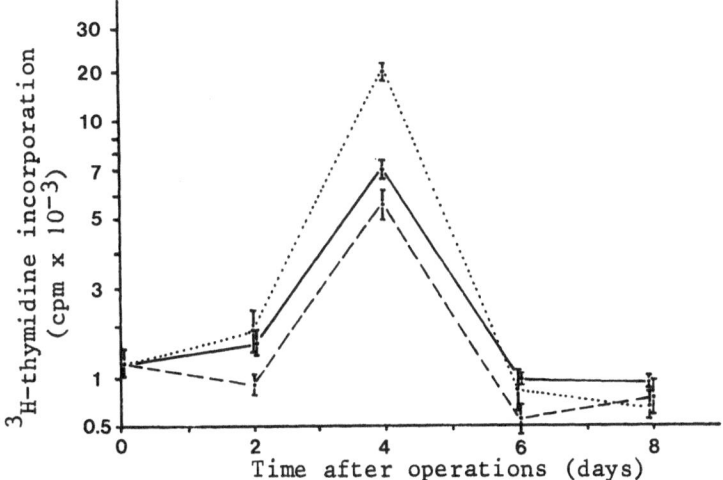

Fig. 1 – Kinetics of first allograft response (·······) and first xenograft response (————) compared to a first wound response (———). At 4 days allograft stimulation is appreciably twice as important as wound stimulation. Each point represents the mean of at least 5 replicas ± SE.

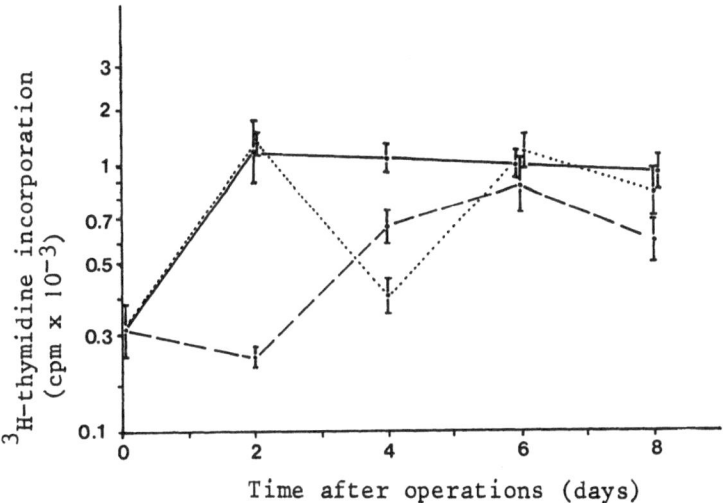

Fig. 2 – Kinetics of second allograft response (·······) and second xenograft response (————) compared to a second wound response (———). Symbols as in Fig. 1.

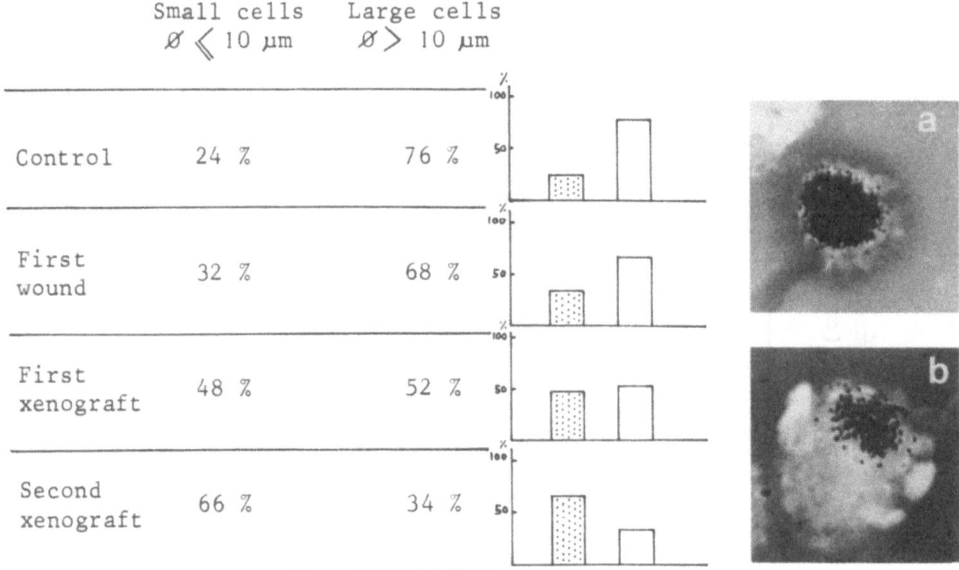

Fig. 3 - Percentages of small and large stimulated leukocytes after a wound, a first xenograft and a second xenograft. On the right, autoradiographs of a typical small cell (a) and large cell (b). Percentage established from cell counts performed on at least 500 labelled cells.

fluorescent staining. All the leukocytes were fluorescent after treatment with tetramethyl-rhodamine-Con A. Chloragocytes exhibited natural fluorescence and it was difficult to determine whether the Con A bound to their surface. For leukocytes, the fluorescence was uniform over the whole cell surface.

DISCUSSION

Graft Stimulation

A graft as well as a wound induced a stimulation of DNA synthesis in leukocytes. The stimulation induced by a graft is slightly higher than the one provoked by a wound. Nevertheless the difference between the kinetic curves of grafts and that of wounds was generally not enough to be significant. This absence of difference is not surprising if we consider that the stimulation measurements were performed on the whole population of leukocytes coming out from the whole worm and not only on the specifically involved population of cells. In contrast a distinction founded on size of leukocytes concerned with the different modalities of stimulation had given interesting results. When only small stimulated cells expressed in percentage of the whole stimulated population were considered a

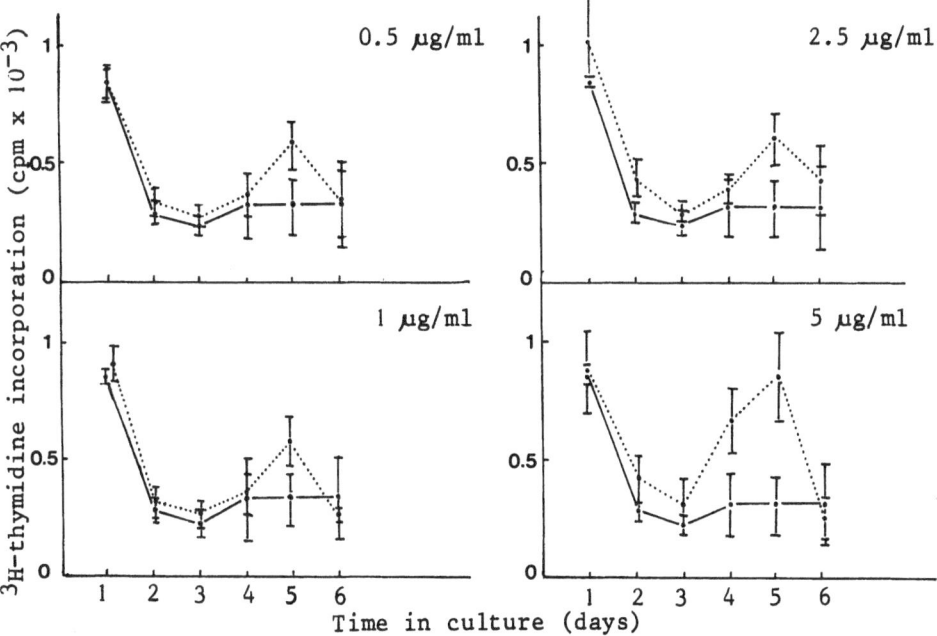

Fig. 4 - Response of normal leukocytes to various doses of Con A.
Kinetics of the response after addition of 0.5 µg/ml, 1 µg/ml, 2.5
µg/ml and 5 µg/ml. Con A pulsed cultures (.....) are compared with
untreated control cultures (——). Symbols as in Fig. 1.

Table 1 - Effects of saccharides on Con A stimulation of leukocytes. The means values $\pm$ SE were based on determination of 2-3
replicas for experiments 1 and 2 and of 5 replicas for experiment 3.
Experiments 1 and 2 were performed with the same pool of cells; experiment 1 pulsed in day 3 to 4, experiment 2 pulsed in day 4 to 5.
Experiment 3 (different pool) pulsed in day 3 to 4.

Con A 5 µg/ml	Saccharides 0.01 M	^{3}H-Thymidine incorporation (cpm) Experiments		
		1	2	3
−	−	764 $\pm$ 637	295 $\pm$ 115	1777 $\pm$ 225
+	−	1986 $\pm$ 697	667 $\pm$ 451	2116 $\pm$ 332
−	α-MM	nd	nd	1501 $\pm$ 133
−	D-Galactose	nd	nd	1462 $\pm$ 207
+	α-MM	919 $\pm$ 485	239 $\pm$ 74	1447 $\pm$ 275
+	D-Galactose	nd	nd	2119 $\pm$ 623

significant difference between graft and wound was noticed. This difference was more important following a second graft. It may be noticed that more important differences would probably be observed if
cell populations near the graft or the wound had been harvested
alone. Previous histological data had established that immunity
could be transfered by leukocytes therefore that leukocytes were
involved in specific recognition. Present preliminary results have
suggested that small leukocytes are selectively stimulated by grafts.
Consequently, it seems that biochemical factors involved in the
specific recognition must be researched at first on these stimulable
small cells.

Con A Stimulation

Like vertebrate lymphocytes, leukocytes of earthworms respond
to soluble Con A by an increase of DNA synthesis. The kinetics of
stimulation are similar by several features in both zoological
groups although the extent of stimulation was much lower in worms
than in vertebrates.

α-MM selectively abolished the effect of Con A on leukocyte
activation in a range of concentration from 0.01 to 0.1 M/l. It seems
that the inhibition was the result of a competition between carbohydrate and binding sites of leukocytes for the specific binding
site of Con A. Lumbricid leukocytes and vertebrate lymphocytes (18)
would have therefore similar cell membrane Con A receptor sites.

In earthworms like in vertebrates, a few stimulated cells have
been found though all the leukocytes seemed able to fix Con A molecules. It may be postulated (19) that the cell receptors initially
binding Con A are unable to induce DNA synthesis. A stimulation of
synthesis would only occur when a second cell receptor has interfered
with the mitogen or with the complex mitogen-first receptor.

In vertebrates, T lymphocytes are optimally stimulated in a
narrow range of mitogen concentrations. In earthworms, an increased
synthesis has only been found for concentrations ranging from 0.5
to 5 μg/ml; concentrations of 10 or of 20 μg/ml had given no stimulation. Despite evident similarities between worms and vertebrates
such as the kinetics of the stimulation, the inhibitory effect of
α-MM or the distribution of cell receptors, the possibility of
convergent phenomena is not excluded and present results require
complementary studies with other mitogens to be phylogenetically
significant.

Phylogenetic Implications

Leukocytes of lumbricids, like vertebrate T lymphocytes, can
be stimulated by graft antigens and by Con A. It has been hypothe-
tized several years ago that some groups of invertebrates could be
able to elicit cellular reactions of immunity and not humoral ones
(20). Then immunologically competent invertebrates would possess
leukocytes sharing some physiological properties with T lymphocytes.
It seems, with references to our work in progress, that earthworm

leukocytes also possess stimulation sites for LPS of E. coli (21).
In vertebrates such sites characterize B lymphocytes.

In concluding remarks, we may state that leukocytes of worms
already possess many biochemical characters of lymphocytes. But they
are more primitive cells which have a lower level of specialisation
as evidenced by previous electron microscopy studies (22). A next
step of our investigations will consist in searching if leukocytes
populations of earthworms show a physiological heterogeneity, similar to that known in lymphocyte populations of vertebrates.

REFERENCES

1. VALEMBOIS, P., Comp. Rend. Acad. Sci. Paris, 257: 3489-90 (1963)

2. DUPRAT, P., Ann. Inst. Pasteur, 113: 867-881 (1967).

3. VALEMBOIS, P., Contemporary Topics Immunobiol., 4: 121-126 (1974)

4. GOWANS, J.L., MAC GREGOR, D.D., COWEN, D.M. and FORD, C.E.,
    Nature London, 196: 651-655 (1962).

5. NOWELL, P.C., Cancer Res., 20: 462-466 (1960).

6. LING, N.R., Lymphocyte stimulation (North Holland Publ. Co.,
    Amsterdan, 1968).

7. PEAVY, D.L., ADLER, W.H. and SMITH, R.T., J. Immunol, 105:
    1453-1458 (1970).

8. JANOSSY, G. and GREAVES, M.F., Clin. exp. Immunol., 9: 483-494
    (1971).

9. AVEL, M., Bull. Biol. France et Belgique, 63: 149-318 (1929).

10. VALEMBOIS, P., ROCH, Ph. and DU PASQUIER, L., Comp. Rend. Acad.
    Sci. Paris, 277: 57-60 (1973).

11. GAY, R., Ann. Epiphyties, 14: 61-75 (1963).

12. BORER, A., Doctoral Thesis, Department Biology, St Bonaventure
    University, N. Y., 1-102 (1968).

13. COOPER, E.L., in Proc. 3d Intern. Colloquium on Invert. Tissue
    Culture, Bratislava, 381-404, June 1971 (1973).

14. AGRAWAL, B.B.L. and GOLDSTEIN, I.J., Biochem. J., 96: 23-25
    (1965).

15. SALPETER, M.M. and BACHMANN, L., J. Cell Biol., 22: 469-476
    (1964).

16. WISSE, E. and TATES, A.D., in Proc. 4th Europ. Reg. Conf.
    Electron Microscopy, Rome, 465-466 (1968).

17. NOVOGRODSKY, A. and KATCHALSKI, E., Biochim. Biophys. Acta, 228:
    579-583 (1971).

18. GOLDSTEIN, I.J., HOLLERMAN, C.E. and SMITH, E.E., Biochem., 4: 876-883 (1965).

19. ANDERSSON, J., SJOBERG, O. and MOLLER, G., Transplant. Rev., 11: 131-177 (1972).

20. GOOD, R.A., J. exp. Med., 119: 105-130 (1964).

21. ROCH, Ph., Doctorat 3me Cycle Biologie n° 1077, Université de Bordeaux 1, 1-70 (1973).

22. VALEMBOIS, P., Bull. Soc. zool. France, 96: 59-72 (1971).

RECOGNITION FACTORS OF THE CRAYFISH AND THE GENERATION OF DIVERSITY

C. R. Jenkin and D. Hardy

Department of Microbiology, The University of Adelaide

Adelaide, South Australia 5000

During the last decade there has been a renewed interest in the mechanisms of immunity in the invertebrates. This has been due partly to the desire of immunologists to find a mechanism in these lower forms that may be an evolutionary precursor to the well defined system in the vertebrates. Approaches to this problem have been basically along two lines. It is now well established that invertebrates may have, in their haemolymph, haemagglutinins to erythrocytes from various species of vertebrates. In certain studies it is clear that these haemagglutinins are functionally analogous to the haemagglutinins present in the sera of vertebrates, for example in their presence, the phagocytosis of erythrocytes is enhanced (1 - 4). A number of investigators have purified haemagglutinins from various species of invertebrates but to date it would appear that there are no structural homologies between these haemagglutinins and the immunoglobulins of the vertebrates (5 - 12). The second approach and the one that we have chosen has been to concentrate primarily on functional analogies and to concern ourselves with the problem of determining whether the recognition of foreign material by phagocytic cells in the invertebrates depends on the reaction of the foreign material with specific proteins as it does in the vertebrates.

The invertebrate that we have chosen to study is the freshwater crayfish (Parachaeraps bicarinatus) which has been reclassified recently as Cherax destructor. In these animals we have studied both in vivo and in vitro the mechanism which enables phagocytic cells to recognise foreign particles such as erythrocytes from various species of vertebrates and various antigenically different strains of bacteria. In all instances we have found that the recognition of foreignness requires the association of the

foreign particle with certain substances in serum that we have
termed recognition factors. These recognition factors which are
trypsin labile may be associated either with the membrane of the
phagocytic cell or free in the haemolymph (4, 13, 14). Cross
adsorption studies have indicated that there is a measure of specificity in this reaction although the specificity appears at first
not to be as fine as that observed with the immunoglobulins of
vertebrates. This facet has been commented on by other workers in
the field (12, 15, 16, 17).

Unlike the vertebrates which are a monophyletic group, the
invertebrates are polyphyletic. In a limited study it would appear
that the recognition factors that we have studied will function
only within the phylum. Thus, for example, whilst haemagglutinins
to sheep erythrocytes from the snail (Helix aspersa) will enhance
phagocytosis of these cells by phagocytes from this animal, they
will not enhance phagocytosis of sheep erythrocytes by phagocytes
from the crayfish and vice versa. However, the haemagglutinin to
sheep erythrocytes from the crab (Ozius truncatus) will enhance the
phagocytosis of sheep erythrocytes by crayfish phagocytic cells (4).

We have extended these studies to determine whether or not
crayfish haemocytes can recognise foreign mammalian cells. One
purpose of this study was to see if we could establish a model that
might be useful in defining the mechanism of graft rejection in the
invertebrates. It is clear from the work of Cooper, and Hildemann
and colleagues, that many invertebrates are capable of rejecting
foreign tissue grafts. The mechanism involves cells and in some
cases it would appear that there is a short term memory to such
biological abuse (18 - 22). However, despite these studies we are
still unaware of the precise mechanism involved in the recognition
of the foreign tissue and the factors that may be released by the
cells attacking the graft which leads to the final rejection.

Possibly the best way of defining this system would be to
devise an in vitro system where the cellular events involved in
attacking a foreign tissue could be quantitated. We have chosen
to study the inter-reaction of crayfish haemocytes with tumour
cells from vertebrates (23). Three cell lines were chosen: an
Ehrlich's ascites tumour (EAT), Krebs II ascites tumour, and HeLa
cells. It was found that haemocyte monolayers from the crayfish
caused a rapid release of ^{51}Cr label from the ascites tumour cells
but were inactive against the HeLa cells. The data illustrated in
Fig. 1 shows this release from the Ehrlich ascites tumour. Staining with trypan blue revealed that a 50%-60% release of ^{51}Cr
indicated that greater than 90% of the tumour cells had been killed.
Experiments carried out with different ratios of haemocytes to
tumour cells established that this cytotoxic reaction was likely to
be a property of the majority of the cells in the haemocyte monolayer (Fig. 2). Further studies showed that the recognition of the

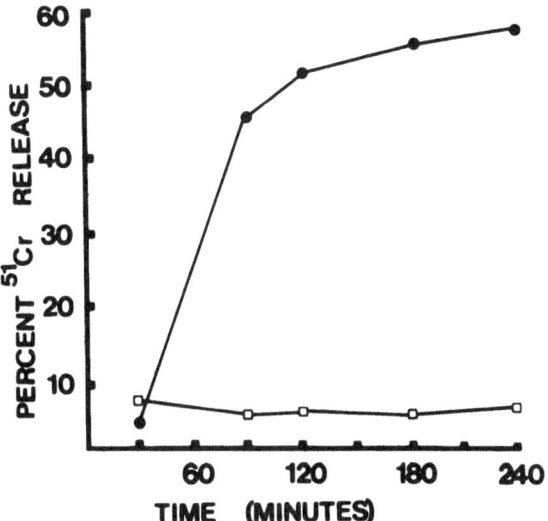

Fig. 1. The cytotoxic action of crayfish haemocytes on ^{51}Cr-labelled EAT cells. ●–● Leighton tubes containing monolayers of crayfish haemocytes. □–□ Leighton tubes containing no haemocytes.

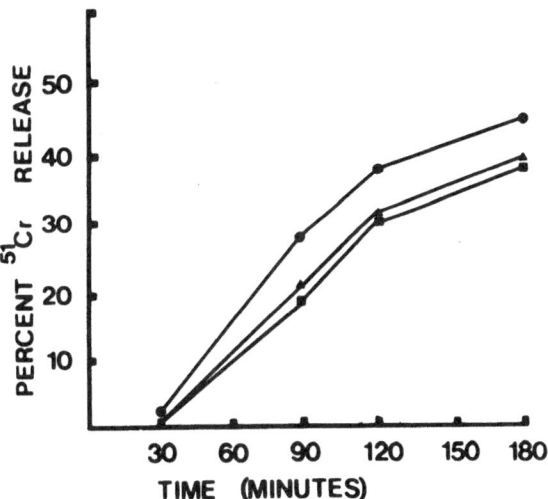

Fig. 2. The effect of varying the ratio of haemocytes to ^{51}Cr-labelled EAT cells on the cytotoxic reaction. ■–■ Leighton tubes containing approx. 1 haemocyte:1 tumour cell. ▲–▲ Leighton tubes containing approx. 2 haemocytes:1 tumour cell. ●–● Leighton tubes containing approx. 20 haemocytes:1 tumour cell.

tumour cells and the consequent cytotoxic events could be abolished by pretreating the haemocytes with trypsin, suggesting that trypsin labile factors associated with the haemocytes were responsible for the recognition of the tumour cell line. Trypsin treatment did not affect apparently other functional activities of the haemocytes since they would phagocytose bacteria readily providing these had been pretreated with haemolymph.

The fact that the haemocytes were not cytotoxic to HeLa cells could be due possibly to one of two reasons; either the haemocytes lacked the necessary receptor sites enabling recognition to take place, or if the recognition system was present the HeLa cells were resistant to the cytotoxic principle(s) released following contact of the two cells. If the first supposition is correct, then it might be possible to demonstrate a cytotoxic reaction if we impose on the HeLa cell an antigen that the haemocyte can recognise. Our previous data have established that haemocytes have on their membranes recognition factors capable of reacting with Salmonella abortus equi.

Recent studies indicate that some of these factors are directed against the lipopolysaccharide component of the 'O' somatic antigen of this strain of bacteria. One of the properties of many lipopolysaccharides from gram-negative bacteria is their ability to adhere to cell membranes. Taking advantage of this property HeLa cells were coated with the lipopolysaccharide from S. abortus equi and added to a monolayer of haemocytes from the crayfish. The data presented in Fig. 3 show that such sensitised HeLa cells are now destroyed by the haemocytes whereas unsensitised cells are not. One might argue that the phenomenon described in this study is similar to that of allogeneic inhibition as delineated by Hellstrom and Hellstrom (24) and Hellstrom, Hellstrom and Motet (25). However, the results obtained with HeLa cells renders this unlikely. In all experiments using cells not sensitised with lipopolysaccharide, cell to cell contact was excellent according to visual examination. It is unlikely therefore that mere histocompatibility differences between the two cell lines could account for the observed cytotoxicity. It would suggest however that the cytotoxicity is dependent on the cells binding together due to a reaction between specific complementary sites rather than by mere membrane contact. We believe these results are important from two aspects. The one is that they demonstrate that cells from the crayfish recognise both erythrocytes, bacteria and tumour cells by a specific recognition system which involves factors either free in the haemolymph or associated with the phagocytic cell membrane. Secondly, the system described may be of value in defining more clearly the mechanism of not only graft rejection in these animals but also rejection of metazoan parasites.

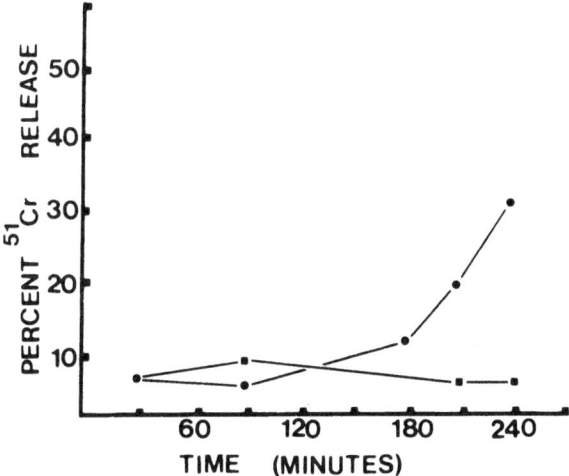

Fig. 3. Effect of haemocytes on HeLa cells. • HeLa cells sensitized with LP. ■ HeLa cells without LP.

Let us consider now the nature of the recognition factors in invertebrates and a possible means by which a generation of diversity may be accomplished within these molecules.

There are considerable differences in the molecular size and weight of the haemagglutinins purified from various species of invertebrates. Thus a haemagglutinin from the oyster (<u>Crassostrea virginicana</u>) has a molecular weight greater than 1,000,000 whilst a haemagglutinin from the snail (<u>Helix pomatia</u>) has a molecular weight of 79,000. However, there is a common feature to all these molecules and that is they may be dissociated into sub-units by a series of different chemical treatments which do not destroy covalent bonds. Furthermore, it would appear that in many cases the agglutination of erythrocytes by these molecules requires the presence of Ca^{++} ions. Indeed the removal of Ca^{++} ions may lead to some dissociation of the molecule into its sub-units (5-12). Recently we have purified the recognition factors from the haemolymph of the crayfish by affinity chromatography and shown them to be antigenically related. Chromatography on calibrated columns using Biogel P-150 and Sephadex S100 have revealed that these molecules have a molecular weight of 81,500 and may be dissociated into sub-units of 13,500 molecular weight. Thus it would appear that the recognition factors against bacteria and erythrocytes in this particular species are molecules composed of six sub-units (26).

There are certain peculiarities of the invertebrate recognition
system that differ it from the system known in the vertebrates,
which we should consider before embarking on hypotheses relating to
the generation of diversity within the molecules involved. Earlier
we have stated that the specificity shown by the haemagglutinins
appears not to be as fine as that displayed by the haemagglutinins
from vertebrates. We have observed this phenomenon with the recognition factors to both erythrocytes and bacteria isolated from the
haemolymph of the crayfish. Cross adsorption experiments with
bacteria that appear antigenically unrelated have shown that adsorb-
ing with the one may remove frequently a considerable proportion of
the titre of the recognition factors against the other. Nevertheless it is apparent from data derived from such cross adsorptions
that in some cases the titre against one strain of bacteria or
erythrocyte is undiminished by adsorption with another. This
indicates a measure of specificity displayed by these molecules.
It is clear also that as far as the crayfish is concerned agglutination of bacteria is unusual and yet by using a modified Coomb's
technique one can show that bacteria which are not agglutinated by
haemolymph have recognition factors adsorbed to their surface.
Two further peculiarities of the crayfish system are that (1) prior
exposure of the animal to erythrocytes or bacteria does not raise
the titre of the recognition factor to these foreign antigens, and
(2) the titre of the recognition factors is remarkably constant
between individuals within this species. This constancy in titre
and inability to induce in general an anamnestic response has been
commented on by other workers in the field (1, 4, 27, 28). Bearing
these peculiarities in mind and the sub-unit structure of these
recognition molecules, we propose the following hypothesis which
might account for them.

If we consider the crayfish there are six sub-units in the
molecule which we can call A, B, C, D, E, F. If we assume that all
six sub-units are made by the same cell, that they differ one from
the other, that they combine in a random fashion and that the combination of A with B engenders a different specificity than A with C,
we can ask the following question: How many different specificities
may be produced by such a random combination?

Whilst we are unaware of the arrangement of the units in the
molecule, we have assumed that it is similar to that of the haemagglutinin to horse erythrocytes that has been purified by
Marchalonis and Edelman (5, 29). A preliminary computer analysis
by one of our colleagues in the Mathematics Department indicates
that one may produce $6 \times 10^3 - 8 \times 10^3$ different specificities (30).

This hypothesis could explain why the titre of a specific
recognition factor is not altered in the invertebrates by prior

exposure to the specific antigen. Since all the cells are producing the same variable specificities, it is not possible to select
and expand a clone of cells producing a specific product as in the
vertebrates and thus increase the product. It would explain also
why the titre of a specific recognition factor does not vary
greatly between individuals within the same species, since one
would expect this if the specificities are produced by a random
combination of basic sub-units.

We have at present two pieces of experimental evidence which
though preliminary would support the above hypothesis. Let us say,
for example, that AB defines the specificity for sheep erythrocytes.
If we adsorb the haemolymph with sheep erythrocytes then we should
remove all AB specificities. However, sub-units A and B will still
exist in other molecules in different combinations with sub-units
C, D, E, F. If we dissociate now the remaining recognition factors
into their sub-units and allow them to recombine at random, we
should in theory regenerate specificity for sheep erythrocytes.
Previous data indicate that the recognition factors of the crayfish
may be partially dissociated in the presence of E.D.T.A. The data
given in Table 1 show that haemolymph following adsorption with
sheep erythrocytes and treatment with E.D.T.A. regains specificity
for sheep erythrocytes after removal of the E.D.T.A. by dialysis
and addition of Ca^{++} ions. Similar results have been obtained
using chicken erythrocytes which show no antigenic cross reaction

Table 1.   Recovery of activity against sheep erythrocytes
           following adsorption of haemolymph with sheep
           erythrocytes and dissociation of the adsorbed
           haemolymph into sub-units

Material used	Haemolytic titre against sheep erythrocytes
Haemolymph	128 units
Haemolymph adsorbed with sheep erythrocytes	0 units
Haemolymph treated overnight with E.D.T.A. dialysed and reconstituted in the presence of tris/Ca^{++} buffer	32 units

with sheep erythrocytes. Adsorption of a partially purified fraction containing the recognition factors gave results similar to that obtained using haemolymph. Further supporting evidence for our hypothesis arises from studies on the synthesis of these recognition factors <u>in vitro</u> by cells harvested from the haemolymph. Briefly the technique involves overlaying a monolayer of haemocytes in tissue culture with a mat of sheep erythrocytes. At different intervals of time the sheep erythrocytes are harvested and after washing are resuspended in a tris/Ca^{++} buffer. To these cells a suitable dilution of a rabbit antiserum specific for the recognition factors is added and the mixture incubated for 60 minutes at 37°C. After this initial period of incubation guinea pig serum as a source of complement is added and incubation continued for a further 45 minutes. The degree of haemolysis is measured by O.D. at 541 mμ. Data presented in Fig. 4 show that over a period of 6 hrs incubation about 80% of the erythrocytes have recognition factors associated with their membranes (31). One might argue that these experiments do not rule out the idea of a clonal theory of one cell producing one specific recognition factor since the factor could diffuse through the medium contacting erythrocytes at a great distance from the source of production. However we think this

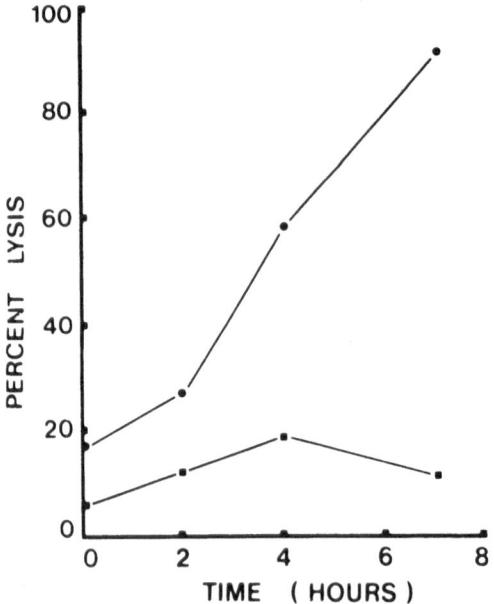

Fig. 4. Production of recognition factors to sheep erythrocytes by haemocytes in tissue culture. •——• Haemocytes incubated with sheep erythrocytes. ■——■ Sheep erythrocytes alone.

unlikely.   On a clonal theory one would expect point sources of production of the recognition factor which would not diffuse away to any great extent, in view of the density of erythrocytes, until the specific sites on the erythrocytes in the immediate area of the producing cell had become saturated.   Once this had occurred, the recognition factor would be free to diffuse in all directions and in our particular tissue culture systems, because of the volume of tissue culture fluid, the dilution effect would be considerable.   In fact we have never been able to measure any activity in the tissue culture fluid prior to harvesting the erythrocytes.   It would seem to us improbable that such a degree of sensitisation as revealed by the Coomb's technique could be due to synthesis of the specific recognition factor by a few cells but rather that a large percentage of the cells in the monolayer are involved in the production.

These results though preliminary support rather than detract from the hypothesis presented here.   However, should further work prove the hypothesis untenable, we shall have learned at least a great deal more regarding the synthesis of these recognition factors and their specificity.

ACKNOWLEDGMENTS

This work was supported by grants from the Australian Research Grants Committee.   Fig. 1 and Fig. 2 were reproduced by permission of the Australian Journal of Experimental Biology and Medical Science.

REFERENCES

1.   Tripp, M.R., J. Invert. Path., 8: 478 (1966).

2.   Stuart, A.E., J. Path. Bact., 96: 401 (1968).

3.   Prowse, R.H. and Tait, N.T., Immunol., 17: 437 (1969).

4.   McKay, D.J. and Jenkin, C.R., Aust.J.exp.Biol.med.Sci., 48:139 (1970).

5.   Marchalonis, J.J. and Edelman, G.H., J. Mol. Biol., 32: 453 (1968).

6.   Acton, R.T., Bennett, J.C., Evans, E.E. and Schrohenloher, R.E., J. Biol. Chem., 244: 4128 (1969).

7.   Hammerstrom, S. and Kabat, E.A., Biochem., 8: 2696 (1969).

8.   Hammerstrom, S., Methods in Enzymology, Vol. XXVIII, Complex
     Carbohydrates, Part B, p.368 (Academic Press, New York, 1972).

9.   Jenkin, C.R. and Rowley, D., Aust. J. exp. Biol. med. Sci., 47:
     129 (1970).

10. Finstad, C.L., Litman, G.W., Finstad, J. and Good, R.A., J.
     Immunol., 108: 1704 (1972).

11. Hall, J.L. and Rowlands, D.T., Biochemistry, 13: 821 (1974).

12. Pauley, G.B., Contemporary Topics in Immunobiology, 4: 241
     (1974).

13. Tyson, C.J. and Jenkin, C.R., Aust. J. exp. Biol. med. Sci., 52:
     341 (1974).

14. Tyson, C.J. and Jenkin, C.R., Aust. J. exp. Biol. med. Sci., 51:
     609 (1974).

15. McKay, D.J., Jenkin, C.R. and Rowley, D., Aust. J. exp. Biol.
     med. Sci., 47: 125 (1969).

16. Tyler, A. and Metz, B., J. exp. Zool., 100: 387 (1945).

17. Tyson, C.J., Stevens, C. and Jenkin, C.R., Unpublished observa-
     tions (1975).

18. Cooper, E.L., Transplantation, 3: 332 (1968).

19. Cooper, E.L., J. exp. Zool., 171: 69 (1969).

20. Duprat, P.C., Transpl. Proc., 2: 222 (1970).

21. Hildemann, W.H., Dix, T.G., and Collins, J.D., Contemporary
     Topics in Immunobiology, 4: 141 (1974).

22. Valembois, P., Contemporary Topics in Immunobiology, 4: 121
     (1974).

23. Tyson, C.J. and Jenkin, C.R., Aust. J. exp. Biol. med. Sci.,
     52: 915 (1974).

24. Hellstrom, K.E. and Hellstrom, I., Iso Antigens and Cell
     Interactions, p.79 (Wister Institute Press, Philadelphia, 1965).

25. Hellstrom, K.E., Hellstrom, I. and Motet, D., Cellular
     Recognition, p.155 (North Holland Publishing Co., Amsterdam,
     1969).

26. Tyson, C.J. and Jenkin, C.R., Unpublished observations (1974).

27. Acton, R.T. and Evans, E.E., In-Vitro, 3: 146 (1968).

28. Cornick, J.W. and Stewart, J.E., J. Invert. Path., 21: 255
    (1973).

29. Fernandez-Moran, H., Marchalonis, J. and Edelman, G.M., J. Mol.
    Biol., 32: 467 (1968).

30. Bhaskaran, S., Unpublished data (1975).

31. Busbridge, W., Unpublished observations (1975).

INVERTEBRATE IMMUNOLOGY

Immunodiscrimination and Integrity of Metazoans

ENDOSYMBIOSIS AND CELLULAR TOLERANCE IN THE HAWAIIAN SOFT CORAL

SARCOTHELIA EDMONDSONI VERRILL

E. H. Mercer and A. P. Singh

University of Hawaii at Hilo

Hilo, HI 96720

SUMMARY

The relationship between the soft coral Sarcothelia edmondsoni Verrill and its symbiotic algae is considered as an early instance of cellular tolerance which can be disturbed by a variety of adverse conditions. The algal cells lie in vesicles deep within the endo-dermal cells of the host and are not subject to digestion. Their expulsion appears to be a reverse translocation to the distal end of the host cell and escape by a form of reversed phagocytosis resem-bling secretion. The cellular mechanisms involved are not clear.

INTRODUCTION

In tracing the phylogeny of a complex highly evolved phenomenon, such as the immunological response, it is necessary to peel away the successive stages of elaboration to reach a presumed primitive state and it can be a matter of opinion as to where one calls a halt. Multicellular associations have one requirement not incumbent upon unicells: they must exclude foreign cells or suffer colonization and become mere mixtures. In this requirement one may trace the origin of the faculty to distinguish self and nonself. The simpler metazoa are more tolerant of foreign cells than are more evolved organisms and symbiosis is common. The coelenterate - algae associa-tion is notable but as found here it is far from simple and already shows evolutionary adaptation with mechanisms for regulating popula-tion ratios that have no counterpart in the evolution of immunologi-cal phenomena.

   This symbiosis between coelenterates and unicellular algae
(zoochlorellae or zooxanthellae) is an ubiquitous, persistent and
obviously ancient association which nevertheless is not obligatory;
the two partners may be separated experimentally and may be maintained each in isolation. When released from the restraints imposed
by the symbiosis, many of the algal cells undergo a transformation
into typical motile dinoflagellates. Motile cells are also released
under natural conditions and may contribute towards maintaining the
algal population in other coelenterate hosts.

   Specificity in accepting algae has been clearly shown in hydra
under well-controlled laboratory conditions[1], which suggests that
something analogous to a cellular recognition exists and that the
symbiotic association has features which may cast light on the nature
of cellular tolerance. Pardy and Muscatine[2] have proposed that the
process be separated for analysis into three phases: contact, endocytosis, and intracellular transportation. To include the phenomenon
we are examining here, the expulsion of algae, which we would regard
as an essential part of the whole cycle of the coelenterate-alga-
dinoflagellate symbiosis, we would add: reverse translocation and
exocytosis as further phases.

   Experimentally it has been noted that various adverse conditions
-- mechanical or chemical trauma, a rise in temperature, changes in
salinity and poor lighting conditions -- promote the mass shedding
of algae. Not all the symbionts are lost as a rule, although this
effect can be produced in hydra[3] which may be totally decolorized
by the loss but remain viable. Evidently the factors which control
the ratio of symbiont mass to host mass are influenced by ambient
conditions and may be presumed to act in some way to maintain an
optimal population ratio. Something is known of the biochemical
traffic between the host cell and symbionts.[4] The algae, while not
essential, are of some survival value to hydra and enhance its
growth rate. The autotrophic photosynthetic symbiont can supplement
the carbohydrate needs of the host during starvation and the removal
of carbohydrate may also assist the algae since it may be of a type
(e.g. maltose) not used by them. It is easy to imagine that some
biochemical feedbacks, operating between the two partners, can work
to maintain a biochemical optimum. Experimental evidence of the
existence of controls is growing and the coelenterate-algal association appears to be an excellent model system in which to study growth
control mechanisms in multicellular systems.

   While biochemical controls may be adequate in conditions which
do not depart too suddenly or markedly from normal, the existence of
the phenomena of mass expulsion of symbionts under traumatic conditions shows that other kinds of control mechanisms can be activated
when needed. Under such conditions the cellular tolerance extended
by the host seems to be suddenly reduced and the alga are recognized
as foreign and promptly expelled from their intracellular niche. In

the expectation that this process will have a structurally recognizable component, we have been investigating it by means of electron microscopy using the small, soft coral Sarcothelia edmondsoni common in coastal Hawaiian waters.[5]

EXPERIMENTAL

Sarcothelia edmondsoni Verrill is a small colonial, soft coral about 0.8 mm in height which forms patches of closely packed polyps on rocks at a depth of a few feet.[5] Characteristically the expanded polyp is a bright purple color making it easily recognizable. The color is due to a superficial layer of small crystals located mostly on the tentacles and upper portions of the animal. The organisms secrete a dense yellowish mat of waxes and mucus which holds the colony together on the rocky supports.

Collection and Maintenance

Small colonies attached to rocks were collected from Hilo Bay and the organisms either used at once or were maintained until needed in small aquaria in the laboratory. Those kept in aquaria shed over a few days the greater part of their superficially placed purple crystals and lost color. The level of illumination was far lower than direct sunlight (about 100-200 foot candles) and many of the alga were lost at the same time. Many polyps could be seen to be shedding alga cells when examined microscopically particularly when disturbed mechanically. Such polyps were selected for fixation in an attempt to obtain instances where the symbiont was in the process of leaving the cells of the host.

Electron Microscopy

Routine methods of "double fixation" were used: 3% glutaraldehyde in 0.05M cacodylate buffer pH 7.2 for 12 hrs was followed by washing in buffer and a further fixation in 2% osmium tetroxide in 0.05M cacodylate for 1 hr. The specimens were then washed in buffer, dehydrated in a graded series of acetone, and embedded in either epon or araldite. The only difficulty met was in stabilizing the animals in an extended state. This was achieved finally by suddenly squirting polyps from a hand syringe with the glutaraldehyde fixative.

Sections were cut on an LKB Ultratome using a diamond knife. They were stained with uranyl acetate and lead citrate and examined in a Zeiss 9 S-2 electron microscope.

FINDINGS AND DISCUSSION

The algal symbionts are located exclusively in intracellular
vacuoles deep within the endodermal digestive cells of the host (see
Figure and Plate I) where they are crowded together with the normal
organelles of the host. They were identified from our electron
micrographs by Drs. J. D. Dodge and D. L. Taylor as <u>Gymnodinium
microadriaticum</u>.[6]

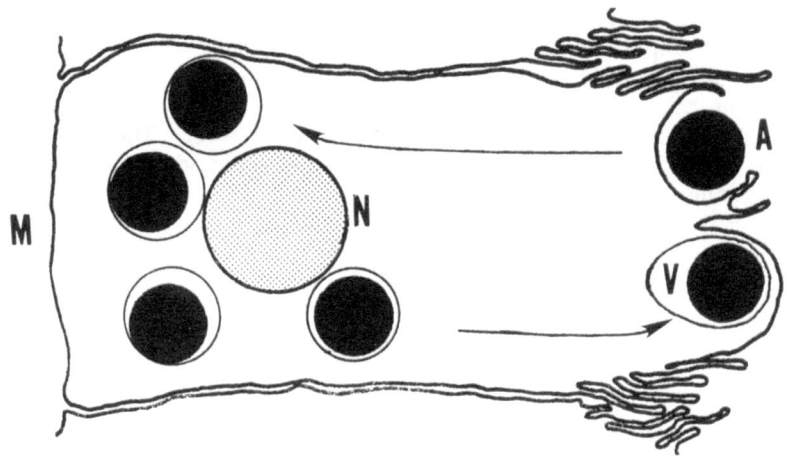

Figure 1. Intracellular location of symbiotic algae cells A and
secretory or lysosomal vacuoles in gastrodermal cell of host
organism and presumed pathways of entry and rejection of symbionts.
N nucleus of host, M mesoglea, V vacuole, A algal cell.

The algal vacuoles are found in close proximity to vacuoles
containing digestive enzymes without any evidence that the two may
interact. The membranes of the digestive vacuole and those enclosing
the symbiont appear identical in thickness and character. We have
not observed any other material in a symbiont's vacuole nor any sign
that digestive enzymes are released into such a vacuole as would
occur were it a phagocytic vacuole. This means that the failure
of the host to treat the algal cell as food and to digest it is to
be ascribed not to a special character or resistance of the algal
cell's own enveloping membranes; it is seated rather in the host's
response or to some peculiarity of the membrane with which it invests
the foreign cell. That is, the membrane of the vacuole enclosing the
symbiont does not seem to have the property of fusing with the membrane of a lysosome in such a way as to permit a transfer of contents
as would occur were it a phagocytic vacuole (see Figure 2).

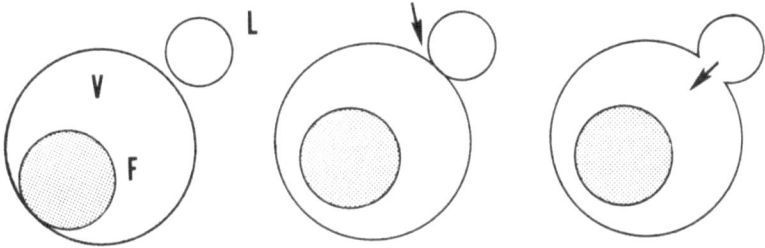

Figure 2. Stages in the formation of a secondary lysosome (digestive vacuole) from a phagocytic vacuole. V initial vacuole containing food fragment, F; L lysosome, containing lytic enzymes. The lysosome membrane fuses with the membrane of the food vacuole and an opening is formed permitting the hydrolytic enzymes to enter.

Tolerance of the symbiont's presence, once it has entered the host cell, seems to be due to the intruder's success in not activating the host's normal response to what in other respects seems a routine phagocytosis (endocytosis) and, on these structural observations, we would suspect that the effect is achieved by some modification in the symbiont's enveloping vacuolar membrane. Turning to the reverse process, the loss of tolerance and the expulsion of the symbiont, in the first place we have not noted anything to suggest that this is in anyway associated with a sudden attempt to digest the alga. That aspect of tolerance persists. What happens is that the algal vacuole migrates towards the apex of the host cell as though it were now being treated as a secretory granule to be released extracellularly. What initiates this intracellular transportation is as obscure as that which on entry causes the symbiont to penetrate deeply into the host cell. It needs also to be noted that in this special process only the symbiont vacuole moves towards the host's surface, the many lipid granules and other organelles remain in situ (Plate I). The expulsion itself is selective.

That the entire process is in other ways not strictly analogous to normal secretion is shown by some structural elaborations which develop at the surface and accompany the expulsion of the symbiont. The normal process of secretion is usually pictured structurally simply as a reversal of phagocytosis (see Figure 1 above). The enclosing membrane of the cell, fuses with it at that point, establishes an opening through which secretion can occur without the continuity of the plasma membrane itself being interrupted.

In Sarcothelia the exposed cell membrane of the gastrodermal cells lining the digestive cavity bear patches of cilia and microvilli and their intercellular contacts usually end in deep clefts choked with microvilli and occasional cilia. Algal cells, still within vacuoles and apparently about to break out, distend the

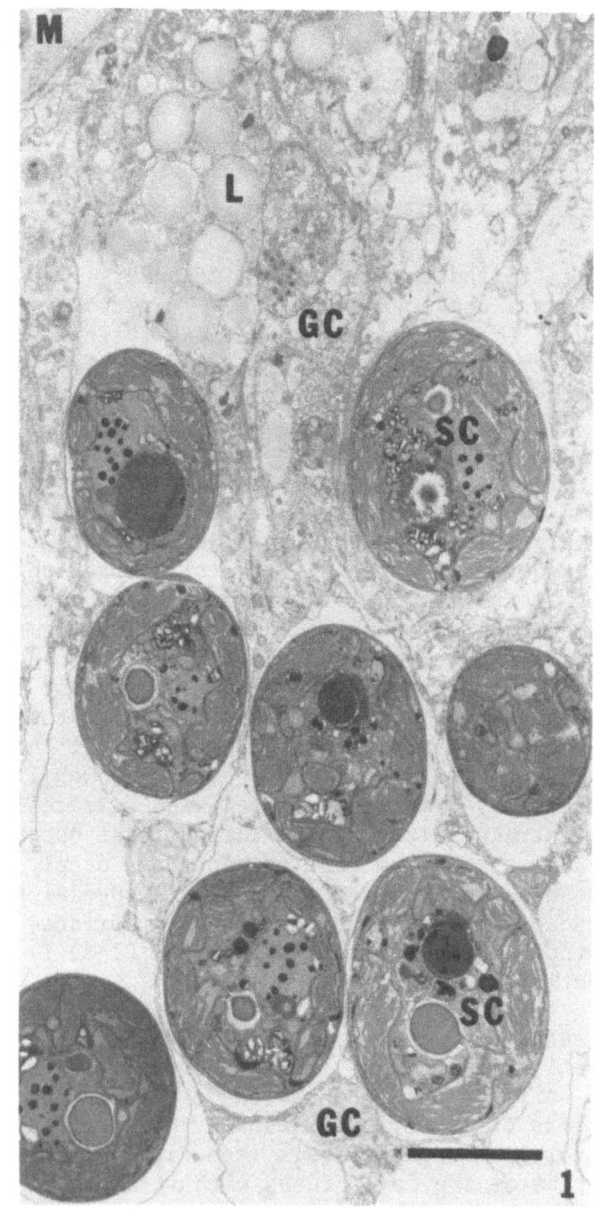

Plate 1. Electronmicrograph of the gastrodermal layer of Sarcothelia showing algal cells SC in intracellular vacuoles, some deep
within the cell, others nearing the free surface in the process
of expulsion. M is mesoglea, L lipid droplet, SC symbiont cell,
GC the cytoplasm of the gastrodermal cell. Line is 5μ long.

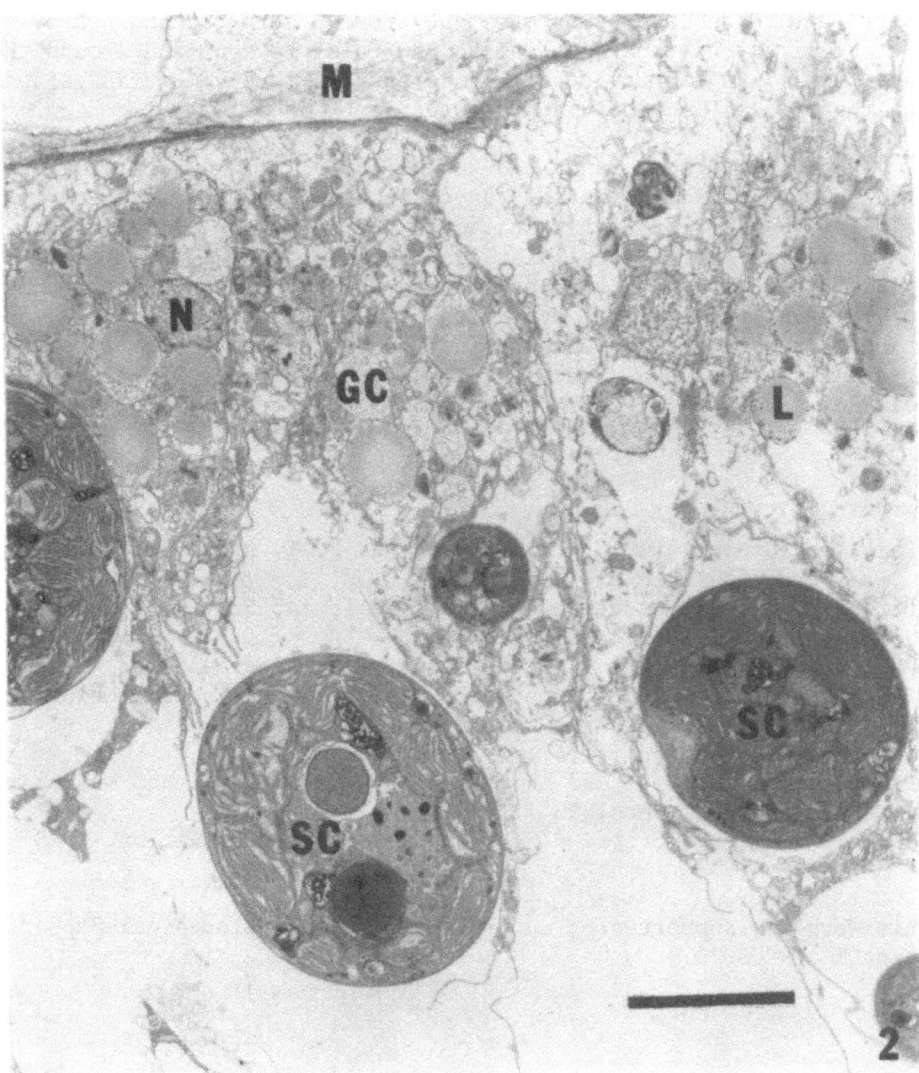

Plate 2. A portion of gastrodermal layer showing algal cells
breaking through the free surface of the gastrodermal cell GC.
N nucleus, M mesoglea, L lipid, and SC symbiont cells. Line is
5µ long.

surface into large tenuous balloons enclosed in two membranes, the external cell membrane and the vacuole membrane. The vacuole seems enlarged and water has perhaps entered which may lead to rupture-- there is no sign of other structural mechanism to aid expulsion. After rupture the enclosing membranes form a deep cup and nearby microvilli extend tapering fingers and folds towards and around the algal cell. An impression of active surface involvement is gained but the process is otherwise obscure.

Both in the acceptance and the rejection of the algal cell by the coelenterate cell there is an elaboration and modification of cellular recognition partly seated in the external cell membranes and partly in the intracellular accommodation of the alien cell. Some of these features are peculiar to this particular system and not relevant to the later evolution of cellular tolerance, however, the pattern of acceptance and rejection has elements clearly capable of elaboration in the direction of the complex interplay between cells of different origins found in more advanced phyla.

REFERENCES

[1]Park, H., Greenblatt, C. L., Mattern, C. F. T. and Merrill, C. R. J. exp. Zool. 164 141-162 (1967).
[2]Pardy, R. L. and Muscatine, L. Biol. Bull. 145 565-579 (1973) and Amer. Zool. 10 513 (1970).
[3]Reviewed by Muscatine, L. Endosymbiosis of Cnidarians and Algae in "Coelenterate Biology" eds. Leonard Muscatine and Howard M. Lenhoff Acad. Press New York (1974) p.179-191.
[4]See references cited in (3).
[5]Edmondson, C. H. Reef and Shore Fauna of Hawaii. Bishop Museum Special Pub., Honolulu (1946).
[6]Singh, A. P. and Mercer, E. H. Submitted for publication (1975).

This work was supported by an N.I.H. Minorities Biomedical Support Grant No. RR08073.

HARD TISSUE TUMORS OF SCLERACTINIAN CORALS

Daniel P. Cheney

Hilo College, University of Hawaii

Hilo, Hawaii 96720

The susceptibility of vertebrates to neoplasia is believed linked to the presence of an immunologic apparatus and a well-developed lymphoid system[1]. Recent observations on invertebrates have revealed the presence of primitive immunologic mechanisms, beginning with the coelenterates[2]. Based on this consideration, even lower invertebrates possess the theoretical capacity to acquire tumors. In this report, I will draw an example from a spontaneous tumor occurring in the scleractinian coral, Acropora formosa (Dana), and relate it to the growth patterns observed in this coral and other coelenterates.

Corals are found in warm, shallow tropical seas. They are nearly all included in the order Scleractinia, with at least 77 known genera[3]. Corals may be solitary or colonial with massive, incrusting or branching forms. Growth is accomplished by an increase in polyp height and diameter. Upon reaching a certain size, polyps undergo asexual division, forming multi-polyp colonies or buds of solitary forms. The most obvious element of this growth is the calcium carbonate exoskeleton laid down by the calcioblastic epithelium. This skeleton is formed by precipitation of calcium carbonate crystals around a framework of chitin or chitin-like substance[4]. The morphology of the skeleton is very stable within species and is an important taxonomic tool.

The rates of growth and calcium deposition are light dependent and markedly influenced by the presence of intracellular algae known as zooxanthellae. The function of the zooxanthellae is not entirely clear but it is obvious that they enhance the rate of skeleton deposition[4]. The absence of zooxanthellae in specimens

which have been starved or held in darkness for extended periods
leads to a cessation of growth and atrophy[5]. Moreover, DNA-
dependent ^{3}H-thymidine uptake is also much reduced when zooxanthellae are absent[6].

In contrast to these examples, corals which have not been
totally deprived of their zooxanthellae normally have limited areas
of rapid growth where these algae are few or lacking. In the
Acropora, growth rates measured by 45-calcium uptake are highest
in the tips, while chlorophyll content, which indicates the
abundance of zooxanthellae, is much reduced[7]. The apical tips and
edge zones of these corals seem to be utilizing nutrients trans-
ported from adjacent areas containing normal numbers of zooxanthellae. However, these areas of enhanced growth have lower densities
than the more mature areas of colonies, indicating a higher rate
of tissue growth in relation to calcium deposition[8].

Histological studies of tissue growth and differentiation in
colonial and solitary hydroids have demonstrated that cell divisions
occur almost uniformly throughout the body column. Morphogenesis
and tissue replacement is facilitated by the differentiation,
dedifferentiation and migration of cells and cell sheets. These
processes do not immediately trigger increased mitotic activity
nor do they require an established population of undifferentiated
cells. Cell divisions are believed to be the consequence of
growth and morphogenesis[9].

This may explain why corals and other coelenterates are able
to respond so rapidly to injury. They are able to reestablish
normal morphology and repair damaged tissue merely by the
rearrangement and movement of cells within the colony. The coral
skeleton undoubtedly plays an important part in these repair
processes, perhaps by providing the template for future skeleton
growth[9].

When corals are subjected to chronic chemical or physical
stresses, such as low oxygen tension, prolonged darkness or
increased temperature, their initial response is to lose the
zooxanthellae. While the exact mechanism of this loss is not
known, there is evidence from microscopic sections that both
epithelia are disrupted when the algae are pushed or pushed out.
Besides zooxanthellae, planula are also expelled or leave their
parents at these times. These sublethal responses are probably
pathologic and not likely to be encountered in the field.

In addition to generalized reactions to injury, corals have
specific behavioral and cellular responses to external stimuli.
Behavioral responses may be observed in xenografts and in reactions
to predators such as juvenile Acanthaster. The acute responses to
xenografts are characterized by the extrusion of mesenterial

filaments, the expansion of polyps of the aggressive species and
the death or continued withdrawal of the subordinate species[10].
The aggressive reactions do not occur in allografts. Instead,
the soft tissues avoid contact and remain viable. After weeks or
months of proximity, grafts are rejected by interfacial cementation.
Corals, therefore, are able to reject or wall off foreign colonies
and render local control over community composition[11].

There are many predators and parasites which have circumvented
the defensive mechanisms of corals. Large predators such as adult
Acanthaster and coralivorous fish appear to ignore or are resistant
to the effects of nematocysts and are able to feed on all but the
most venomous of corals. Gall crabs establish themselves within
the protection of the colony by physically inducing coral growth
around them. Corals contain an abundance of boring algae,
sponges, urchins and microorganisms, some of which are found only
in living colonies. The zooxanthellae are intracellular symbionts,
necessary for coral survival and actively cultured by hermatypic
species.

True parasites are generally uncommon and are usually macroscopic organisms which may be lumped under the class of "fouling"
organisms. An exception are trematode metacercariae of
Plagioporous sp. encysted in polyps of the coral, Porites spp.
from Hawaii[12]. The cysts appear grossly as pinkish nodules 3 to 5
mm in diameter, raised 1 to 2 mm above the surface of the colony.
The nodules are fragile and the metacercariae are easily dissected
from the gastrovascular cavity. The only observed histological
alterations are the compressed epithelial cells and pavemented
cyst walls in the few cases when the cyst had apparently perforated
the gastrovascular cavity. Thus cellular response is usually
lacking, cytology is probably normal, and zooxanthellae are
reduced. Despite the abundance of nodules on affected colonies
(up to 300-400 per m^2), there does not appear to be any morbidity
associated with them. Cysts are frequently overgrown with new
tissue imparting a "lumpy" appearance to heavily infested coralla
(Figure 1).

In 1971 on the island of Guam, Mariana Islands, we began
noting atypical colonies of Acropora formosa. This coral forms
large anastomizing colonies 1 to 30 meters in diameter and is
distributed in shallow protected waters throughout the Indo-Pacific.
The atypical growths or "tumors" appeared to be true neoplasms and
not just hyperplastic responses to macroscopic organisms. Our
initial research objective was to describe the gross and cellular
morphology and the ecology of the Acropora formosa tumors as
potential neoplasms.

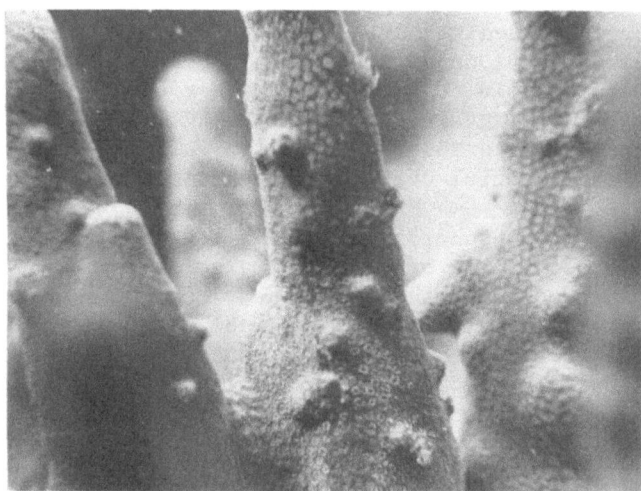

Figure 1. Nodules on <u>Porites</u> <u>compressa</u> caused by encysted meta-
cercaria of the trematode, <u>Plagioporus</u> sp. Specimens
were photographed at Honaunau, Hawaii.

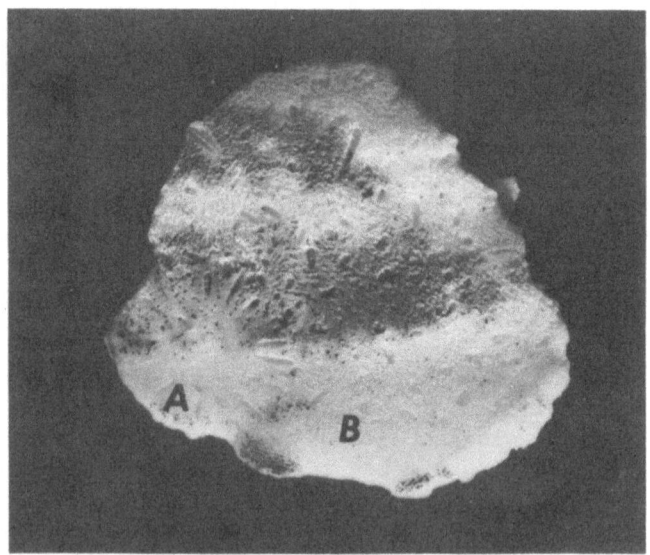

Figure 2. Section through branch (A) and tumor (B) from <u>Acropora</u>
<u>formosa</u>. Approximately life size.

METHODS AND MATERIALS

Field work on A. formosa tumors was conducted on Guam while the author was at the University of Guam Marine Laboratory. Most observations were made from mid-1970 to early-1973 in two colonies which were continuously producing abnormalities during the study period. Recently (mid-1975) similar colonies were studied in Enewetak. The first colony (Piti Lagoon) was located in a fringing reef lagoon in approximately 2 m of water. This colony was 3 m in diameter and 1 m high and was surrounded by a normal lagoon flat community. The second colony or group of colonies (Cocos Lagoon) was 35 m in diameter and 3 m high in about 5 m of water. This colony clump was surrounded by sand channels and normal appearing A. formosa colonies. Each colony was observed at weekly to monthly intervals. Measurements and photographs were taken in situ of selected abnormalities, normal branches on abnormal colonies and normal branches of adjacent, normal appearing colonies. These data were taken for 10 months from the Piti Lagoon colony with 12 data points and for 3 months on the Cocos Lagoon colony with 3 data points. Linear growth measurements in the Cocos Lagoon colony were supplemented by measuring DNA-dependent ^{3}H-thymidine incorporation. The label was introduced in situ into glass jars containing branch sections. The sections were then processed for scintillation counting[6]. Material for microscopic observation was fixed in 10% seawater formalin, decalcified in 10% nitric acid in 70% ethyl alcohol. It was then paraffin embedded, sectioned at 7 μm and stained with hematoxylin and eosin or PAS.

RESULTS

Acropora formosa tumors have been observed on Guam and Saipan in the Marianas, Palau and Ponape in the Carolines, and Enewetak in the Marshalls. They have also been seen around Lizard Island on the Great Barrier Reef. Similar growths have been seen in the Caribbean (Land and Bak, personal communications). Surveys around Guam indicate that the distribution of tumorous colonies on the island is irregular and affected colonies are generally rare. No obvious environmental factors are associated with the occurrence of tumors. The growth form and mode of growth for the Piti Lagoon and Cocos Lagoon colonies were the same. The Piti Lagoon colony exhibited a uniform coverage of abnormalities, but on the large Cocos Lagoon colony, most of the abnormalities were located on one quadrant with densities of 80 to 550 per m^2. The distribution of tumors was patchy and confined to a single colony or group of colonies.

Tumors measure 3 to 90 mm in maximum diameter. They usually occur in multiples on a single branch (up to 30). Growth in the early stages is characterized by a whitish, somewhat raised nodule,

sometimes but not always surrounding a small corallite or polyp.
The larger nodules may take on a smooth, dome-shaped appearance
with corallites much reduced in size and number. A second growth
form frequently appears in which the surface of the tumor is
covered with abundant pleomorphic corallites lying haphazardly
over the surface. In larger and probably older tumors the corallites are numerous but usually flattened and confluent with the
surface.

Closer inspection of the surface of the tumors and hard
tissue sections reveals significant differences in the structure
of the skeleton vs normal material. The normal A. formosa branch
has extensive skeletal material uniting the corallites (coenosteum).
This coenosteum is porous and consists of horizontal and vertical
laminae, more or less radially arranged and becoming denser and
almost rock-like near the center or core of the branch. The
polyps grow radially around the periphery of the branch (Figure 2-a).
This ordered structure is lacking in the tumorous sections (Figure
2-b). These are characterized by a diffuse, reticulated and highly
porous coenosteum with little or no increase in density toward the
center of the tumor mass. The polyps are randomly scattered
throughout the tumor and are quite variable in both size and shape.
They do not seem to be otherwise atypical, however. The density of
normal branch skeleton is 2.52 $\pm$ 1.86 S.D. g/cm^3, while the
density of the tumor mass is 1.13 $\pm$ .05 S.D. g/cm^3 (significant
difference at $P \leq 0.01$). Thus, the tumors have a relatively low
amount of calcium deposition per unit volume when compared with
the normal branches.

No marked cellular alterations are seen in light microscope
sections of tumors. The coenosarc epiderm is not as tall as the
normal, the endoderm is limited to a single layer of cuboidal cells
and zooxanthellae are few or lacking. In general, the coenosarc
is extensive and deep and probably spreads throughout the tumor
mass. In contrast, the coenosarc of normal mature Acropora tissue
is only a few millimeters deep. PAS reactions were similar in both
normal and abnormal colonies with the mesoglea and the cells
surrounding zooxanthellae strongly PAS positive. In no case,
either after extensive probing, trypsin or protease digestion of
coral tissue, or observation of sections in approximately 40
tumors did I observe any agent which could be implicated in their
formation.

Despite the normal cellular picture of the Acropora tumors,
the rate of growth and influence in colony growth is significant.
Data on length increments of tumors, and branches from normal and
abnormal colonies are summarized in Table I. Tumor growth
includes, of course, a significant volume increment when compared
with linear branch growth, but these data were unreliable. The
reduced growth of branches next to the tumor compared with those

on non-tumor areas of the same colony or on normal colonies, indicates that tumors are drawing nutrients from nearby normal tissue in a manner which may be equivalent to the growth of apical polyps[7]. This implies that tumor growth is accommodated by the reduction of growth in the colony or at least part of the colony. Thymidine labeling also indicated that DNA-thymidine uptake was of the same order of magnitude in the tumors as the tips of the colonies and higher than normal branch segments.

TABLE I. Growth rates (mm/day) of branches of <u>Acropora formosa</u> from Guam. All measurements are based on length increments.

Piti Lagoon (5/71 to 3/72)	$\bar{X}$	S.E.	n
Total sample period - 294 days			
Tumors	0.006 $\pm$ 0.002		3
Branches next to tumors	0.010 $\pm$ 0.003		5
Cocos Lagoon (11/72 to 3/73)			
Total sample period - 90 days			
Tumors	0.053 $\pm$ 0.012		3
Branches next to tumors	0.095 $\pm$ 0.018		4
Branches on non-tumorous part of same colony	0.500 $\pm$ -----		2
Branches on normal colony	0.263 $\pm$ 0.015		4

The photographic studies support the measurement data. These photos show the progression of tumor development and formation of new tumors on previously unaffected branches. Rapid tumor progression is demonstrated in Figure 3-a & b, where new tumors can be seen to arise from clear areas further out along the branch. At least one of these new tumors appeared to arise from an area clear of pre-existing corallites. The pleomorphic nodules (Figure 4-a & b) presented a bizarre picture of polyp growth. Very little expression of normal corallite morphology can be seen. The lack of growth in the adjacent branch is clearly seen in this figure.

A progressive necrosis of central surface areas and the invasion of these areas with filamentous algae was observed in larger

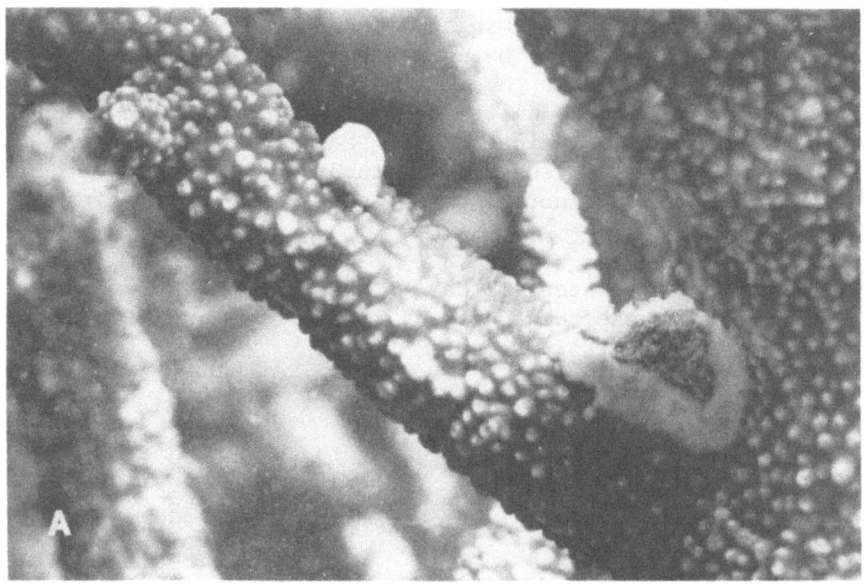

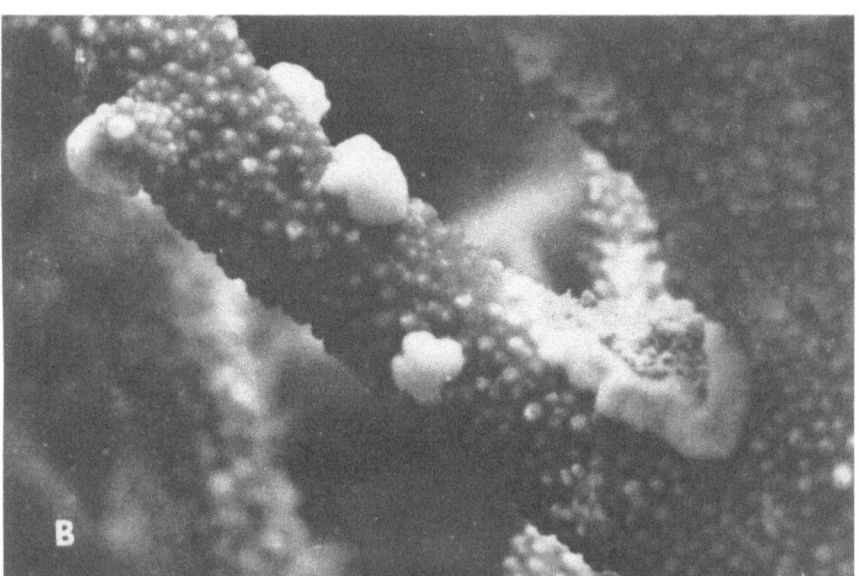

Figure 3.   Smooth growth form tumors on <u>Acropora formosa</u>.   Time
            span between upper (A) and lower (B) plates is 43 days.

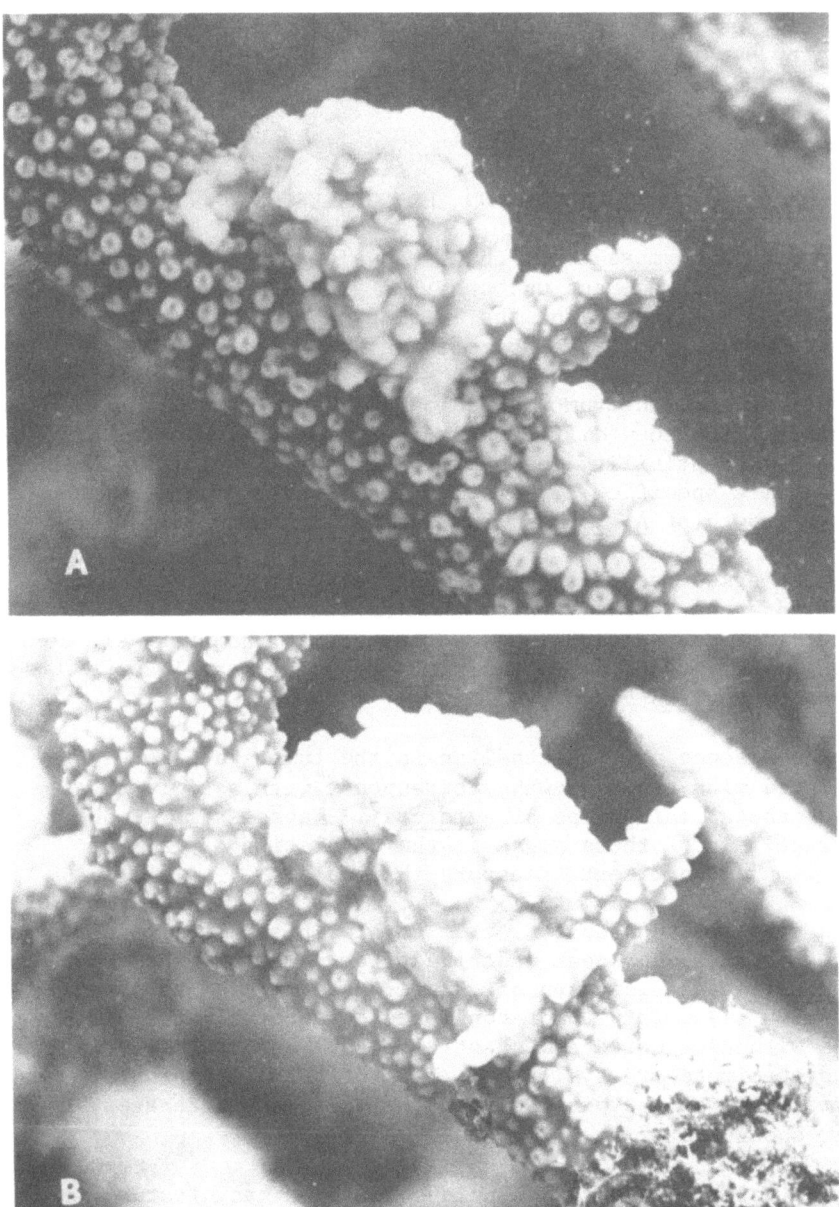

Figure 4. An irregular tumor on <u>Acropora</u> <u>formosa</u>. Time span
between upper (A) and lower (B) plates is 115 days.
Note the lack of growth in the adjacent branch tip.

smooth growth forms (Figure 3). Usually the algae infiltration
leads to erosion of the central tumor mass. In addition, invasive-
like growth was seen in some of the tumors. This resulted in
death of underlying tissues with adhesion of the tumor mass to the
overgrown tissue.

DISCUSSION AND CONCLUSIONS

Acropora formosa tumors have many features of true neoplasms
with rapid, abnormal and uncontrolled growth. It is apparent that
they do not retain or lack the etiologic agents associated with
galls and other similar abnormalities known for corals, but we
cannot discount the influence of smaller metazoans or microbes.
It is clear that the tumorous colonies have a patchy distribution
suggesting that they differ in some way from neighboring colonies
in their susceptibility to tumor formation. Since the tumors are
also species specific, at least on Guam, the growth form and
mode of growth of A. formosa may facilitate tumor development.

The marked reduction of zooxanthellae in tumors compared with
normal adjacent tissue is also seen in the nodules caused by
metacercarial cysts on Porites. These cysts, however, are confined
to single polyps and are broadly distributed on at least two
species of Porites[12].

The absence of zooxanthellae in the tumors and nodules,
correlated with rapid growth, corresponds with a similar pattern
seen on the apical polyps of Acropora[7]. These examples question
the exact role of these algae in the regulation of calcium
deposition and nutrient transport in corals.

A presumptive neoplasm from corals, possibly similar to the
Porites nodules, has been described from a museum specimen of
Madrepora kauaiensis taken off Kauai, Hawaiian Islands in the
early 1900's[13]. This tumor consisted of abnormal and enlarged
polyps with disordered and chaotic septa. Unfortunately, no
living specimens are available. For further discussion of these
abnormalities and atypical growths of other coelenterates, the
reader should refer to a review by Sparks[14].

The Acropora tumors are unique but have many features common
to similar tumors found in higher animals. They are useful
experimental models with many questions relating to their formation
and cytology yet to be answered. The absence of observable
pathology at the cellular level seems to preclude classifying
these tumors clinically as neoplasms. On the other hand, the
tendency of the tumors to be invasive (or competitive), to
possibly metastasize and to be nutrient dependent suggest that
they are indeed, in the biological sense, neoplastic.

LITERATURE CITED

1. Good, R. A. and Finstad, S., National Cancer Institute Monograph, 31:41 (1969).

2. Hildemann, W. H., Nature, 250:116 (1974).

3. Wells, J. W., U. S. Geological Survey Professional Paper, 260-1 (1954).

4. Chapman, G., The Skeletal System, p. 93-128, In: L. Muscatine and H. M. Lenhoff, eds., Coelenterate Biology (Academic Press, New York, 1974).

5. Franzisket, L., Intern Rev. Gesamten Hydrobiol., 55:1 (1970).

6. Cheney, D. P., Proc. Second Intern. Symposium on Coral Reefs, Vol I, 69 (1974).

7. Pearse, V. B. and Muscatine, L., Biol. Bull., 141:350 (1971).

8. Barnes, D. J. and Taylor D. L., Helgolander wiss. Meeresunters, 24:284 (1973).

9. Campbell, R. D., Development, p. 179-210, In: L. Muscatine and H. M. Lenhoff, eds., Coelenterate Biology (Academic Press, New York, 1974).

10. Lang, J., Bull. Mar. Sci., 23:260 (1973).

11. Hildemann, W. H., Linthicum, D. S., and Vann, D. C., Immunogenetics, 2: 269 (1975).

12. Cheng, T. C. and Wong, A. K. L., J. Invert. Pathol., 23:303 (1974).

13. Squires, D. F., Science, 148:503 (1965).

14. Sparks, A. K., Invertebrate Pathology (Academic Press, New York, 1972).

THE DISCRIMINATORY CAPACITY OF PHAGOCYTIC CELLS IN THE CHITON (Liolophura gaimardi)

R. Crichton and K.J. Lafferty

John Curtin School of Medical Research, P.O. Box 334, Canberra A.C.T., Australia 2601, and Webb-Waring Lung Institute, University of Colorado Medical Center, 4200 East Ninth Avenue, Denver, Colorado 80220, U.S.A.

INTRODUCTION

In the chiton (Liolophura gaimardi) phagocytic cells are responsible for the removal of foreign material from the haemolymph (1). These cells occur as mobile cells in the haemolymph and are also found as fixed cells lining haemolymph spaces throughout the animal. The neuropedal sinus contains a spongy network of phago-cytic cells which forms a phagocytic organ that filters haemolymph as it moves along these major haemolymph channels.

In this study we have attempted to measure the capacity of this invertebrate phagocytic system to discriminate between a number of haemocyanins that show differing degrees of immunochemical relation-ship to the test animal's own haemocyanin. The results of this study show that the chiton has the capacity to discriminate between molecules that are structurally related and that these animals can rank these proteins in an order of foreignness that corresponds to their immunochemical relationship. We also present evidence that foreign protein recognition is mediated by specific recognition units.

MATERIALS AND METHODS

Animals were collected and maintained in marine aquaria as previously described (1). The procedure for injection of foreign

89

proteins and the collection of haemolymph samples was also as
described previously (1). Isolation of Chiton Haemocyanin: Haemocyanin was obtained by the passage of haemolymph over Sepharose 6B
(Pharmacia, Sweden) columns equilibrated with Tris buffer (0.01 M
Tris, 0.1 M NaCl, 0.01 M CaCl$_2$, pH 7.5). This procedure resolved
two major protein peaks, one of which had the blue pigment characteristic of haemocyanin. This peak was concentrated and rechromato-
graphed to give the final haemocyanin preparation. Each preparation
was checked for homogeneity by electrophoresis and immunodiffusion,
and the purified proteins were characterized as haemocyanin by
spectral analysis of both the oxygenated and the deoxygenated
protein (2). Protein radioiodination and estimation: Radioiodination was carried out using chloramine T essentially as described
by Hunter and Greenwood (3). Protein estimations were carried out
using the method of Lowry et al (4). Protein bound iodine was
estimated by counting material precipitated at 4° by 8.2% trichlor-
acetic acid. Cellulose acetate electrophoresis was carried out as
described by Fazekas et al (5). Immunodiffusion: Double diffusion
in agar was performed by the Ouchterlony method (6) at 4°. The
supporting medium was 1% Noble agar (Difco) in Tris buffer (0.01 M
Tris, 0.1 M NaCl, 0.01 M CaCl$_2$, pH 7.5).

RESULTS

Elimination of Protein from the Haemolymph of the Chiton

        Previous studies (1) have shown that the chiton can discrimi-
nate between proteins of its own haemolymph and bovine serum albumin
(BSA). Twelve hours after injection, 85% of the BSA was removed
from the circulation while only 10% of the labelled homologous
protein was removed in this time. The BSA was taken up by fixed
phagocytic cells and was particularly prominent in phagocytic cells
of the neuropedal sinus. To quantitate this ability of the chiton
to discriminate between different proteins in a way that would allow
us to compare the elimination of both proteins in the same animal,
we carried out double labelling experiments.

        In these experiments, the homologous haemolymph protein was
labelled with ^{125}I and the test protein was labelled with ^{131}I.
Both proteins were injected into the test animal simultaneously.
By measuring the amount of each isotope in the haemolymph at any
given time, we could estimate the rate at which the test protein is
removed relative to the homologous protein. The difference between
the percentage of the test protein removed and the percentage of the
homologous protein removed we have called an index of discrimination.
Using this method we can compare the ability of the chiton to
recognize a number of different proteins on a relative basis. In
the following analysis, we make the assumption that the greater this

index the greater are the recognizable differences between the test protein and homologous protein.

Fig. 1 shows the discrimination curve obtained in chitons injected with BSA and homologous haemolymph protein. This data shows that the chiton can readily discriminate between homologous haemolymph protein and BSA. However there are considerable physical differences between these proteins, and physical factors such as molecular change are known to influence the interaction of proteins with phagocytic cells (7). In an attempt to overcome this problem we carried out further experiments in which we compared the ability of the chiton to discriminate between a number of different haemocyanins.

Discrimination between Immunochemically Related
and Unrelated Haemocyanins

Haemocyanin was isolated from three closely related chiton

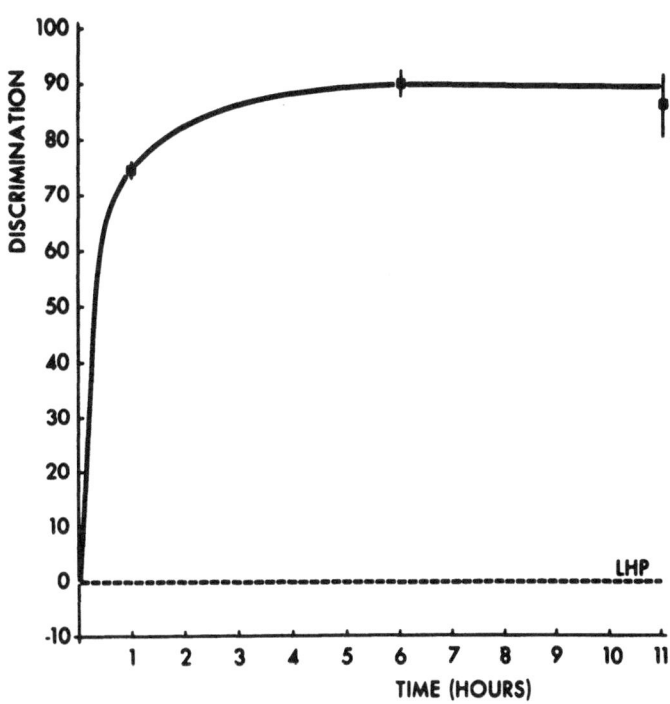

Fig. 1. Discrimination curve showing the clearance of 0.25 mgm ^{131}I-BSA (upper curve) relative to 0.25 mgm ^{125}I labelled <u>Liolophura</u> haemolymph protein (LHP, lower broken line). Each point is the mean of values obtained in 4 animals and the vertical lines show the standard error of the mean.

species (Liolophura, Ischnoradsia and Poneroplax). These proteins
were electrophoretically homogenous and had identical mobilities
(Fig. 2a). The three haemocyanins cross react immunochemically
when tested with pooled rabbit anti-Liolophura haemolymph serum,
indicating that they share common antigenic determinants (Fig. 2b).
A very faint precipitin arc was seen with keyhole limpet (Megathura
crenulata) haemocyanin, but no cross reactions were observed with
the crayfish (Jasus lalandii) haemocyanin (Fig. 2b). Comparison of
the intensity of the precipitin line produced by Poneroplax haemocyanin and Ischnoradisia haemocyanin, and the rate of spur formation
at the junction of these lines with Liolophura protein indicated
that Ischnoradisia protein was more closely related to Liolophura
protein than was Poneroplax haemocyanin.

Using the relative discrimination assay, we compared the
ability of the chiton (Liolophura gaimardi) to discriminate between
Liolophura haemocyanin and each of the other haemocyanins. Fig. 3
shows the results of these studies. This data shows that the chiton
can recognize degrees of foreignness, and that Ischnoradisia,
Poneroplax, keyhole limpet and crayfish haemocyanins were recognized

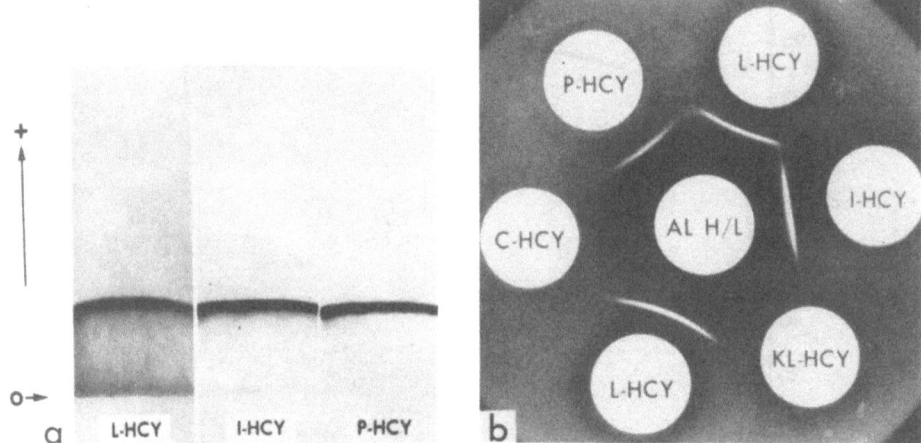

Fig. 2a. Cellulose acetate electrophoresis of Liolophura (L-HCY),
Ischnoradisia (I-HCY) and Poneroplax (P-HCY) haemocyanin. Electrophoresis was carried out in Tris HCl pH 7.5 at 4⁰ for 12 hours,
with a potential gradient of 3.5 volts/cm. (0, origin; + anode).

Fib. 2b. Double diffusion in agar showing the relationship between
Liolophura (L-HCY), Ischnoradisia (I-HCY), Poneroplax (P-HCY),
keyhole limpet (KL-HCY) and crayfish (C-HCY) haemocyanin. The
central well contained antiserum raised against Liolophura haemolymph
(AL H/L). All haemocyanin preparations contained 5.0 mgm protein/ml.
The plate was developed for 3 days at 4⁰.

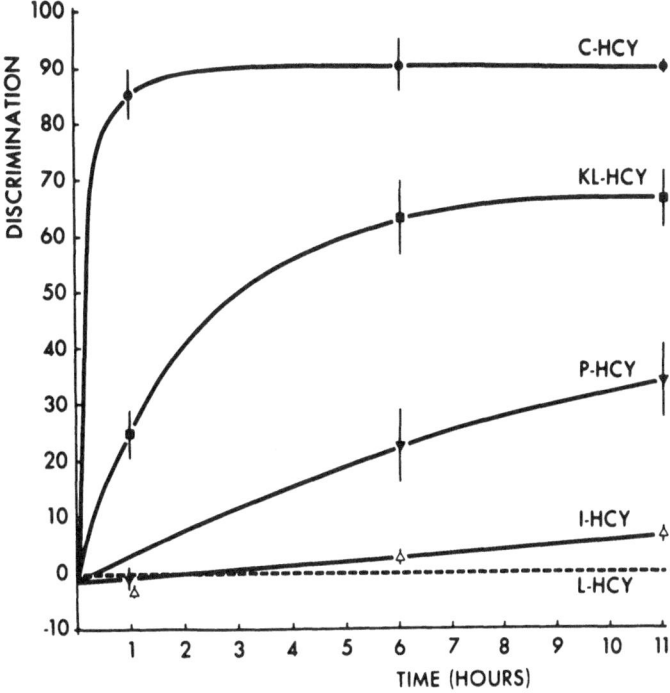

Fig. 3. Discrimination curves showing the rate of clearance of
Ischnoradisia (I-HCY), *Poneroplex* (P-HCY), keyhole limpet (KL-HCY)
and crayfish (C-HCY) haemocyanin, relative to the clearance of
Liolophura haemocyanin (L-HCY). Groups of animals were injected
simultaneously with 0.25 mgm ^{125}I-labelled L-HCY and 0.25 mgm ^{131}I-
labelled test haemocyanin. Each point is the mean value obtained
in groups of 4 animals and the vertical lines show the standard
error of the mean.

in that order, as being increasingly foreign. This observation
parallels the observed immunochemical relationship between the five
haemocyanins studied.

Specific Inhibition of the Recognition System

When chitons are injected with a relatively large dose of cold
HSA (25 mgm) one hour before a test dose (0.25 mgm) of labelled
protein is used to determine the elimination rate, there is a marked
inhibition of the rate at which the labelled protein is removed from
the haemolymph (Table 1). This inhibition shows a degree of
specificity. Animals pretreated with the same dose of HSA eliminate
Poneroplax haemocyanin at the same rate as uninjected controls.
However the elimination of labelled BSA is inhibited in a similar

TABLE 1

Specific Inhibition of the Recognition System

Animal Pretreatment	Index of Discrimination (11 hrs.)		
	Test Protein		
	HSA	BSA	P-HCY
Nil	88.4 + 1.6*	94.8 + 3.5	34.8 + 6.8
25 mgm HSA	35.3 + 3.1	28.1 + 6.5	31.2 + 4.5

*Standard error of mean obtained from groups of 4 animals

manner to HSA. Thus it would appear possible to competitively inhibit the removal of one protein without affecting the removal of an unrelated molecule.

DISCUSSION

In this paper we have shown that the chiton phagocytic system can distinguish between haemocyanin molecules that are similar physicochemically and which are antigenically related. Differences in the rate of clearance of Ischnoradisia and Poneroplax haemocyanin relative to the homologous Liolophura protein can only be attributed to minor structural differences between these proteins. Thus, the chiton phagocytic system is capable of recognizing structural differences whose magnitude is comparable with differences detected by serological techniques. Moreover, the greater the structural differences between the homologous and the test haemocyanin, the more rapidly these molecules are cleared from the haemolymph. Although the physicochemical properties of keyhole limpet haemocyanin and crayfish haemocyanin were not investigated in this study, the former protein is reported to have similar sedimentation properties to other molluscan haemocyanins (8). Crayfish haemocyanin, in common with other crustacean haemocyanins is built on an entirely different subunit structure (9). In the case of this protein, major differences in size and/or charge may also influence the rate at which the protein is removed from the haemolymph.

This capacity of the chiton to recognize relatively minor structural differences between proteins and to rank such molecules in order of their degree of relatedness to the homologous protein, suggests that these animals possess a recognition system that consists of independent recognition units with a diverse range of specificity. This proposition is further supported by inhibition studies. The fact that HSA, in high concentration, can inhibit the removal of a test dose of labelled HSA from the haemolymph but has no effect on the rate at which Poneroplax haemocyanin is removed from the circulation, can only mean that distinct recognition units are involved in the elimination of these two proteins. In mammalian systems, such specific blockade of the reticuloendothelial system has been shown to be due to the removal of serum opsonins (10). In chiton we have no evidence to say whether the recognition units are humoral or cell bound factors. Limits in the resolving power of this system are shown by the fact that HSA inhibits to a similar extent the removal of both HSA and BSA. In view of the physical and immunochemical similarity between HSA and BSA (11) it is not surprising that the chiton is unable to discriminate between these proteins.

Relevance to Immunologic Phylogeny

The above data provides evidence for a non-self recognition system in an invertebrate, that is based on a diverse library of recognition units. This system has a discriminatory capacity that is comparable to that of vertebrate antibody. However the general characteristic of the invertebrates is their failure to show an adaptive humoral response. While there is some evidence of short term memory in the allograft response of some annelids and echinoderms (12), it is unlikely that the specific adaptive response, so characteristic of the vertebrates, is widespread amongst the invertebrates.

Allogeneic interactions may form a link between the immune reactivity of vertebrates and invertebrates. Vertebrate allogeneic interactions are complex; these reactions have both a specific adaptive component and a nonadaptive component. Adaptive responses are seen when one follows the generation of specific cytotoxic cells in mixed leucocyte cultures (13). However, as we have pointed out before (14), cells other than immunocompetent can respond in allogeneic interactions, and in such cases the response does not result in proliferation and differentiation of specific immunocytes. It is for this reason that these responses are not adaptive. This dual reactivity of vertebrate allogeneic interactions is described by the following reaction sequences (15):

$$\text{Sag} + {}^{I}\text{Rab} \xrightarrow[(2)]{(1)} {}^{I}\text{R'ab} \qquad \text{(A)}$$

$$\text{Sa}^{+} + {}^{h}\text{Ra}^{-} \xrightarrow[(2)]{} {}^{h}\text{R'a}^{-} \qquad \text{(B)}$$

Reaction (A) describes the adaptive response in which a stimulator cell (S) carrying antigen (ag) interacts with an immunocompetent responsive cell (^{I}Rab) through its specific receptor (ab). The

binding of ag to the receptor on the responsive cell delivers
signal 1 to this cell, and the intimate cell contact resulting from
this interaction allows the stimulator cell to provide signal 2 to
the responsive cell; this signal is an inductive signal which in
combination with signal 1 results in the production of the activated
immunocyte (^{I}R'ab). Such a sequence would describe the activation
of specific T-cells in mixed leucocyte culture. Reaction (B)
applies to the activation of immature blood cells (^{h}Ra$^-$). These
cells are activated by signal 2 alone (15) and the surface contact
is mediated by the a$^+$/a$^-$ interaction. The question to be answered
concerns the nature of this a$^+$/a$^-$ interaction. We have considered
the case where a$^+$ is an ab like receptor and a$^-$ is an antigen on
the surface of the responsive cell (15). While this assumption
explains many of the observed phenomena it does not adequately
explain certain proliferative reactions, such as that seen when
adult F$_1$ leucocytes cause the activation of embryonic parental strain
spleen cells (14).

Hildemann has recently suggested that reactions of the (B)
type may be a vestige of invertebrate alloreactivity of the type
seen in certain colonial ascidians (12). Oka's study of the
genetics of tunicate alloreactivity suggest that genes controlling
fusibility of colonial ascidians are the same as the genes that
prevent self-fertilization (16). Fusion occurs between colonies of
the same genetic constitution but fertilization does not. Within
a given population, these fertility/fusibility genes appear to be
polymorphic, the population contains multiple alleles F$_1$, F$_2$ ------.
The function of these genes, at least in the case of fertilization,
is to prevent the intimate cellular cooperation of fertilization,
a reaction involving both cytoplasmic and nuclear interactions.
Thus the F factors may be considered as <u>inhibitors of intimate cell
interaction</u> (inhibitors for short). If we assume that factors
analogous to these invertebrate inhibitors are responsible for the
control of interactions of the type shown in reaction (B), we
have a situation where the delivery of signal 2, thought to result
from the cytoplasmic interaction between S and the responder cell
(16), would be inhibited when the interacting cells are of the same
genotype, but would be facilitated when cells differing at this
locus come into contact. These interactions can be written as
follows:

$$SF_1 + {}^hRF_1 \quad\text{------}\quad \text{No interaction} \quad\quad (C)$$

$$SF_2 + {}^hRF_1 \quad\text{------}\quad {}^hRF_1 \quad \text{(activation of the} \quad (D)$$
$$\text{responder cell)}$$

Here F$_1$ and F$_2$ represent the vertebrate analogues of the invertebrate
fertility factors.

There is now a growing body of evidence that the most efficient S cell in vertebrate allogeneic interactions is the macrophage (17-19). The prime function of the F marker on the macrophage may be to allow this cell to signal other blood cells (inflammatory cells) and specific immunocytes when foreign agents have entered the organism, and to prevent such responses under normal conditions. How could such F factors exert such a control function in a system where both the stimulator and the responder carry the same F product (say, F_1)? This could only come about if the binding of antigen to the macrophage in some way alters the phenotypic expression of its F factor. Antigen may interact with the surface F factor in such a way that the F_1 antigen complex is now phenotypically equivalent to F_2 or some other F factor. Such an event would release the macrophage from the restriction that forbids the activation of syngeneic cells and such macrophages would act as an inflammatory focus. Such a "non-specific" inflammatory mechanism could operate in both invertebrate and vertebrate animals. It may also be this type of blood cell activation that is responsible for the incompatibility observed when attempts are made to fuse tunicate colonies of different F genotype. In this context it is interesting to note that colony specificity is not seen in all compound ascidians but appears to be a feature of those ascidians in which fusion of test and/or blood vessels occur (20).

The above scheme provides a link between vertebrate and invertebrate immune reactivity. Both systems may make use of two separate recognition systems.

(1) Non-clonally distributed self compatibility markers (F inhibitors) which when modified by antigen set in motion the inflammatory sequence; a process that is not antigen specific.

(2) A diverse library of specific recognition units required for a fine degree of self not-self discrimination.

The development at the vertebrate level is the expression of a specific adaptive response. According to the above system, this development occurred when the specific recognition units were linked to the immunocyte surface in such a way that the stimulating cell could deliver signal 1 in conjunction with signal 2, thus providing a mechanism for the specific expansion of immunocyte clones.

REFERENCES

1. Crichton, R., Killby, V.A.A. and Lafferty, K.J., Aust. J. exp. Biol. med. Sci., 51: 357 (1973).

2. Heirwegh, K., Burginon, H. and Lontie, R., Biochim. Biophys. Acta, 48: 517 (1961).

3. Hunter, W.M. and Greenwood, F.C., Nature, 194: 495 (1962).

4. Lowry, O.H., Rosebrough, N.J., Farr, A.L. and Randell, R.J.,
    J. Biol. Chem., 193: 265 (1951).

5. Fazekas de St. Groth, S., Webster, R.G. and Datyner, A.,
    Biochim. Biophys. Acta, 71: 377 (1963).

6. Ouchterlony, D., Acta Path. Micro. Scand., 32: 231 (1953).

7. Lafferty, K.J. and Dickson, M., Aust. J. exp. Biol. med. Sci.,
    49: 167 (1971).

8. Tornabene, T. and Bartel, A.H., Tex. Rep. Biol. Med. 20: 683
    (1962).

9. Moore, C.H., Henderson, R.W. and Nichol, L.W., Biochemistry,
    7: 4075 (1968).

10. Jenkin, C.R. and Rowley, D., J. exp. Med., 114: 363 (1961).

11. Weigle, W.O., J. Immunol., 87: 599 (1961).

12. Hildemann, W.H., Nature, 250: 116 (1974).

13. MacDonald, H.R., Cerottini, J-C. and Brunner, K.T., J. exp. Med.
    140: 1511 (1974).

14. Lafferty, K.J., Walker, K.Z., Scollay, R.G. and Killby, V.A.A.,
    Transplant. Rev. 12: 198 (1972).

15. Lafferty, K.J. and Cunningham, A.J., Aust. J. exp. Biol. med.
    Sci., 53: 27 (1975).

16. Oka, H., Profiles of Japanese Science and Scientists, 198 pp.
    (Kodansha, Tokyo, 1970).

17. Rode, H.N. and Gordon, J., Cellular Immunology, 13: 87 (1974).

18. Greineder, D.K. and Rosenthal, A.S., J. Immunol., 114: 1541
    (1975).

19. Talmage, D.W. and Hemmingsen, H., J. Allergy and Clin. Immunology
    (in press 1975).

20. Mukai, H. and Watanabe, H., Biol. Bull., 147: 411 (1974).

    This work was supported in part by U.S. Public Health Service
Grant CA 13419 and a Fellowship from the International Union Against
Cancer.

INVERTEBRATE IMMUNOLOGY

Allogeneic Incompatibility
and Transplantation Immunity

DIRECT EVIDENCE OF HETEROLYSIS OF GORGONIAN TARGET CELLS

Jacques L. Theodor and Jacqueline Carriere
Laboratoire Arago, 66650 Banyuls sur mer, France

The level of the lysis of a gorgonian target explant following a contact with a xenogeneic or with an allogeneic killer explant is directly related with the time during which this contact is maintained. This level is also dependent on the mass ratio between the killer explant and the target explant; but only to a certain extent. When, in order to emphasize this mass effect, a target is sandwiched between two killer explants during three hours or more, the resulting lysis is, surprisingly, quite low (only 16% of the target volume lyse under sandwich conditions vs 85% in usual superimposition - target on killer-conditions). The hypothesis was put forward that the observed lytic process required the intervention of cells in normal physiological condition. By means of some system implicating a synthesis in the target explant, surviving cells destroy the cells that have been hit by a toxic (killer) factor. It was also demonstrated by a 14C valine incorporation test that one or two minutes of xenogeneic contact between killer and target explants were sufficient to inflict a measurable damage to target cells (1). The following experiments bring direct evidence adding support to the hypothesis that the lysis of the target cells is a consequence not of the autolysis of these cells, but of their heterolysis by other cells in the target explant (strictly speaking there is autolysis of the target explant, but heterolysis of the target cells). This phenomenon could not appear when all or most of the target cells were dead; as in the sandwich conditions.

Four series of target explants (Lophogorgia sarmentosa) are induced by contact with xenogeneic killer explants (Eunicella stricta); for two (a, b) of these series, the targets are

superimposed on killer explants and for the other two (c, d), the
targets are sandwiched between two killer explants (1). After a
7 hour induction the target explants are separated from the killer
explants. The targets of series (a) and (c) are simply placed in
the usual culture medium, whereas each of the targets of series
(b) and (d) are superimposed on autologous (i.e. from the same
specimen of Lophogorgia sarmentosa) explants having the size of a
killer explant. Controls include non-induced target explants.
The values, measured macroscopically, and expressed as a percentage
of the volume of the explants, are shown in Table I (A and B).
They have been divided in two groups: A - results of all 8 experiments; thus 8 x 40 target explants in each of the four (a-d) series,
plus 60 control explants (e) in each experiment, B - the average
results for three of these experiments where lysis of the controls
(e) exceeded 50%.

TABLE I. LYSIS OF TARGET EXPLANT CELLS
WITH THE ACTIVITY OF HEALTHY CELLS

		A (all experiments)	B (control level over 50%)
(a)	Superimposed target explants; thereafter separated.	74	77
(b)	Superimposed target explants; separated and placed on autologous explants.	84	89
(c)	Sandwiched target explants; thereafter separated.	40	23
(d)	Sandwiched target explants; separated and placed on autologous explants.	78	78
(e)	Controls (non induced explants).	44	78

The results of Table IA show that whether the cells of the
superimposed targets are "assisted" (b) in their lysis or not, (a)
the levels of lysis are approximately the same. In (c) the explants
do not lyse more than the controls. This particular result was
expected as a consequence of the usual sandwich effect. In (d)
where the lysis is assisted by the action of autologous cells the
destruction is about equal to that of the superimposed targets.
These results demonstrate the activity of the healthy autologous
cells in the lysis of (d) target explants: a feature characteristic

of heterolysis. Consequently such results confirm the proposition that there is no resulting lysis if all or most of the cells of a target explant are hit by the cytotoxic factor. In three of these experiments (Table IB) the considerably higher natural lysis of control explants (average 78 vs 44, an already high figure, in Table IA) is the consequence of an unusually poor physiological condition of the explants. Even under these particular conditions in Table IB, the level of the lysis is low in the (c) explants. This last result suggests that the toxic factor as "transmitted" from the killer explant to the target explant, has such a drastic effect on the target cells that it prevents or at least retards the occurrence of natural lysis (23% in the (c) explants; 78% for the natural lysis of the controls).

The explant situation in which a contact is forced between the explants is an experimental one. It is essentially different from the confrontation between antagonistic tissues under the natural circumstances. Histocompatibility is proposed to have biological significance in organisms permanently attached to the substrate, such as stony corals, horny corals, bryozoans and tunicates (2). A natural confrontation of tissues of such invertebrates is the consequence of their eventual growth, one towards the other. The distance separating these tissues is controlled by the incompatible organisms themselves. In the explant situation the contact between the explants is an experimental artifact. Whether the results obtained in vitro do or do not reflect some aspects of the process of invertebrate histoincompatibility in nature remains to be shown.

REFERENCES

1. Theodor, J. L. and Senelar, R., Cytotoxic Interaction Between Gorgonian Explants: Mode of Action. Cell. Immunol. (in press, 1975).

2. Theodor, J. L., Recherche, 57: 573 (1975).

IMMUNOINCOMPATIBILITY REACTIONS IN CORALS (COELENTERATA)

W. H. Hildemann[1], D. S. Linthicum[2], and D. C. Vann[3]

[1]Hilo College, University of Hawaii at Hilo, [2]Department of Pathology, University of California, San Diego, [3]Department of Genetics, School of Medicine, University of Hawaii at Manoa

Immunorecognition of allogeneic tissue followed by incompatibility reactions now appears characteristic of the Coelenterata or Cnidaria. Indeed, allogeneic incompatibility has been described in controlled experiments with colonial hydroids (1, 2), anthozoans (3), gorgonians (4) and reef-building corals (5). Although the various antagonistic reactions observed appear quasi-immunological in character, the sequential mechanisms of reactivity remain unknown. Coral allografts and even xenografts may persist in intimate soft-tissue contact for prolonged periods before sensitization leads to tissue destruction (5). However, in certain interspecific combinations, early unidirectional tissue killing may occur, suggestive of non-immunological aggression. Both specific and non-specific defense mechanisms may function depending on the circumstances.

The components of supposed rudimentary immunocompetence in invertebrates (6) are poorly understood. Our initial focus on corals was intended to define the range of reactions in the category of transplantation immunity in this heterogeneous group of lower metazoans. Evaluation of naturally-occurring isogenic, allogeneic, and xenogeneic reactions among coral species of Enewetak Atoll was undertaken during 1974 in conjunction with experimental tissue transplantation in selected donor-recipient combinations. The illustrated and detailed results of this pioneering study have been presented elsewhere (5). Some further insights and an overview are proffered here.

ISOGRAFT AND ALLOGRAFT REACTIONS

Naturally-occurring graftings. Any of many species of coral

105

with colonies exhibiting confluent branches can be identified as examples of compatible isografting or successful syngeneic grafts. The tissue organization including corallites and zooxanthellae in contact zones is normal grossly and microscopically. This complete compatibility persists, even when intracolony branches have been broken off and then refused at odd angles, because the soft tissues share the same genetic (antigenic) composition. Such compatible, intracolony isografts were commonly recorded for at least 9 species of staghorn corals (Acropora) plus species in three other genera (Helipora, Pocillopora and Porites) at Enewetak Atoll. This fusion is a concomitant of normal intracolony growth and serves among other functions to sustain the structural integrity of the whole colony against wave action. Under the stereomicroscope, abundant isograft connections showed normal zooxanthellae patterns and soft tissue characteristics in three quite different species in vivo - Acropora formosa, Heliopora coerules, and Pocillopora verrucosa. Each species of reef-building coral has distinctive zooxanthellae or at least a distinctive pattern of these unicellular, symbiotic algae throughout the superficial soft tissues. Why each coral species will accept or fail to reject only certain zooxanthellae is another unanswered question of foreign agent recognition.

In toto, living coral reefs display a veritable cornucopia of natural isografts. Since diverse species of corals also coexist in close proximity, the integrity of each species, if not each clonal colony, requires recognition signals to preclude random tissue fusion. Intercolony allografts, though difficult to identify in reef communities, were consistently found to be incompatible in several species. Acropora nasuta, which usually grow as large table corals with quite separate bases anchoring each colony, exhibited allogeneic incompatibility by a contact zone of bluish-white cementation devoid of soft tissue and polyps (Figure 1). Hard tissue fusion with concomitant separation of soft tissues was also observed at intercolony connections of A. formosa. Similarly, a narrow zone of calcareous cementation was found to separate allogeneic colonies of the heavy-fingered coral, Pocillopora grandis.

Experimental graftings. Evidence of rudimentary immunocompetence in coelenterates was first forthcoming from experiments with the hydroid Hydractinia echinata (1, 2). Allogeneic colonies failed to fuse when grown in contact, while clonally-derived colonies grew together compatibly. Moreover, two incompatible colonies in direct contact induced hyperplastic growth with subsequent regression at the interface. Breeding experiments revealed a complex genetic control of these histoincompatibility reactions, but the underlying immune or antagonistic responses still await definition.

Since thriving coral requires running sea water with natural plankton, temperature and lighting, care was taken with experimental coral in the present studies to avoid overheating, drying, or other

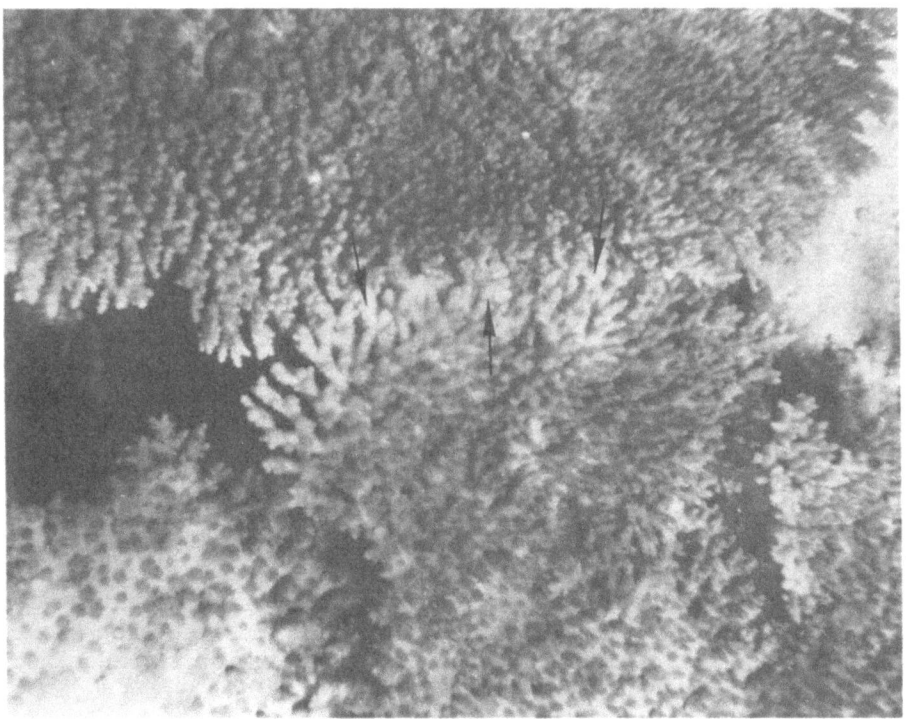

Fig. 1. Naturally-occurring allogeneic incompatibility in _Acropora nasuta_ marked by arrows pointing to contact zone cementation between two large "table-top" specimens viewed from above.

insults. Graftings were done by firmly tying 5-7 cm. pieces or branches of living coral together using 6-0 monofilament nylon. Coral pieces can be cleanly cut with heavy bone shears. Graftings should be done in sea water under a cool lamp in a manner that gently achieves multiple points of surface contact between soft tissues. Control isografts and experimental allografts were done on the same days and were subsequently kept under the same running sea water conditions. Each reciprocal donor-recipient pair was identified by a labeled plastic tag attached to the monofilament loop holding the pair together. Problems of infection or parasitism occurred only with _Porites andrewsii_ which produces considerable mucus leading to deposition of aquatic debris; this is preventable by maintaining a quite vigorous flow of sea water. Little is yet known about infectious diseases in reef corals (7), but their potential introduction at sites of experimental trauma or grafting must be taken seriously.

Some 30 pairs of allografts and 14 pairs of control isografts
were performed in Acropora formosa and were scored up to 20 days
under the stereomicroscope. Specimens for histologic examination
were fixed, decalcified and sectioned as previously described (5).
No evidence of inflammation or antagonistic responses appeared at
points of isograft contact which yielded compatible soft tissue
fusion after 3-4 days. Even gaps as wide as 2-3 mm between isograft pieces resulted in normal tissue union by outgrowth within
8 days. Confluent brown zooxanthellae in the normal pattern were
observed at all points of contact. A similar picture of isograft
compatibility was observed in joinings of Acropora loripes, a
yellow-pigmented species. The persistent contact of naturally-
occurring isografts leads to confluent cementation and soft tissue
fusion. By contrast, a contact avoidance reaction was evident among
A. formosa allografts where soft tissues did not fuse across narrow
gaps of 1 mm or less. In areas of direct physical contact between
allogeneic corallites, soft tissue fusion with localized hyperplasia
did occur, but no blanching or tissue destruction was visible during
18-20 days after grafting. Moreover, a normal pattern of zooxanthellae persisted in contact areas during this early period. Chronic
incompatibility of naturally-occurring allografts in A. formosa is
evidenced by a demarcation zone of cementation lacking confluent soft
tissue. This allogeneic contact incompatibility must develop slowly;
further long-term experiments are planned to determine the sequence
and timing of events.

Multiple pairs of isografts and allografts were also studied in
Porites andrewsii. Compatible fusion of isografts was apparent after
7-8 days, whereas allografts exhibited tissue fusion only where
physical contact was enforced. However, no soft tissue destruction
consequent upon allogeneic contact was discernible during an 18 day
observation period. As in A. formosa, a much longer experimental
period will be required to characterize slow manifestations of allogeneic incompatibility. Four pairs of Fungia fungites, a common
disc-shaped, solitary coral, tied in allogeneic contact displayed no
adverse reactions during a 10-day period of daily observation, but
naturally-occurring allografts accidently forced into prolonged contact sometimes showed blanching suggestive of transplantation immunity. Since the ambient water temperature at Enewetak was already a
warm 28°-30°C, no acceleration of first-set reactions appears possible by raising the temperature.

The mild reactions of transplantation alloimmunity may be tentatively characterized as 1) early contact avoidance reaction and 2)
late allogeneic contact incompatibility (Figure 2). In A. formosa,
most extensively studied so far, there is allogeneic tissue contact
avoidance wherever possible, absence of tissue death despite 18-20
days of enforced contact, but later contact zone cementation separating allogeneic soft tissues.

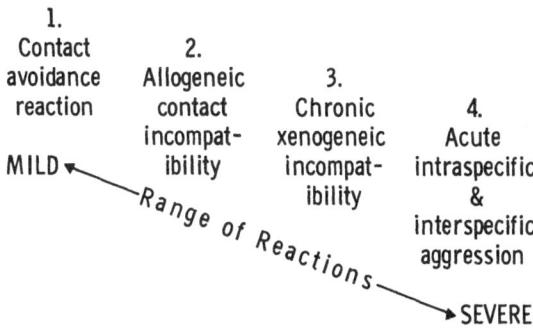

TRANSPLANTATION IMMUNITY IN COELENTERATES

Fig. 2. Four levels of "immunoreactivity" ranging from mild to severe are discernible, especially in scleractinian corals.

XENOGRAFT REACTIONS

Chronic xenogeneic incompatibility. Some 24 interspecific combinations of naturally-occurring, incompatible xenografts were found cemented together on various Enewetak reefs (5). Despite close proximity and firm calcareous interconnection, actual soft tissue fusion between different coral species was not observed. In crowded reef communities then, species integrity is maintained either by contact avoidance during coral growth or by active cementation where contact has accidently occurred. This secretion of a thin wall of "cementum" which eventually leads to soft tissue separation invites detailed investigation. Grossly, this cementum appears similar to that normally formed for coral attachment to a base of rock or dead coral. Among numerous incompatible combinations involving diverse Acropora species, neither partner appears to gain at the expense of the other when both are large pieces or colonies. In some situations, however, a unidirectional injury or overgrowth of one species by another has been observed. The yellow fire coral, Millepora platyphylla, frequently overgrows A. formosa progressively at Enewetak.

Intrageneric grafts made between six pairs of Acropora acuminata and Acropora formosa yielded avoidance reactions across all narrow-gaps, while coenenchyme in direct contact showed little or no fusion by 6 days. Blanching at the interfaces occurred in all pairs at about 9 days, but extended only about 2 mm to either side. Consistent occurrence of the contact avoidance reaction by xenogeneic corallites in proximity was also found in multiple experimental pairings each of A. formosa vs. P. andrewsii, A. formosa vs. Turbinaria danae, and A. loripes vs. P. andrewsii. Contact injury was not discernible in these latter three combinations during 10 days of daily observation. Again, longer-term studies will have to be undertaken to characterize the slow and apparently localized reactions of incompatibility.

Acute aggressive reactions. Pioneering studies of acute interspecific aggression among various Caribbean and eastern Pacific
species of corals have recently been reported by Lang (8) and Porter
(9). According to Lang, "when polyps of different corals touch, the
species which are "stronger" aggressors extrude mesenterial filaments
over their "less aggressive" neighbors, dissolving those tissues
within reach by extracoelenteric forms of digestion" (8). Highly
aggressive species were concentrated in the suborder Faviina (Mussids,
Meandrinids and Faviids), but there appeared to be a hierarchical
structure to the interactions of different species in particular
communities. Such aggression was reported to occur within 1-12 hours
of physical contact and tissue killing could be followed by aggressor
overgrowth of the exposed skeleton. Our own study of one "dominant
aggressor" species at Enewetak summarized below indicates a more complex range of reactions from severe to slight to none. This contra-
dicts the conception of a sequentially structured hierarchy at least
at the genus/species level of recognition.

Our experimental "aggressor" was Fungia fungites, a solitary,
free-living coral that extends its soft tissue mantle nocturnally
for 2 cm or more from a discus-shaped skeleton (Figure 3). Xenograft
reactions mounted by F. fungites against three genera represented by
nine species of corals were tested by multiple pairings in each interspecific combination. Individual Fungia and similar sized colonies
from four species of Acropora, three species of Pocillopora, and two
species of Porites were apposed on tagged, wooden tongue depressors
with monofilament nylon. Unidirectional injury of differing severity
induced by F. fungites led to contact zone blanching with destruction
of zooxanthellae and polyps at 2 days ($\sim$ 50 hours) in Acropora
rotumana, Pocillopora elegans, and Pocillopora eydouxi. This early
tissue damage progressed on subsequent days, most extensively in A.
rotumana, but remained within 6 mm of the interface with the two
Pocillopora species even after 7 days. After one week, only a slight
blanching reaction was evident at P. andrewsii interfaces, while the
remaining five species - A. formosa, A. humilis, A. nasuta, Porites
lopata, and Pocillopora verrucosa - showed no evidence of injury or
acute incompatibility.

Note that the timing of these killing reactions involved 2-7
days rather than just a few hours as reported for several Jamaican
hermatypic corals (8). Quite probably, different mechanisms of
recognition and responsiveness may function depending on the species
combination involved. Incidentally, multiple pairs of intrageneric
xenografts between individual F. fungites and F. echinata yielded
no tissue injury to either species during a week of testing. Although
F. fungites is clearly capable of damaging foreign species, the high
degree of discrimination evident at both xenogeneic and allogeneic

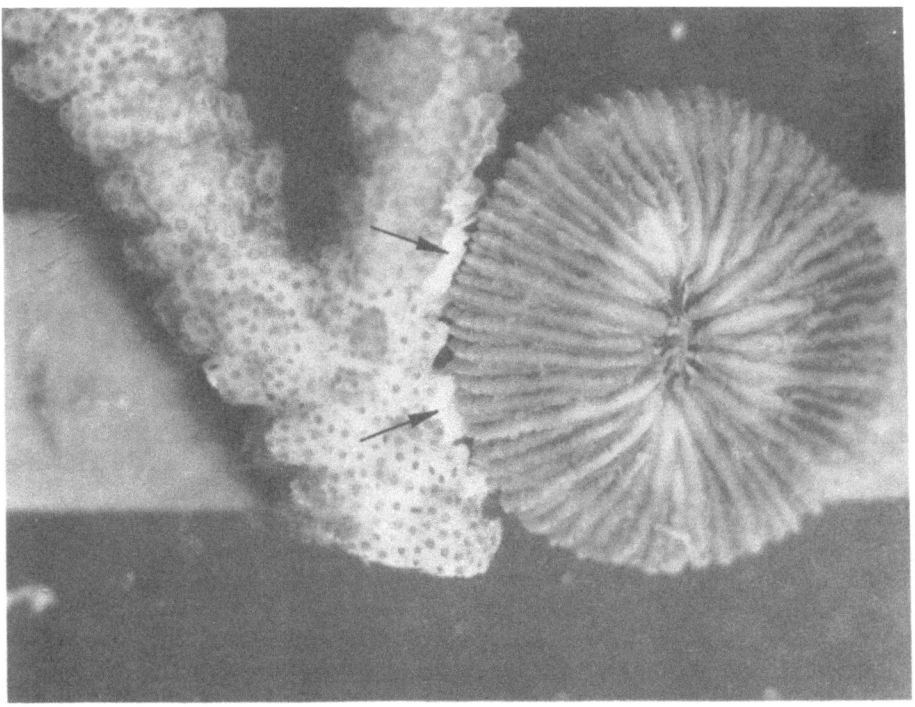

Figure 3. Acute interspecific "aggression" of Fungia fungites (right) against Pocillopora elegans (left) is illustrated by unilateral blanching (arrows) of P. elegans at interface after 2-3 days of contact.

levels of recognition and host resistance invites much further study. The most useful indicators of graft viability versus rejection in these several reef coral studies were (a) allogeneic or xenogeneic contact avoidance/inhibition evident by failure of soft tissues to fuse or grow across small gaps; (b) persistence or disappearance of pigmented zooxanthellae in coenenchyme at contact points and (c) hyperplasia/blanching/necrosis of coenenchyme in allogeneic or xenogeneic contact areas.

Acute agression in coelenterates associated with allogeneic as well as xenogeneic recognition was recently described in a sea anemone, Anthopleura elegantissima (3). Actual contact between allogeneic non-clonemates appears necessary for an aggressive response which involves discharge of ectodermal nematocysts into the body of the victim. Such attacks could be evoked by contact with non-clonemates or another anthozoan species, but not by isogenic clonemates, hydrozoans, predator or prey species, or inert objects. Intraspecific and interspecific aggressive reactions elicited within minutes or hours after first contact could of course represent non-immunological antagonism despite the high degree of specific recognition required. Nevertheless, the possibility of specific sensitization of these animals indigenous to a densely populated, intertidal environment has not been ruled out. In any event, the combined evidence at hand is consistent with the general assumption of specific immunorecognition in coelenterates leading to early or late manifestations of incompatibility.

CONCEPTS OF INVERTEBRATE IMMUNOPHYLOGENY

Newer studies of immunodiscrimination and cell-mediated immunity in various invertebrates, including coelenterates, are admirably summarized by other authors elsewhere in this volume. Quite different interpretations of similar evidence have been put forward which one of us has previously tried to reconcile in a limited way (10). Such apt terms as "specific immunity" or "immunocompetence" in describing given invertebrate responses need not commit the user to the far more sweeping assumption of a continuous phylogenetic progression in immune mechanisms extending from primitive invertebrates to advanced vertebrates. However, the long-standing, converse notion that all invertebrates lack specific immunological capability must now be rejected as untenable.

Immunorecognition, broadly defined, is already evident at the metazoan level of coelenterates where reactions of transplantation immunity range from mild allogeneic contact incompatibility to severe intraspecific and interspecific aggression (Figure 2). Even intact allogeneic colonies of sponges may also show specific contact incompatibility, but without apparent cytotoxic antagonism (11). Our identification of four categories of reactions in coelenterates under the heading of transplantation immunity is not meant to imply separate mechanisms necessarily. The recognition signals, receptors, effector cell types, and molecular pathways involved, all remain to be determined in future work. The contact avoidance reaction despite soft tissue proximity was consistently seen as early as 2-3 days after grafting as a prelude to both allogeneic contact incompatibility and chronic xenogeneic incompatibility at sites of forced contact. The avoidance reaction suggests a sensitive recognition of foreignness which precedes antagonistic reactions requiring a longer period of contact sensitization.

Neither we nor others have yet undertaken experiments to test for a specific memory component in the apparent sensitization process. Evidence concerning the nature and timing of late reactions of allogeneic incompatibility preceding interfacial termination of soft tissue contact in scleractinian corals is needed first. The acute aggression reactions distinguished by both very early occurrence and unidirectional killing appear to result from release of either mesenterial enzymes or nematocyst toxins. However, the recognition signals or cell-surface receptors triggering these attacks can show remarkable specificity. Thus, the common denominator among the diverse reactions of transplantation-type immunity in coelenterates may be cell-surface immunorecognition with exquisite discrimination. The molecular specificity for such recognition could reside in histocompatibility antigens (12) or in constituent polypeptide chains with variable regions equivalent to antigen-recognizing molecules on the cell surface. No immunoglobulin or beta-2-microglobulin as such have yet been detected on invertebrate cells, but the negative evidence is thin. Beta-2-microglobulin is a polypeptide chain associated with histocompatibility antigens, is present on the surface of most cell types, and is probably present in all vertebrates if not invertebrates (13).

Primordial cell-mediated immunity revealed by specific allograft rejection with at least short-term memory has been demonstrated in certain advanced invertebrates - annelids (14) and echinoderms (15). Allogeneic incompatibility is also characteristic of colonial tunicates (16). Mobilization of lymphocytes and other differentiated leukocytes in orthotopic integumentary allografts undergoing chronic rejection was found in the solitary tunicate Ciona (17), but critical tests for immunologic memory in protochordates remain to be accomplished. Several levels of recognition and reaction to foreignness are now discernible in phylogenetic progression (10). The immune system of advanced vertebrates may represent highly specialized versions of more general systems of receptors. Immunologic specificity and memory may both be viewed as adaptively evolving characteristics. Histocompatibility systems and transplantation-type immunity now appear fundamentally similar all the way from coelenterates to mammals.

ACKNOWLEDGEMENTS

This work was supported by NIH research grant AI-07970 to W. H. Hildemann and by the Mid-Pacific Marine Laboratory, a branch of the Hawaii Institute of Marine Biology, University of Hawaii.

REFERENCES

1. Hauenschild, C., Z. Naturforsch., 11: 132 (1956).
2. Ivker, F.B., Biol. Bull. 143: 162 (1972).
3. Francis, L., Biol. Bull. 144: 73 (1973)
4. Theodor, J.L., Nature, 227: 690 (1970).
5. Hildemann, W.H., Linthicum, D.S. and Vann, D.C., Immunogenetics, in press.

6. Hildemann, W.H. and Reddy, A.L., Federation Proc. 32:2188 (1973).

7. Garrett, P. and Ducklow, H., Nature, 253: 349 (1975).

8. Lang, J., Bull. Marine Sci., 23: 260 (1973).

9. Porter, J.W., Science, 186: 543 (1974).

10. Hildemann, W.H., Nature, 250: 116 (1974).

11. Van de Vyver, G., Ann. Emb. Morph., 3: 251 (1970).

12. Edelman, G.M., in Cellular Selection and Regulation in the
    Immune Response, p. 1 (Raven Press, New York, 1974).

13. Cunningham, B.A. and Berggard, I., Transplant. Rev., 21: 3 (1974).

14. Hostetter, R.K. and Cooper, E.L., Cellular Immunol., 9: 384(1973).

15. Karp, R.D. and Hildemann, W.H., this volume.

16. Tanaka, K. and Watanabe, H., Cellular Immunol., 7: 410 (1973).

17. Reddy, A.L., Bryan, B. and Hildemann, W.H., Immunogenetics, 1:
    584 (1975).

ALLOGENEIC DISTINCTION IN *Botryllus primigenus*

AND IN OTHER COLONIAL ASCIDIANS

Kunio Tanaka

Department of Pharmacology, Kitasato
University School of Medicine
Sagamihara, Kanagawa, 228, Japan

INTRODUCTION

Certain species of colonial ascidians have colony specificity or the ability to distinguish self colonies from not-self colonies within the same species. In *Botryllus primigenus*, when a colony recognizes another as belonging to the self strain, both colonies fuse with each other to form one colony (designated as "fusion"). On the contrary, when colonies of a not-self strain come into contact, they do not fuse, and a necrotic zone occurs at the contact surface between the two colonies (designated as "nonfusion").

These phenomena were first observed by Bancroft (1903) and further studies have been performed by a Japanese group. The genetic control of the fusibility of *Botryllus p.* was demonstrated by Oka and Watanabe (1957, 1960) and Oka (1970), and they proposed the following hypotheses: (1) Each colony in nature is heterozygotic with respect to the gene governing fusibility; (2) the gene is represented by a series of alleles like the S gene governing selfincompatibility in flowering plants; (3) colonies containing at least one gene in common are fusible with one another. Their proposal was introduced by Burnet (1971, 1974) with interest from the view point of the evolution of immunity.

The alteration of fusibility was demonstrated by Mukai (1967), using the techniques of fusion and reseparation and this was the first attempt to analyse the mechanisms of fusibility. Further detailed observations (Tanaka and Watanabe, 1972, 1973; Tanaka, 1973) showed that cells and humoral factors may participate at least partly in "nonfusion" reaction, which consist of two steps, specific and nonspecific.

COLONY SPECIFICITY IN ASCIDIANS

The Presence of Colony Specificity

In *Botryllus p.*(Tanaka and Watanabe, 1973; Mukai and Watanabe, 1974), when two pieces derived from the same colony were contraposed at the growing edges, they fused completely and formed a common vascular system through extension of the ampullae which are ending of the vascular system and embedded in the tunic of the growing edges of the colonies (Fig. 1-1). Even if the faced edges were cut artificially, the fusion of two pieces occurred in the same way. This phenomenon was designated as "fusion". On the contrary, when pieces were obtained from different colonies within the natural population, the contact of the pieces usually resulted in necrosis at the contact area, whether at the natural growing edges or the artificially cut surfaces. This phenomenon was designated as "rejection". In either case, whether showing "fusion" or "rejection", however, the fusion of the tunics preceeded the connection or rejection of the vascular system.

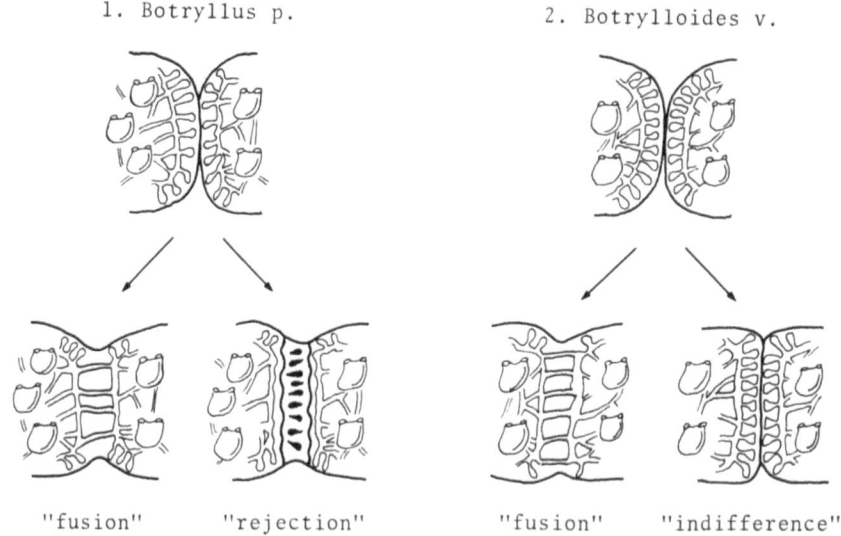

Fig. 1. An illustration of the results of fusion experiments in *Botryllus p.*(left) and *Botrylloides v.*(right). *Botryllus* showed "fusion" or "rejection" and *Botrylloides* showed "fusion" or "indifference". The contact of two pieces was performed at normal growing edges.

In *Botrylloides violaceus* (Tanaka and Watanabe, 1973; Mukai
and Watanabe, 1974), showed that "fusion" or "rejection" was demonstrated at the cut surfaces in the same manner as in *Botryllus*.
When normal growing edges were used, however, a different phenomenon was observed at the contact area (Fig. 1-2). In most cases,
using colonies derived from the natural population, the ampullae of
the two colonies pressed against each other for several days, while
the boundaries between the two colonies seemed to remain distinct.
Subsequently, they gradually regressed but neither rejection nor
fusion of the tunics was observed. This phenomenon was designated
as "indifference". When pieces were taken from the same colony,
"fusion" was always observed at the contact area.

In fusion experiments with six other colonial ascidians, although there were some differences in details among the species,
the behavior of the two pieces could be assigned into either one
of the above three categories. The results of fusion experiments
by several investigators are summarized in Table 1.

The same phenomena, as described above, in *Botryllus* colonies
were further confirmed recently by Mukai and Watanabe (1974) using
Symplegma reptans and *Didemnum moseleyi*.

Fusion experiments with *Perophora orientalis* (Mukai and
Watanabe, 1974; Tanaka, unpublished data) and *Polycitor mutabilis*
(Oka and Usui, 1944) showed that contact by two colonies with artificially cut surfaces always resulted in "fusion", whereas contact
by naturally growing edges resulted in "indifference" in all combinations, including pieces derived from the same colony.

Amaroucium constellatum seems to show an intermediate type of
fusibility, resembling *Botrylloides* in contact between growing
edges, and *Perophora* in contact between cut surfaces. According
to Freeman (1970), colonies originating from tadpoles, collected
at random, showed the above designated "indifference" at the growing edges, whereas two pieces derived from the same colony showed
"fusion". Transplanted zooids were always acceptable, suggesting
"fusion" at the cut surface.

Metandrocarpa sp., a species found in Friday Harbor, USA, has
very interesting features of fusibility (personal communication from
Watanabe). This ascidian constructs its colony in a dendriform.
When the growing tip of a branch comes into contact with another
branch of the self colony, the tip, including the asexually developing zooid, gradually degenerates and disappears within several days.
On the contrary, tips of branches originating from different colonies are able to overlap each other without distinguishable change
in the contact area. This unique phenomenon suggests that *Metandrocarpa* colonies would manifest syngeneic inhibition in some stage of
their development.

Table 1. Summary representation of fusion experiments

Species	Results of contact between		References[a]
	growing edges	cut surfaces	
Botryllus primigenus	F or R	F or R[b]	1, 2
Symplegma reptans	F or R	F or R	2
Didemnum moseleyi	F or R	F or R	2
Botrylloides violaceus	F or I	F or R	1, 2
Amaroucium constellatum	F or I	F[c]	3
Perophora orientalis	I	F	2
Polycitor mutabilis	I	F	4
Metandrocarpa sp.	R[d] or I	–[e]	5
Xenogeneic combination	I	I	2

a) 1. Tanaka and Watanabe, 1973. 2. Mukai and Watanabe, 1974.
    3. Freeman, 1970. 4. Oka and Usui, 1944. 5. Watanabe, un-
    published.
b) Abbreviation; F, "Fusion"; R, "Rejection" and I, "Indiffer-
    ence".
c) Transplanted zooid was always acceptable.
d) Rejection occurred in a self colony.
e) No experiment took place.

        Xenogeneic combinations showed only "indifference", as re-
ported by Mukai and Watanabe (1974).

        The significance of these three categories, "fusion", "re-
jection" and "indifference", should be considered in relation to
allogeneic distinction in colonial ascidians.

        Species such as *Botryllus*, *Symplegma* and *Didemnum*, showing
"fusion" or "rejection" as a result of contact at the growing edges
demonstrate that the outer membrane of the tunic may be lysed, probably by enzymatic reaction. Thus, allogeneic distinction is not
performed at the membrane level. To maintain individuality, factors
included in the tunic exert allogeneic inhibition in these species.
Perophora and *Polycitor* belong to a second type which lacks allogeneic distinction. The individuality of each colony may be maintained
only by the outer membrane of the tunic. The species in this type
seem to have no enzyme for lysing the outer membrane of the tunic.

        Botrylloides and *Amaroucium* are the species showing another
unique type, in which allotype is distinguished at the site of the

outer membrane. The distinction may be performed by enzyme specificity at the contact area. Besides the ability to distinguish,
Botrylloides also possesses factors in the tunic to induce allogeneic inhibition at the artificially cut contact surfaces. *Amaroucium*, however, does not seem to possess this factor in the tunic,
because the transplantation of zooids is always acceptable in any
combination.

Occurrence Rate of "Fusion" in the Natural Population

The occurrence rate of "fusion" among colonies in the natural
population was examined on the two species, *Botryllus p.* and *Botrylloides v.* In *Botryllus*, 45 colonies taken from two stations (N
and S)(Tanaka and Watanabe, 1973) and 30 colonies from three stations (N, T and S)(Mukai and Watanabe, 1975a) were tested for
their reciprocal fusibility. As shown in Table 2, "fusion" occurred at a small rate, 1.1 percent among 990 combinations and 4.8 percent among 435 combinations.

It was also found that, in an experiment described as follows
(Tanaka, unpublished data), *Botryllus* colonies did not change their
fusibility during long term culture. Four F_1 colonies obtained by
sexual reproduction were cultured for about 600 days. The colonies,
which consisted of two sets of nonfusible and four sets of fusible
combinations, maintained exactly their original fusibility after
passing through approximately 120 cycles of asexual generation
during this period.

Table 2.   Occurrence rate of "fusion" in *Botryllus p.*

	Combinations of station	Numbers of combinations of colonies	Numbers of fusible combinations	Occurrence rate (%)
a)	N – N	300	6	2.0
	S – S	190	1	0.5
	N – S	500	4	0.8
	Total	990	11	1.1
b)	N – N	45	3	6.7
	T – T	45	3	6.7
	S – S	45	3	6.7
	N – T	100	5	5.0
	N – S	100	3	3.0
	T – S	100	4	4.0
	Total	435	21	4.8

a) According to Tanaka and Watanabe, 1973.
b) According to Mukai and Watanabe, 1975.

The occurrence rate of fusion in *Botrylloides* colonies was observed by Mukai and Watanabe (1975b). The results showed that 31 out of 190 reciprocal combinations (16.3%) were fusible, and the percentages among stations ranged from 8.9 to 28.9 percent.

Histoincompatibility in Solitary Ascidians

In comparison with the colony specificity described above, it seems to be interesting to examine histoincompatibility of solitary ascidians. But there are a very few reports examining the histo-incompatibility of solitary ascidians, since the transplantation of their tissue is technically very difficult.

Anderson (1971) reported that *Molgula manhattensis* did not exhibit allogeneic recognition, because autograft and allograft were rejected equally in the same manner.

On the contrary, a preliminary experiment with another solitary ascidian, *Halocynthia hirgendorfi*, indicated that histoincompatibility might be present in cultured hemolymph cells, although tissue grafting was not performed (Tanaka, unpublished data). The results of this experiment were as follows. In two out of nine combinations among six animals, amino acid-^{14}C incorporation into the cells after a 48 hr-culture was higher by 25–35 percent in the mixed

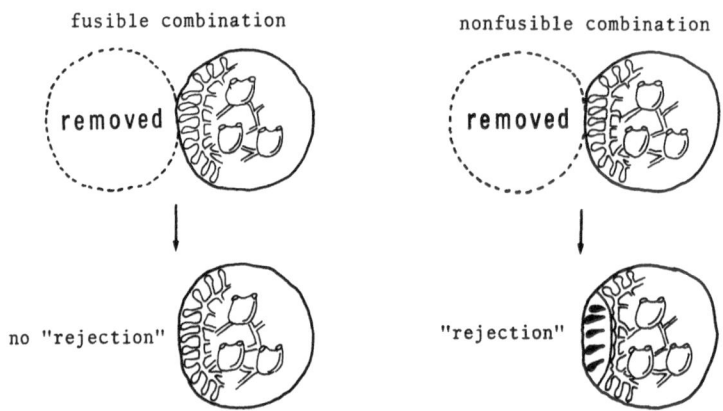

Fig. 2. Schematic representations of the effects of contact after removal of the opposite colony in the experiment with *Botryllus*. In fusible combination, no significant effects were recognized, but in nonfusible combination, "nonfusion" reaction went on at the area which had been contacted and this area was rejected. The removal was performed after the fusion of tunic.

cultures than in the control cultures. In the other seven combinations, incorporation was at the same level in both the mixed and
the control cultures. It will remain uncertain, however, whether
or not this solitary ascidian exhibits real allogeneic recognition,
until the culture methods for ascidian cells are well established,
and other combinations among sisters and many other combinations
among the natural population are tested.

FEATURES OF "NONFUSION" REACTION IN *Botryllus*

The Irreversibility of the "Nonfusion" Reaction

The irreversibility of the "nonfusion" reaction in *Botryllus* p.
was tested by the technique of removing one colony from the other
after contact (Tanaka and Watanabe, 1973). The results in nonfusible
combinations show that when the removal was made after the fusion
of tunics, the "nonfusion" reaction continued irreversibly at the
same speed and in the same way as in nontreated cases, whereas no
sign of "nonfusion" reaction was observed on the removal before
the fusion of the tunics (Fig. 2, right). On the other hand, the results in fusible combinations did not show such an effect as "nonfusion" reaction when the removal was performed after the fusion
of tunics (Fig. 2, left).

Involvement of Humoral and Cellular
Factors in "Nonfusion" Reaction

It was of interest to know what roles cells and humoral factors would play in "nonfusion" reaction. Therefore, experiments
were performed *in vivo* as shown in Fig. 3 (Tanaka and Watanabe,
1972; Tanaka, 1973). Using three strains of F_1 colonies, AC, BC
and BD, a piece from each strain was placed side by side on a glass
slide in the following order, AC-BC-BD, and the growing edges of
the colonies faced each other at proper intervals.

AC and BD colonies are not fusible, so the hemolymphs of the
two colonies can not mix in the natural way. However, when a BC
colony was placed between an AC and BD colony, the hemolymphs of AC
and BD were mixed within the vessel of the BC colony after the
establishment of connections on both sides (AC-BC-BD).

The vascular system of the BC colony did not always fuse with
those of the AC and BD colonies simultaneously because of different
speeds of growth of the three colonies. When the fusion at both
sides occurred almost at the same time, the hemolymphs of the AC
and BD colonies flowed into the BC colony through the opening of
the fused vascular systems. The mixture of hemolymphs of the two
colonies led to the formation of clusters of hemolymph cells

(aggregation or agglutination?) within the vessels at the middle
region of the BC colony and at the contact regions of both sides
within a few hours. Subsequently, the vessels in the three regions
gradually constricted to stop the hemolymph flow and these regions
were finally necrotized.

Histological and electronmicroscopic findings showed that
granular amoebocytes and brown cells were dominant in the cell clusters. The test cells of the BC colony neighboring the necrotizing
vessels were destroyed and thin filaments were formed around them,
in spite of the fact that this BC colony is fusible with both the
AC and BC colonies. These findings in the tunic were essentially
the same as those of the typical "nonfusion" reaction. After one
day, however, new vascular connections were usually observed to
occur at only one of either side of the colonies(Fig. 3, Tf1 = Tf2).

If the fusion of the vascular vessels at one side of the contacts was established earlier than that at the other side(e.g. AC-
BC earlier than BC-BD), the BC colony received hemolymphs from only
the AC colony before the later fusion took place at the other side.

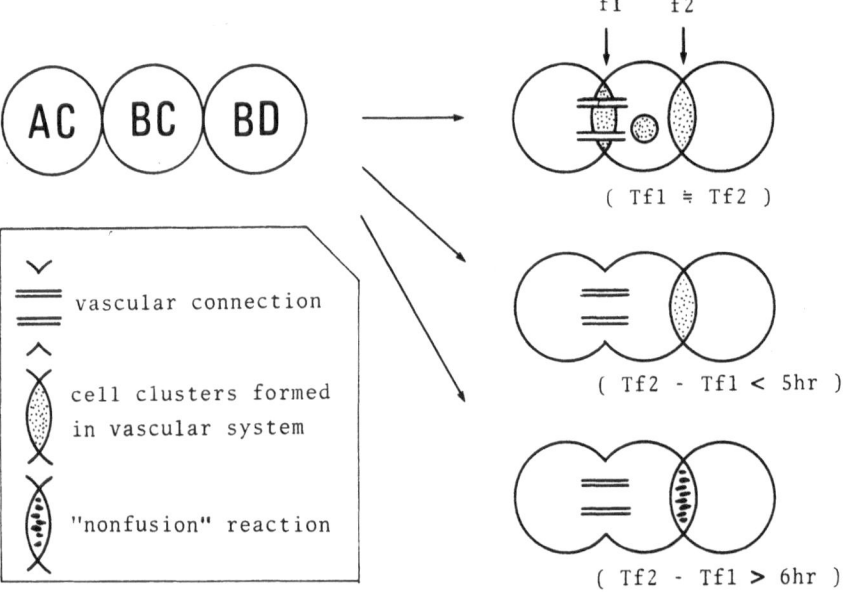

Fig. 3. Results obtained by experiments using three F_1 colonies
are represented schematically. Abbreviations; f1, earlier fusion;
f2, later fusion; Tf1, time of earlier fusion; Tf2, time of later
fusion. See text for details.

After the later vascular fusion of BC-BD was established, the hemolymphs from the BD immediately met those of the AC causing the hemolymph cells to cluster and stop the flowage within the connecting
vessels in the later fused region(Fig.3, Tf2 - Tf1 < 5 hr). The
length of the period between the establishment of the later vascular connection and the stoppage of hemolymph flow was reversely
proportional to the length of the time difference between the
earlier and later fusion.

Over six hours after the establishment of the vascular connection at one side, no connection was observed at the other side and
a typical "nonfusion" reaction occurred (Fig. 3, Tf2 - Tf1 > 6 hr).

From the facts described above, the following conclusions
could be drawn: (1) The hemolymph contains the colony specific
factors, cellular and/or humoral factors. The onset of "nonfusion"
reaction depends on the concentration of the factors. (2) After
the specific reaction, the colony non-specific factors may be released to constrict vessels and to destroy the test cells of a
fusible colony. (3) The colony specific factors of the AC colony
enter the BC colony and diffuse through the vessel wall into the
tunic of the BC colony. When the concentration of the factors in
the tunic becomes high enough, they attack the nonfusible colony
(BD) to cause the "nonfusion" reaction. (4) The factors are assumed to be humoral because active movement of cells through vessel walls into the tunic was not observed.

CONCLUSION

Colonial ascidians examined have the ability to distinguish
self or not-self. The distinction appears to be done at two levels;
the outer membrane of the tunic and active allogeneic inhibition.

The experiments with *Botryllus p.* and *Botrylloides v.* colonies
in the natural population suggest the presence of a various number
of phenotypes governing fusibility, although the precise numbers
are not known at the present time.

Besides colonial ascidians, allogeneic recognition of a solitary ascidian was suggested in *Halocynthia h.*, but further investigation is certainly necessary before drawing definite conclusions.
Possible detection of allogeneic recognition in a mixed culture of
hemolymph cells from ascidians might facilitate a comparison with
that of the vertebrate from the view point of immunologic phylogeny.

"Nonfusion" reaction in *Botryllus p.* is considered to be a successive combination of a type of allogeneic inhibition, which is
induced by colony specific factors, and a type of inflammatory
reaction, which is induced by colony non-specific factors.

REFERENCES

Anderson, R.S., 1971, Cellular responses to foreign bodies in the
    tunicate *Molgula manhattensis* (Dekay), Biol. Bull. 141: 91-98.
Bancroft, F.W., 1903, Variation and fusion of colonies in compound
    ascidian, Proc. Calif. Acad. Sci. Series 3, 3: 137-186.
Burnet, F.M., 1971, "Self-recognition" in colonial marine forms and
    flowering plants in relation to the evolution of immunity,
    Nature (London) 232: 230-235.
Burnet, F.M., 1974, Invertebrate precursors to immune responses,
    in: Contemporary Topics in Immunology vol. 4 Invertebrate
    Immunology (E.L. Cooper, ed) pp. 13-24. Plenum press.
Freeman, G., 1970, Transplantation specificity in echinoderms and
    lower chordates, Transplant. Proc. 2: 236-239.
Mukai, H., 1967, Experimental alternation of fusibility in compound
    ascidians, Sci. Rep. Tokyo Kyoiku Daigaku, B13: 51-73.
Mukai, H. and Watanabe, H., 1974, On the occurrence of colony speci-
    ficity in some compound ascidians, Biol. Bull. 147: 411-421.
Mukai, H. and Watanabe, H., 1975a, Distribution of fusion incom-
    patibility types in natural populations of the compound asci-
    dian, *Botryllus primigenus*, Proc. Japan Acad. 51: 44-47.
Mukai, H. and Watanabe, H., 1975b, Fusibility of colonies in natu-
    ral populations of the compound ascidian, *Botrylloides viola-
    ceus*, Proc. Japan Acad. 51: 48-50.
Oka, H., 1970, Colony specificity in compound ascidians. The gene-
    tic control of fusibility, in: Profiles of Japanese Science
    and Scientists (H. Yukawa, ed) pp. 195-206, Kodansha, Tokyo.
Oka, H. and Usui, M., 1944, On the growth and propagation of the
    colonies in *Polycitor mutabilis* (Ascidiae compositae), Sci.
    Rep. Tokyo Bunrika Daigaku, B: 23-53.
Oka, H. and Watanabe, H., 1957, Colony-specificity in compound
    ascidians as tested by fusion experiments (a preliminary
    report). Proc. Japan Acad. 33: 657-659.
Oka, H. and Watanabe, H., 1960, Problems of colony-specificity in
    compound ascidians, Bull. Mar. Biol. Stat. Asamushi 10: 153-
    155.
Tanaka, K. and Watanabe, H., 1972, Involvement of cellular and
    humoral factors in "nonfusion" reaction (NFR) of *Botryllus
    primigenus*, a compound ascidian, Proc. IInd An. Meet. Japan
    Soc. Immunol. 101-103. (in Japanese)
Tanaka, K. and Watanabe, H., 1973, Allogeneic inhibition in a com-
    pound ascidian, *Botryllus primigenus* Oka. I. Processes and
    features of "nonfusion" reaction, Cell. Immunol. 7: 410-426.
Tanaka, K., 1973, Allogeneic inhibition in a compound ascidian,
    Botryllus primigenus Oka. II. Cellular and humoral responses
    in "nonfusion" reaction, Cell. Immunol. 7: 427-443.

INVERTEBRATE IMMUNOLOGY

Primordial Cell-Mediated
Immunity and Memory

CHARACTERISTICS OF CELL-MEDIATED IMMUNITY AND MEMORY IN ANNELIDS

Edwin L. Cooper
Department of Anatomy
School of Medicine, University of California
Los Angeles, California 90024

INTRODUCTION

To search for the phylogenesis of foreign tissue graft rejection we have utilized the common garden earthworm extensively.
Whereas earthworms never destroy self-tissue or autografts, they
are fully capable of rejecting foreign or not-self tissue allografts (1-5) or xenografts (6). At 15°C, single first-set xenografts exchanged between Lumbricus terrestris and Eisenia foetida
are destroyed at approximately 25-35 days. After a first-set graft
is destroyed at 15°C, immunologic memory is demonstrable by re-
grafting the hosts with a second transplant from the original donor
of the first-graft. Both positive and negative memory are demonstrable. Positive memory occurs when second-set transplants are
rejected significantly faster than first-sets. By contrast, a
lesser percentage of worms have grafts that show prolonged survival
indicating negative memory. However, if repeat second-sets are
performed at 15°C, five days after transplanting a first-set,
during the induction phase of the immune response, there is no
dissociation into positive and negative memory. Instead, both
first- and second-set grafts are destroyed faster than a single
graft (7). It appears therefore that at the evolutionary level of
annelid worms, foreign transplant rejection is specific and the
mechanism includes a memory component. Memory is one characteristic of adaptive immunity as defined for vertebrates (8).

Recently, we have shown that coelomocytes are important in mediating tissue graft rejection (9, 10). Coelomocytes accumulate at

graft sites after transplantation and increase significantly in response to xenografts but not to autografts. When quantitated microscopically, this behavior of coelomocytes reveals an anamnestic or memory response. Moreover, when the destruction of grafts is tabulated grossly, there is memory.

Since earthworms are like poikilothermic vertebrates, their physiologic reactions are temperature dependent. When host worms are maintained at a temperature of $20^{\circ}-21^{\circ}C$, anamnesis occurs without dissociation into positive and negative components. This important temperature variable prompted a re-analysis of earlier preliminary observations to determine if classical memory is demonstrable. After the destruction of a first transplant, could host worms destroy repeat second grafts as positive accelerated rejections, but not as prolonged survivors?

ASSESSMENT OF GRAFT REJECTION

Those grafts considered to be well healed grossly show certain characteristics of viability. When the worms move, grafts contract and expand in concert with the surrounding host tissue and the direction sometimes depends upon the graft's orientation. For example, in deliberately reoriented grafts, with segments now perpendicular to the anterior-posterior axis, lateral to lateral contraction occurs when the worms move anteriorly. Moreover, grafts often respond to touch by immediate contraction and during this same and subsequent period, xenografts and autografts can be "rubbed" with a moistened cotton-tipped stick without disturbance. Autograft controls on worms bearing xenografts or alone on different hosts provide convenient comparisons. They are never destroyed.

All grafts are observed every other day after 48 hours until external features of rejection appear. Thereafter daily observations are made revealing signs of rejection of several types. Occasionally grafts are swollen and blanched followed later by melanocyte breakdown. Pigment thus provides a reliable marker for assessing graft viability especially obvious in _Eisenia_ whose segments are colored with alternating reddish brown and white stripes. Thus, the breakdown of dark stripes is a means of watching progressive stages of graft rejection. This condition usually prevails until complete rejection when there is identifiable necrosis, edema, complete blanching and rapid resorption. Other longer survivors rarely show this reaction. Instead, these grafts continue to decrease in size with gradual depigmentation and graft dissolution.

LACK OF DESTRUCTION OF SELF-TISSUE (AUTOGRAFTS) IN EARTHWORMS

To test the earthworm's capacity to reject grafts specifically and to show immunologic memory, several experiments were undertaken. First, earthworms recognize <u>self</u> tissue and regardless of genera, (<u>Allolobophora</u>, <u>Lumbricus</u> and <u>Eisenia</u>), no autografts are ever destroyed, confirming unequivocally, the rule that self-tissue is always accepted (Figure 1, Table 1). There is a mild and insignificant coelomocyte reaction to autografts, undoubtedly non-specific and related to wound healing and repair.

CROSS REACTIVITY OF CLOSELY RELATED ANTIGENS AS REVEALED BY REJECTION OF FIRST-SET XENOGRAFTS AT 15°C

The three genera, <u>Allolobophora</u>, <u>Lumbricus</u> and <u>Eisenia</u> are all members of the same family (Lumbricidae) and would be expected therefore to share a number of common histocompatibility antigens. Using <u>Lumbricus</u> as host and <u>Eisenia</u> and <u>Allolobophora</u> as donors, one can test for the existance of closely related antigens (Table 1). If both transplants are performed simultaneously, two completely independent survival times are obtained: <u>Eisenia</u> (42 days) and <u>Allolobophora</u> (72 days). Quite the reverse occurs if <u>Eisenia</u> is transplanted first, followed by an <u>Allolobophora</u> graft after a 5 day interval. Both survival times become significantly curtailed to 35 days for <u>Eisenia</u> but much more significantly at

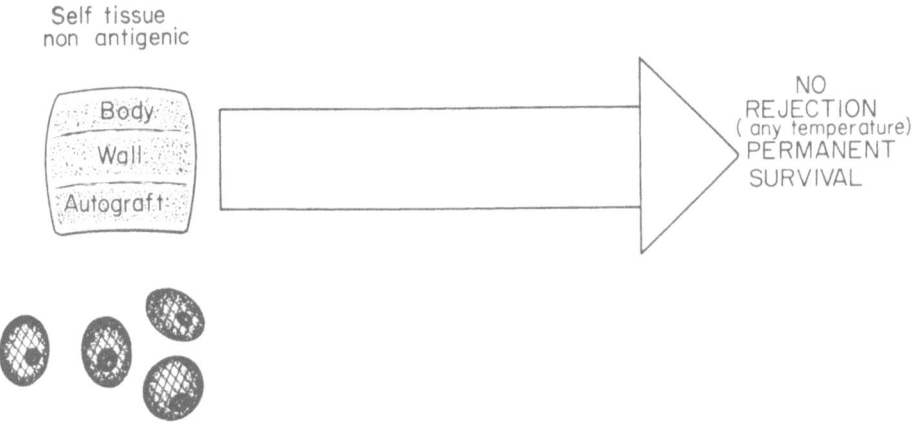

Figure 1. Self tissue or autografts are non-antigenic and therefore are never destroyed at any temperature. The cross hatched coelomocytes are not activated by autografts.

Table 1. Lack of Autograft Destruction, Specificity of First-Set Xenograft Rejection and Interruption of the Immune Inductive Phase In Earthworms

Group and Donor–Host Combination (at 15°C)	Number of Earthworms	Mean Survival Time (in days)
Allolobophora (Autograft)	60	no rejection
Lumbricus (Autograft)	85	no rejection
Eisenia (Autograft)	75	no rejection
Eisenia → Lumbricus + Allolobophora (Xenografts)	38	E → L 42.1 A → L 72.3
Eisenia →+5 Lumbricus + Allolobophora (Xenografts)	34	E → L 35.3 A → L 49.3
Allolobophora →+5 Lumbricus + Eisenia (Xenografts)	18	A → L 73.5 E → L 35.1

+ values indicate number of days between 1st set grafting and 2nd set grafting.

49 days for Allolobophora. This suggests that the Eisenia graft
primed the host so that coelomocytes reacted faster to both transplants. In the opposite direction, a first-set Allolobophora graft
does not prime. If it is followed five days later by an Eisenia
graft, the survival time for Allolobophora is 73 days and for
Eisenia 35 days. Apparently the histocompatibility differences are
greater between Eisenia and Lumbricus than between Allolobophora
and Lumbricus.

INTERRUPTION OF THE INDUCTIVE PHASE LEADING TO ACCELERATED
REJECTION OF BOTH FIRST- AND SECOND-SET TRANSPLANTS AT 15°C

Antigenic differences between Eisenia and Lumbricus are
stronger than Allolobophora and Lumbricus, as reflected by a shorter
survival time of 35 days (Figure 2). Furthermore, the response to
a first graft from Eisenia is specific so that if a second set from
the same donor is performed at 5 days post first-set grafting, the
inductive phase of the immune response is interrupted leading to a
significant accelerated rejection of first- and second-set grafts
at about 15 and 17 days. This does not occur when two different
but closely related antigens (i.e. Allolobophora and Eisenia) are
grafted during the inductive phase. Allolobophora does not prime
the host significantly as does Eisenia (Table 1; Figure 2); it
probably does not represent a true memory response.

DISSOCIATION OF THE MEMORY RESPONSE AT 15°C

When first-set xenografts are transplanted from Eisenia to
Lumbricus, first-set grafts are destroyed. To test for memory,
not to interrupt the inductive phase, second-set transplants are
grafted after the first-sets are destroyed. The worms can be
divided into two major groups and a third minor group based on the
kinds of second-set responses that are induced. Those which are
accelerated with respect to first-set survival times are termed
positive responders and the others, that show prolonged survival,
are termed negative responders (Figure 3). This reaction is
attributed to either short-term memory or to another factor,
temperature.

CLASSICAL IMMUNOLOGIC MEMORY DEMONSTRABLE IN EARTHWORMS
TO SECOND-SET XENOGRAFTS AT 20 ± 1°C

Like poikilothermic vertebrates, invertebrate physiologic
responses are sensitive to environmental temperature. At lower

First Antigen   Second Antigen   MEMORY
                               5 days post I°   ?
                                                                  15°C
                                                               Equivalent
                                                                Primary
                                                                  and
                                                                Secondary
                                                                Rejection

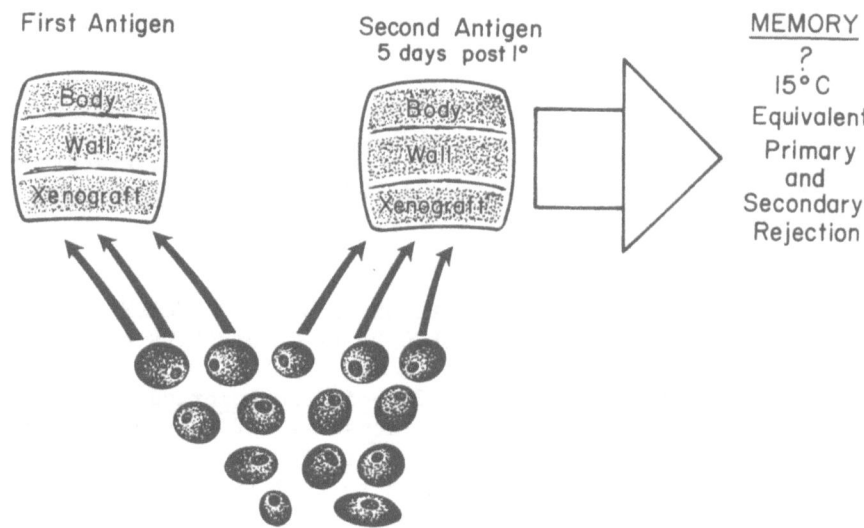

Figure 2. Interruption of the inductive phase. In one group, Lumbricus hosts were grafted with first-set Eisenia grafts at 15°C. If a second-set is transplanted five days after a first-set graft, during the inductive phase, both grafts are destroyed significantly faster than single first sets. This is not interpreted as a true memory response.

temperatures immune responses are slowed but they are accelerated at higher temperatures. At 15°C, the ranges of first-set responses are wide, thus, any second-set reactions are correspondingly offset, leading to a large proportion of accelerated rejections (positive responders) and prolonged survivors (negative responders), opposite extremes that result in dissociation of the anamnestic response (11). However, if the temperature is raised to $20° \pm 1°C$, first-set rejection times are not wide spread but are compressed. Therefore, second-set grafts performed after first-set grafts are destroyed, yield all accelerated rejections, the classical memory response (Figure 4). Undoubtedly this higher temperature constitutes one that is optimal for effecting earthworm cell mediated immune responses. This is demonstrable when observing the gross aspects of graft rejection and even typical anamnesis occurs at the coelomocyte level. Coelomocytes increase in response to xenografts, (not-self) but they do not after transplanting an autograft (self). Immunologic memory can occur in earthworms. Thus cell mediated immune responses have ancestral origins among the invertebrates.

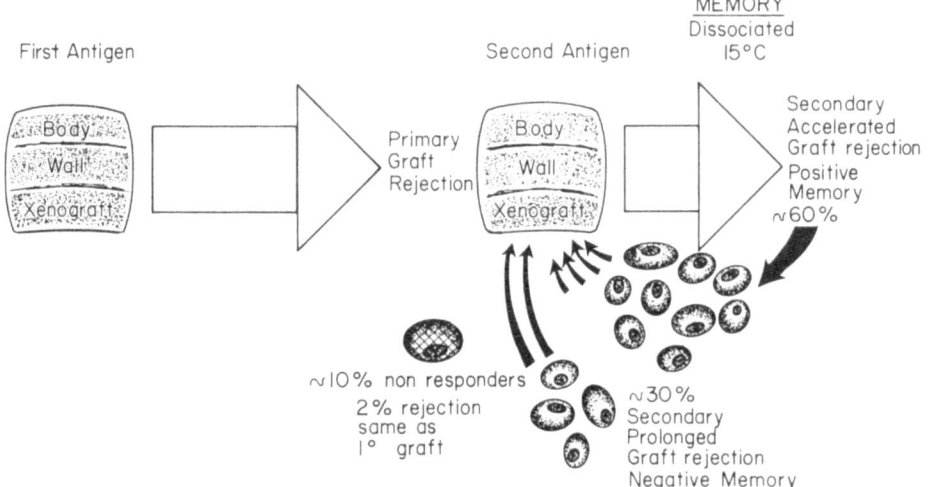

Figure 3. Diagram illustrating dissociation of memory responses at 15°C. When second-set grafts are performed after first-set grafts are destroyed, at least two major groups of responders result. The greatest percentage of second-set grafts are rejected faster than another second group which is prolonged. A third group shows second-set rejections equal to first-sets.

DISCUSSION

At least two invertebrate groups have been studied rigorously with regard to graft rejection: the annelids and the echinoderms. It is the annelids which have been studied more extensively to define those parameters accompanying graft rejection. Hildemann and Reddy (1973) have recently defined all defense reactions among the simplest invertebrates and even some vertebrate responses as quasi-immuno-recognition. The response is modified considerably more in the earthworm, an annelid, and an advanced invertebrate. Because any animal inferior to the annelids would be expected to only recognize foreign material, they would not be expected to show advanced types of responses such as specificity and memory. According to Burnet (1968) present day immune mechanisms evolved from an ancestral invertebrate wandering cell which recognizes and reacts to antigen. Earthworm coelomocytes are indeed capable of recognizing and reacting to an antigen. Following reaction to an antigen, two additional characteristics are demonstrable: both specificity and memory. Of major significance, the demonstration

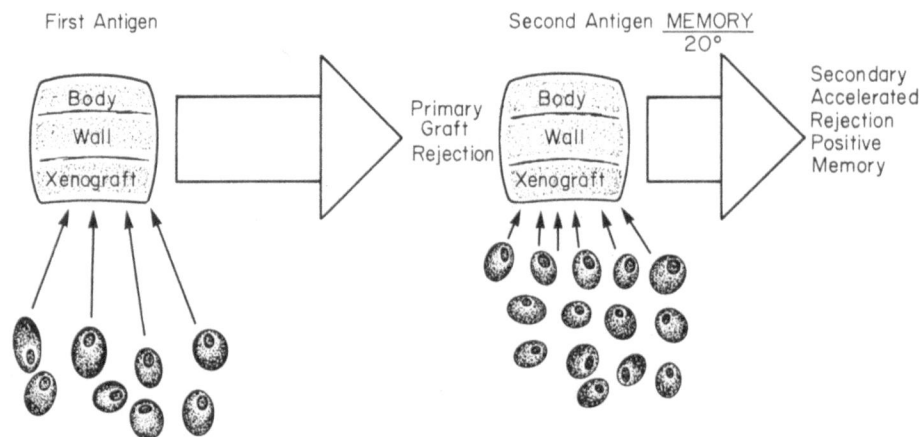

Figure 4. At 20 $\pm$ 1°C, first-set grafts are destroyed at
approximately 25 days. In another group, if second-sets are
performed after first-sets are destroyed the second-set survival
time is curtailed significantly indicating a true anamnestic
response, not an interruption of the inductive phase nor a
dissociation of the memory response. This is a true accelerated
secondary response to a second-set xenograft. Note that the
coelomocytes react faster to a second graft than to the first graft.

of memory is strongly dependent on temperature. We can therefore
conclude that memory in the immune system, like that in neurons of
the nervous system had origins traceable to the invertebrates.

Simply defined, memory in the immune system means that after
challenge or immunization with antigen A an animal then becomes
immune by activities and inherent capacities of its immune cells
or immunocytes. They make contact with the antigen which may cause
them to divide later. Thus immune information can be passed on to
subsequent daughter cells by mitosis. That these cells will
respond to a second antigen (A), with heightened reactivity, implies
both specificity and memory. The experiments described herein
support this view for the earthworm.

The importance of this work reveals that earthworms produce
accelerated second-set responses to tissue antigens after initial
priming of hosts. This interesting observation for comparative
immunology, coupled with previous information on the behavior of
earthworm coelomocytes reveals the coelomocyte as a prime example
of Burnet's hypothetical invertebrate wandering cell that recognizes and reacts to antigen. This cell is the ancestor of diverse

vertebrate immunocytes such as lymphocytes and plasma cells that reject foreign grafts and produce antibodies (12). Contrary to recent views, specific immunologic memory in earthworms supports the hypothesis that the basic capacity to recognize foreignness, to do it specifically, and to show memory, developed phylogenetically among the invertebrates and not among the primitive vertebrates (13). In fact, the primordial immune cell may be an invertebrate relative of the vertebrate T lymphocyte that mediates cellular immunity such as graft rejection (14).

ACKNOWLEDGEMENTS

Supported in part by NSF grant GB-17767, NIH grant 1R01 HD09333-01, and a grant from the Brown-Hazen Corporation. Send all reprint requests to E. L. Cooper.

REFERENCES

1. Valembois, P., C. R. Acad. Sci., Paris, 257: 3489-3490 (1963).

2. Duprat, P., C. R. Acad. Sci., Paris, 259: 4177-4180 (1964).

3. Cooper, E. L., Am. Zool., 5: 254 (1965).

4. Cooper, E. L., J. Exptl. Zool., 171: 69-73 (1969a).

5. Cooper, E. L. and Rubilotta, L. M., Transplantation, 8: 220-223 (1969).

6. Cooper, E. L., Transplantation, 6: 322-337 (1968).

7. Cooper, E. L., Science, 166: 1414-1415 (1969b).

8. Hildemann, W. H. and Reddy, A. L., Fed. Proc., 32: 2188-2194 (1973).

9. Hostetter, R. K. and Cooper, E. L., Immunol. Comm., 1: 155-183 (1972).

10. Hostetter, R. K. and Cooper, E. L., Cell. Immun., 9: 384-392 (1973).

11. Winger, L. A. and Cooper, E. L., Am. Zool., 9: 352 (1969).

12. Burnet, F. M., Nature, 218: 426-430 (1968).

13. Burnet, F. M., Immunological Surveillance (Pergamon, Oxford, London, New York, Toronto, Sydney, 1970).

14. Cooper, E. L., in Phylogeny of Immunity (Blackwell Oxford, in press, 1974).

SPECIFIC REJECTION OF INTEGUMENTARY ALLOGRAFTS BY THE SEA STAR

Dermasterias imbricata

Richard D. Karp[1] and W. H. Hildemann[2]

Department of Microbiology and Immunology, and Dental
Research Institute, University of California, Los
Angeles, California 90024

The origins of well-developed adaptive cell-mediated immune
responses in vertebrates would seem to reside among the invertebrates. The work supporting this contention has been extensively
reviewed elsewhere (3, 7). Since the immune responsiveness of
vertebrates appears to have gone through a step-wise evolutionary
development, one would not expect to find specific adaptive immunity
widespread throughout all phylums of invertebrates. Indeed, there
are few reports in the literature of what appear to be specific cell-
mediated immune responses among invertebrates. The studies of Cooper
(1) and that of Duprat (2) showed that annelids are capable of
specific transplantation immunity with at least short-term memory.
Reddy et al. (6) have recently presented evidence that tunicates at
the protochordate level are also capable of specific allograft rejection. The data of Hildemann and Dix (4) suggest that at least
one representative of the echinoderms, the sea cucumber Cucumaria
tricolor, can reject allografts with development of heightened secondary responsiveness. This preliminary study stimulated our further
interest in characterizing the immunological potentialities at this
level of phylogeny. Thus, we have undertaken extensive studies utilizing the sea star Dermasterias imbricata (class Asteroidea), to ascertain whether or not these animals possess an adaptive immune response as evidenced by specific rejection of integumentary allografts.

[1]Present Address: Department of Biological Sciences, University of
Cincinnati, Cincinnati, Ohio 45221. [2]Present Address: Hilo College,
University of Hawaii, Hilo, Hawaii 96720.

ALLOGRAFTING PROCEDURES

The sea star Dermasterias imbricata is a deep sea echinoderm preferring colder temperatures. The animals used in this study were collected off the coast of southern California by Pacific Bio-Marine Supply Co., of Venice, Calif. The sea stars were housed in tanks of recirculating sea water maintained at a temperature of $14-16^{\circ}C$, and fed assorted fish ad libitum. Animals were randomly paired and grafted using the following surgical procedures: A soft plastic template overlay was utilized to allow all integumentary grafts to be cut a uniform square size. A no. 11 surgical scalpel blade was used to outline the graft, and then a no. 15 scalpel blade served to cut it free from subcutaneous connective tissue. Grafts were sutured in place, in each of four corners, with 6-0 monofilament nylon. Animals were individually numbered by suturing single loops of 4-0 monofilament nylon through the integument of appropriate arms. First-set animals received a 5x5 mm full-thickness autograft on one arm, and a 5x5 mm full-thickness allograft, from its partner, on the next consecutive arm relative to the madreporite. Sutures were removed after one week, since the grafts were well healed in by this time. Second- and third-set grafts were placed on animals within one week of rejection of the preceding graft. Each subsequent graft was placed on the next consecutive arm from the last graft to avoid the possible occurrence of non-specific reactions due to local tissue injury. At the same time of second- and third-set grafting, some of the animals received unrelated third party allografts as a further indicator of specificity.

Animals were scored once a week by inspection of grafts under a stereomicroscope. The criteria used for rejection were loss of normal pigmentation (either blanching or darkening discoloration), fibrotic disorganization of tissue, edema and necrosis. Grafts were scored as completely rejected when total disappearance of normal pigmentation occurred. One or more of the other criteria usually accompanied this end point. Biopsies of autografts and allografts, along with adjacent normal tissue, were taken for histological study. The tissues were fixed in 10% formalin (in sterile sea water), dehydrated, and embedded in wax using standard procedures. Sections were stained with hemotoxylin and eosin. Median survival times (MST) with their 95% confidence limits were calculated using the Litchfield nomographic method (5), which takes into account allografts not rejected.

SPECIFIC REACTIVITY TO ALLOGRAFTS

Seventy sea stars (35 pairs) received first-set allografts as well as control autografts (Table 1). Seventeen of these animals rejected their first-set allografts with a MST of 213 days and 95%

Table 1: Reactions to first-, second-, and third-set allografts.

Allografts	No. animals rejecting graft	No. indefinite survivors	Non-scorable[a]	No. in progress
First-set	17	5[b]	37	11
Second-set	5	2[c]	3	1
Third-set	4	–	–	–

[a]Animals died either before total rejection of graft or before reaching indefinite survival status (i.e., fully viable after 300 days)

[b]Showing no signs of rejection >300 days.

[c]Showing no signs of rejection >110 days.

confidence limits of 170-266 days (Fig. 1). Five others showed no signs of rejecting their grafts after 300 days, and 37 died of various causes during prolonged observation before they could be scored definitively one way or the other. Eleven experimental animals are still being scored at this writing. None of the autografts showed any signs of being rejected, nor were any lost for technical reasons. In fact, autografts generally healed in so well that it was difficult to discern even a suture line after one month (Fig. 2). First-set grafts that had been rejected lost their normal pigmentation by either total blanching or darkening of their usual coloration, with the accompaniment of a cloudy appearance or hyperplasia due to fibrous disorganization of the tissue (Fig. 3). First-set grafts were not usually sloughed, but rather contracted, gradually leading to resorpion by the host in many instances.

Histological comparison of the allograft at the end point of zero survival with the adjacent, normal recipient tissue reveals the destruction of the allograft cytoarchitecture (Figs. 4 and 5). The long columnar cells which predominate in the normal dermis are no longer in evidence in rejecting allografts, but have been displaced by a heavy cellular infiltrate comprised of small lymphocyte-like cells and large phagocytic cells. Deposition of fibrous material was also observed. Autografts, on the other hand, could not be distinguished from normal adjacent tissue (Fig. 6).

The rejection of second-set allografts was far more intense than that of first-set allografts, and greatly accelerated. The MST was 44.2 days with 95% confidence limits of 17.7-110.5 days (Fig. 1). This

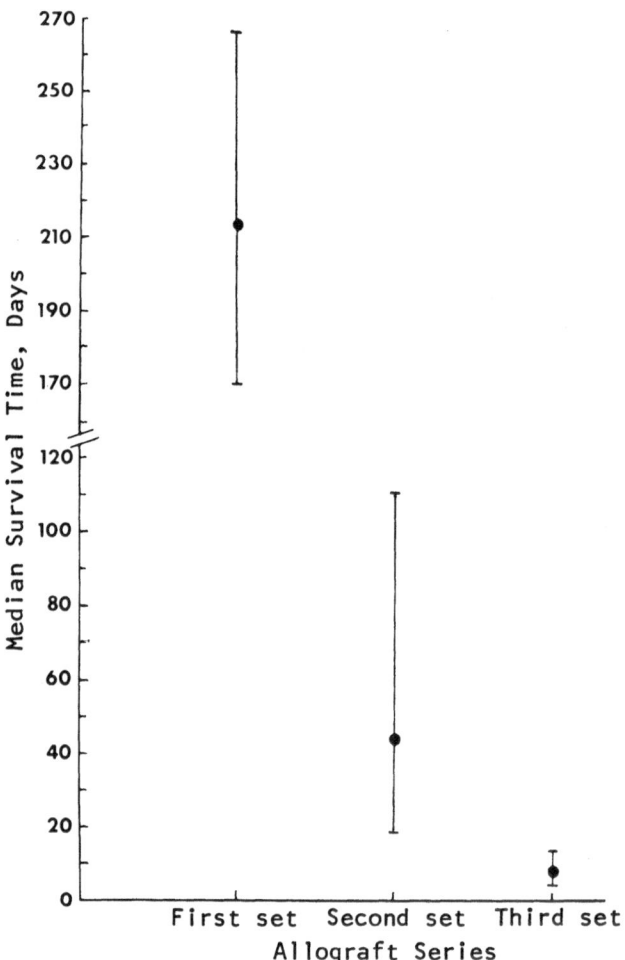

Figure 1: Median survival times of allografts with 95% confidence limits.

represents a significant reduction in survival time over that of first-set allografts. Of the 11 second-set grafts performed (Table 1), 5 were rejected, 2 have retained their grafts beyond 110 days with no signs of rejection, 3 died before they reached a scorable conclusion and one is still under observation. Grafts undergoing rejection displayed edematous swelling, had large areas of necrosis, and were eventually sloughed.

Histological examination of rejected second-set allografts revealed that there had been total disruption of the tissue due to a heavy infiltration of large phagocytic cells, small lymphocyte-like cells and deposits of fibrous material (Fig. 8). The normal recipient tissue adjacent to the allograft had a normal appearance (Fig.7).

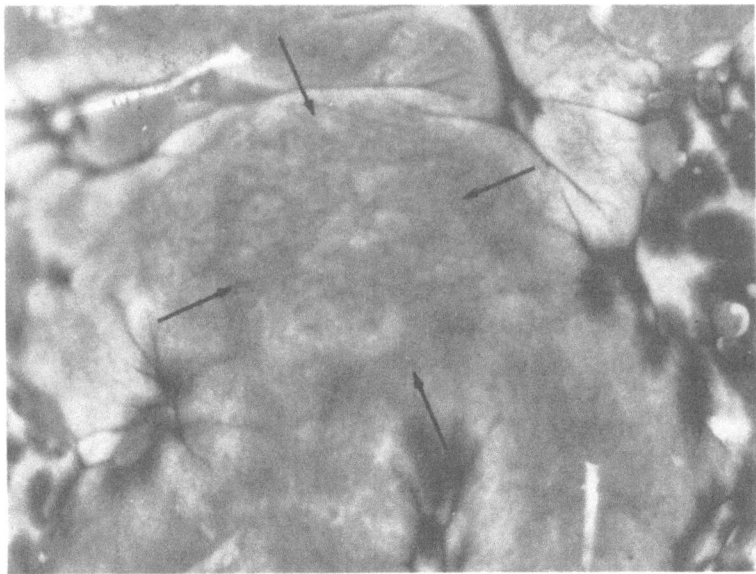

Figure 2: Autograft 190 days post-grafting. Arrows indicate margins of graft. 8.7x.

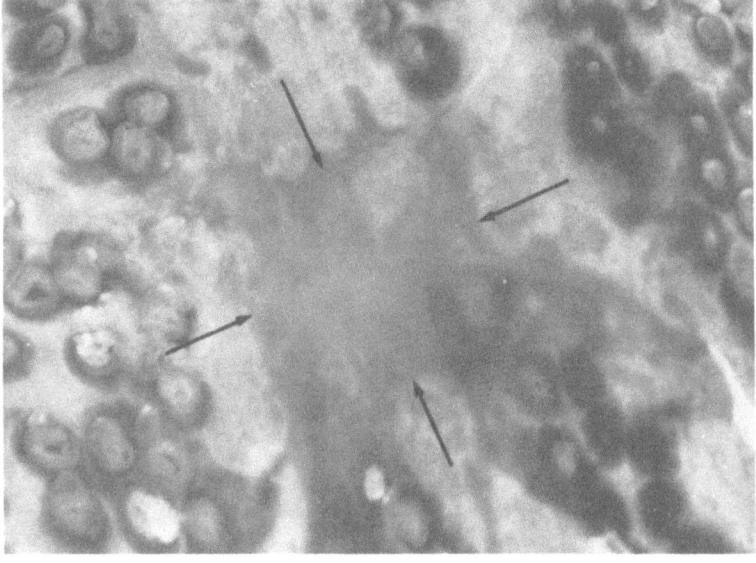

Figure 3: First-set allograft rejected 165 days post-grafting. Note darkening discoloration of normal pigment characteristic of slcwly mobilized first-set reactions. Arrows indicate margins of graft. 8.7x.

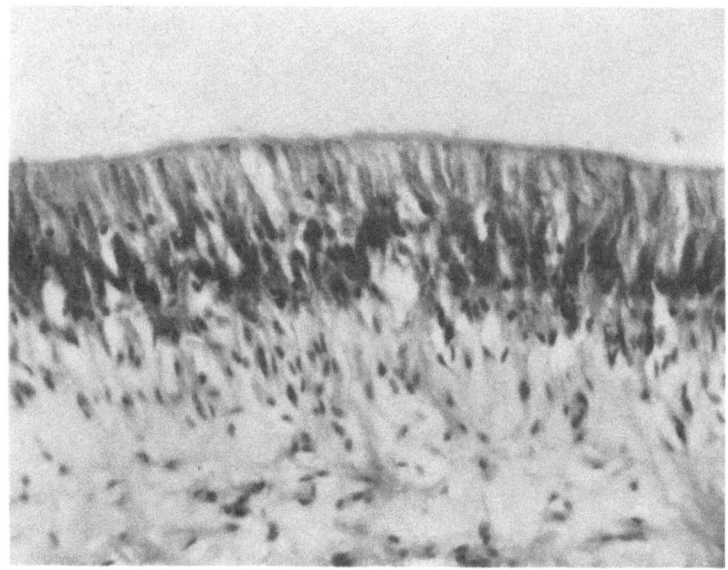

Figure 4: Normal recipient tissue laterally adjacent to a first-set allograft rejected 196 days post-grafting. Hematoxylin and eosin. 470x.

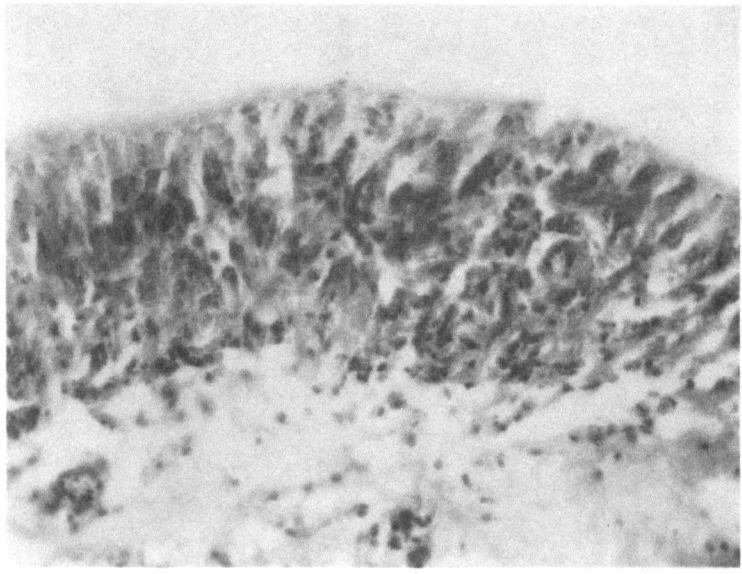

Figure 5: First-set allograft rejected 196 days post-grafting. Note cell infiltration associated with tissue disorganization. Hematoxylin and eosin. 470x.

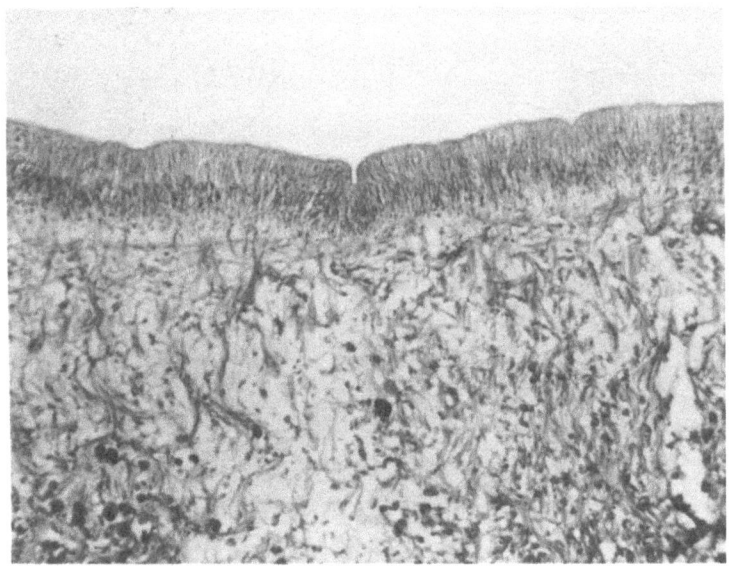

Figure 6: Autograft 102 days post-grafting. Low power scan depicting similar cytoarchitecture between autograft and adjacent normal tissue. Hematoxylin and eosin.   120x.

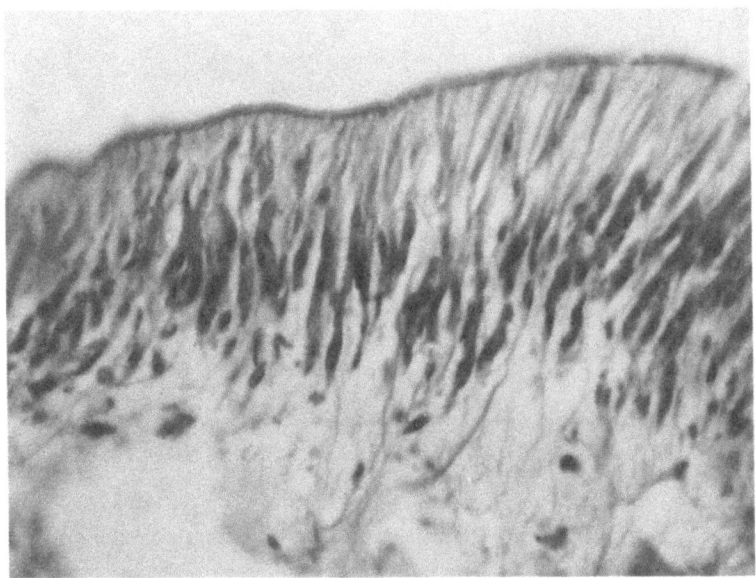

Figure 7: Normal recipient tissue laterally adjacent to second-set allograft rejected 28 days post-grafting. Hematoxylin and eosin. 470x.

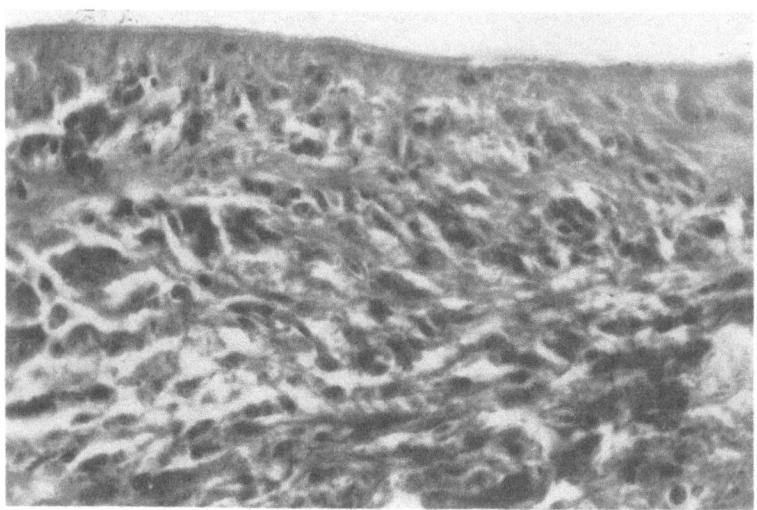

Figure 8: Second-set allograft rejected 28 days post-grafting. Note deposits of fibrous material and disruption of normal tissue organization. Hematoxylin and eosin. 470x.

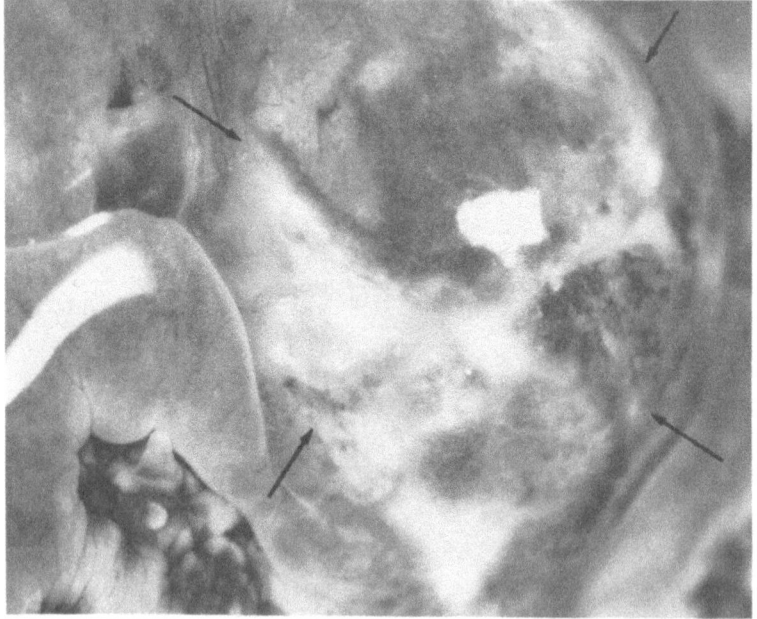

Figure 9: Third-set allograft rejected 9 days post-grafting. Note edematous swelling and large white patches of necrosis. Arrows indcate margins of graft. 8.7x.

All four of the third-set allografts were rejected, and had a MST of only 8 days with 95% confidence limits of 4.7-13.6 days (Fig. 1). This falls into the acute range of reactivity and is a significant increase in the rate of rejection over that of second-set allografts. The gross observations of the rejection phenomenon revealed that these third-set grafts underwent edematous swelling, necrosis and sloughing in quick succession (Fig. 9). Histologically, the picture was much the same as that for second-set grafts. The reaction was characterized by a heavy cellular infiltrate and deposition of fibrous material, whereas normal adjacent recipient tissue was unaffected.

Third-party allograft data, summarized in Table 2, supports an assumption of alloantigenic polymorphism in _Dermasterias_ leading to individually specific allograft sensitization. One animal, still under observation, rejected its second-set allograft in 15 days, but has shown no signs of rejecting a third-party allograft, placed at the same time as the second-set graft, after more than 100 days postgrafting. The four sea stars that had third-set allografts received third-party allografts as soon as their third-set grafts reached the zero end point of survival. One of these animals rejected its third-set graft in 5 days, but died only 15 days after receiving the third-party graft. Two other sea stars rejected their third-set grafts in 9 and 18 days, but both died 47 days after third-party grafting. At the time of death, there were no signs of rejection of any of these third-party grafts. The latter two animals had survival times for their third-party grafts well beyond the range for third-set rejection. The third-party graft on the fourth animal in this group has survived for more than 300 days without being rejected.

Table 2: Differential reactions to repeat and third-party allografts.

Repeat allografts	Times of rejection (days)	Survival times (days) of respective third-party allografts		
Second-set	15	>100		
Third-set	5, 9, 18, 11	>15[+],	>47[+],	>47[+], >300

[+]Died with fully viable allograft.

ADAPTIVE CELL-MEDIATED IMMUNITY IN SEA STARS

The results from these studies with the sea star Dermasterias
imbricata show that this advanced invertebrate possesses a well-
developed, adaptive cell-mediated immune capability. This was reflected in the chronic rejection of most integumentary allografts
with a high degree of specificity. There was also at least a short-
term immunological memory component to this transplantation immunity.
The specificity of the reaction was demonstrated by the greatly in-
tensified and increasingly accelerated rejection of second- and
third-set allografts. Furthermore, the prolonged survival of unrelated third-party allografts showed that the accelerated rejection
of previous repeat allografts was not a consequence of non-specific
events.

The prolonged chronicity characterizing first-set rejection
supports the assumption of very weak alloantigenic differences in sea
stars. The existence of weak histocompatibility barriers is further
supported by the finding that five animals failed to reject their
first-set allografts even after more than 300 days. Evidently, some
animals from this large population possess either extremely weak or
very few alloantigens. Alternatively, the library of genes governing
cell-mediated immunity in the recipients may be quite restricted.
Apart from the quality of antigens involved and the inherent responsiveness of the recipient, the step-wise sequence of cell-mediated
reactivity including recognition of foreignness, antigen processing,
activation, and proliferation and maturation of immunocytes must also
be considered. In any event, no major histocompatibility system or
locus has yet evolved at this level of invertebrate phylogeny (4).

Allograft rejection was characterized by loss of pigmentation,
edema and necrosis. First-set allografts appeared to contract and
eventually be resorbed by the recipient, whereas second- and third-
set grafts were usually sloughed. Histological examination revealed that the usual organization of the dermis was disrupted by
the infiltration of small lymphocyte-like cells and large phagocytic
cells. Deposits of fibrous material were also in evidence. Further
characterization of the cell types involved is in progress.

Throughout these experiments, animals were maintained at 14-16°C.
Since this species of sea star dies very quickly when the water temperature is above 16°C, the temperature dependence of these reactions
could not be determined. However, tropical sea cucumbers and sea stars
also exhibit similarly slow first-set allograft reactions even at
25°C (4). Conversely, Dermasterias sea stars are physiologically
capable of prompt or acute rejection as revealed by the early third-
set allograft reactions taking place at the lower temperatures of 14-
16°C. Thus, the rate or vigor of allograft reactivity in echinoderms
appears far more dependent on the temperature during the afferent or

sensitization phase than during the later efferent or target-cell killing phase.

The present studies have shown that the discriminating adaptive responses of cell-mediated immunity found in vertebrates have an analog among the echinoderms. Whether the reactions reported represent rudiments of T-cell function as associated with lymphocytes in vertebrates remains to be seen. Since echinoderms are thought to be directly ancestral to the vertebrates, apparent collaboration between lymphocyte-like cells and phagocytic cells in advanced invertebrates is not surprising (6). Hopefully, future studies to characterize effector cell functions, duration of immunological memory, and nature of the cell surface receptors mediating specific recognition should shed more light on unanswered questions.

ACKNOWLEDGEMENTS

This research was supported by NIH grant AI-07970. Dr. Karp was a recipient of an NIH postdoctoral fellowship 5T01 AI 00431, and a Celeste Durand Rogers postdoctoral fellowship.

REFERENCES

1. Cooper, E.L., Transpl. Proc. 2: 216 (1970).
2. Duprat, P.C., Transpl. Proc. 2: 222 (1970).
3. Hildemann, W.H., In: Transplantation Antigens - Markers of Biological Individuality. Eds. B. D. Kahan and R. A. Reisfeld. Academic Press, New York, 538 pp. (1972).
4. Hildemann, W.H. and Dix, T.G., Transplantation 15: 624 (1972).
5. Litchfield, J.T., J. Pharmacol. Exptl. Therapeut. 97: 399 (1949).
6. Reddy, A.L., Bryan, B. and Hildemann, W.H., Immunogenetics 1: 584 (1975).
7. Tam, M.R., Reddy, A.L., Karp, R.D. and Hildemann, W.H., In: Comparative Immunology. Ed. J.J. Marchalonis, Blackwell Press, in press.

VERTEBRATE IMMUNOLOGY

Structure and Functions
of Antibodies

PRELIMINARY STRUCTURAL CHARACTERIZATION OF PACIFIC HAGFISH IMMUNO-GLOBULIN

A. E. De Ioannes[1] and W. H. Hildemann[2]

Department of Microbiology and Immunology and Dental
Research Institute, University of California at Los
Angeles

The immune capacities of primitive fishes of the class Agnatha, the lamprey and the hagfish, have been under study for nearly a decade. Early results from Good and his collaborators suggested that lampreys, but not hagfish, possessed an adaptive immune response (1, 2). However, subsequent work of Linthicum and Hildemann (3) and Hildemann and Thoenes (4, 5) showed that hagfish (Eptatretus stoutii) could also respond specifically to certain immunogens and could reject allografts under appropriate conditions.

The structure of antibodies evoked in lampreys is still unclear. Marchalonis and Edelman (6) using bacteriophage f_2 as an antigen were able to isolate and characterize immunoglobulin peaks of 14 S and 6.6 S, composed of light chains (22,000 daltons) and heavy chains (70,000 daltons) but lacking interchain disulfide bonds. However, when partial amino acid composition and aminoterminal sequencing were done, lamprey immunoglobulin resembled classical Ig (6). Later, Litman et al. (7), using Brucella abortus as an antigen, found a very specific and inducible Ig in lampreys which was very different from any other described. They proposed a four chain model which assumed a native parent molecule of 320,000 daltons that spontaneously dissociated into subunits of approximately 150,000 daltons and 75,000 daltons. No data for amino acid composition were reported, but the spectrum of circular dichroism found was very far from any mammalian or other immunoglobulin previously described (8).

Present address: [1]Departamento de Biologia Celular, Laboratorio de
Microbiologia e Immunologia, Universidad Catolica de Chile, Santiago; [2]Hilo College, University of Hawaii at Hilo.

Hildemann and collaborators (3, 5) found a specific and inducible antibody response against both particulate antigens (sheep red cells) and soluble antigens (keyhole limpet hemocyanin) in hagfishes, but only at relatively high temperature (18 to 19°C) and after prolonged immunization. On the basis of serum fractionation with Sephadex G-200, immunoelectrophoresis and sedimentation coefficients, they suggested that this antibody was similar to IgM, but further physicochemical characterization was not done. Recently, we have undertaken further physicochemical and immunochemical characterization of hagfish antibodies. Experimental results described in the present report indicate the presence of an unusual immunoglobulin in hagfish, unlike the classical IgM found in sharks (9). Indeed, Pacific hagfish evidently have only light chain and non-heavy chain components arranged in a structure different from either of the models previously proposed for lamprey immunoglobulin (6, 7).

MATERIALS AND METHODS

Hagfish. Adult hagfish (E. stoutii), purchased from Pacific Bio-Marine Supply Co., Venice, California and ranging in length from 20 to 40 cm, were used in these studies. The animals were acclimatized to a large aquarium with circulating, filtered sea water and were held at 14°C-15°C throughout the experiments. Hagfish were kept in the dark and provided with opaque plastic tubing for shelter, since these animals are photophobic and bottom-dwelling. Animals subjected to bleedings were fed twice a month with fresh, homogenized beef liver by oral insertion of a plastic catheter into the gut. Normal hagfish feed spontaneously and gorge themselves, but experimentally traumatized animals are wary and may require forced-feeding.

Anesthesia and bleeding. Tricaine methane sulfonate (Finquel of Ayerst Labs., Inc., New York, N.Y.) was the most suitable anesthetic and took effect within 30 min. When the animals were placed on a slant board, blood flowed into the tail sinus by gravity; then bleeding could be easily accomplished using a 2 or 3 ml syringe with a 25 gauge needle. Blood from 15 to 20 animals involved in each experiment was often pooled. The blood was allowed to clot overnight at 4°C. The clot and remaining blood cells were removed by low speed centrifugation and the serum was either employed fresh or kept at -20°C until needed.

Serum fractionation. For ultracentrifugal separation, the serum was centrifuged at 1200 g for 30 min at 4°C. The crude pellet was discarded and the supernatant was ultracentrifuged at 50,000 rpm in a Beckman 50 Ti rotor (polycarbonate tubes filled with 5.4 ml of serum) for three hours at 4°C. The supernatant containing lipoproteins and low molecular weight proteins was discarded. The pellet, which was enriched in high molecular weight proteins, was allowed to

dissolve overnight at 4°C in 0.2 M NaCl in 0.05 M tris/HCl buffer
at pH 8.0, containing 1 mM EDTA and 0.02% sodium azide (standard
buffer). After the pellet was redissolved, any insoluble material
in minute quantity was removed by low speed centrifugation. For
sucrose gradient separations by ultracentrifugation, the following
procedure was employed: A Sw 50.1 Beckman rotor was used with 5 ml
cellulose acetate tubes at a speed of 50,000 rpm at 10°C for 6 hours.
A continuous, linear gradient from 10% (w/v) to 45% (w/v) sucrose
in the standard buffer solution was used. One-half ml of the redissolved ultracentrifuge pellet (2% protein concentration) was
layered on the top of the gradient. After the run was completed,
fractions of 0.2 ml were collected and each fraction was diluted to
1 ml with buffer. Protein concentration throughout the gradient was
spectrophotometrically determined at 280 mμ.

Column chromatography. For ion exchange chromatography, diethyl-
aminoethyl cellulose (DE-52) contained in a column 0.9 cm in diameter and 30 cm long was used. The column was equilibrated with
starting buffer of 0.05 M tris/HCl, pH 8.0 at 22°C. Whole serum,
fractions from ultracentrifuge pellets, or high molecular weight
fractions from sucrose gradients were dialyzed against starting
buffer before application to the column. Proteins were eluted
with a continuous linear gradient of NaCl from 0.0 to 0.4 M in the
starting buffer. Sepharose 6B gel filtration was done on a Sephadex (#K-15/100 Pharmacia, Uppsala, Sweden) column using upward flow
adaptors and equilibrated with standard buffer. Sample volume was 2
ml, and using a flow rate of 6 to 7 ml/hr, fractions of approximately
3 ml were collected; the elution profile was recorded in a LKB Uvicord
at 280 mμ. All operations were performed at 22°C. Reconcentration of
serum fractions was performed by negative pressure dialysis.

Electrophoresis and immunodiffusion. Immunoelectrophoretic
analysis of the serum fractions was performed by the usual micro-
technique using 25 x 75 mm glass microscope slides on an LKB immunoelectrophoresis apparatus (3, 10). Anti-whole hagfish serum was
produced in adult New Zealand white rabbits after 3 inoculations each
of 1.0 ml of whole hagfish serum emulsified in an equal amount of complete Freund's adjuvant. Injections were made into the footpads and
subcutaneously (SC) 3 weeks apart. A booster injection of whole hagfish serum (aqueous, SC) was given after 3 months. The rabbits were
bled 10 days after the last immunization. Double (Ouchterlony)
immunodiffusion was performed using 25 x 75 mm microscope slides.
Three ml of a 1% agarose gel was used with isotonic hagfish solution
(i.e., phosphate buffered saline with 1.2% NaCl at pH 7.4).

Sodium dodecyl sulfate (SDS) acrylamide electrophoresis was performed by the technique described by Laemmeli (11, 12). Twelve percent acrylamide was used in the running gel with isobutanol (13)
instead of distilled water as a layering agent. Samples were previously dialysed against sample buffer overnight before electrophor-

esis was performed. Samples to be reduced were dissolved in 0.0625
M tris/HCl at pH 6.8, with 15% glycerol, 5% 2-mercaptoethanol, and 3%
SDS, and then quickly heated to 90°C for 2 to 3 min. A small amount
of bromophenol blue was added to the sample to act as a dye marker.
Standard peptides of known molecular weight used to characterize the
system were: bovine serum albumin (BSA), human 7 S IgG heavy and light
chains, chicken ovalbumin (OA). The standards used were also run in
SDS acrylamide as described above. At the end of each run, gels were
fixed and stained with 0.2% Coomassie Brilliant Blue in 50% methanol
and 10% acetic acid for 2 hours. Gels were then destained with 50%
methanol and 10% acetic acid solution overnight in a BioRad Destainer.
Relative migration on the horizontal axis was plotted against molecular weight on the vertical axis as a semi-log plot. The linear
regression was calculated by the method of least squares.

RESULTS

Purification of hagfish immunoglobulin. Hagfish serum was fractionated by preparative ultracentrifugation as a preliminary step in
the isolation of the immunoglobulin. Although the serum analyzed
was obtained from a pool of unimmunized animals, the general hagfish
serum pattern as studied in immunized animals (3, 5) enabled the
ready identification of the Ig-containing fractions. The ultracentrifuge pellet was allowed to dissolve in buffer overnight and was then
layered on a sucrose gradient. The sucrose gradient pattern is shown
in Fig. 1. The high molecular weight fraction (Peak I) was pooled and
reconcentrated, and further purified by ion exchange chromatography
(DE-52). The first peak containing the Ig fraction as previously described (5) was eluted from DE 52 with 0.1 M NaCl as illustrated in Fig.
2B. Peak I was pooled and reconcentrated; when this fraction was
analysed on an analytic Sepharose 6B column, only one peak was found
(Fig. 2A). Ouchterlony analysis showed one main band and traces of
impurities when tested against antiwhole hagfish serum (Fig. 3).

Polypeptide analysis of the hagfish Ig fraction. Hagfish Ig, as
purified above, was subjected to SDS-acrylamide electrophoresis on
12% acrylamide gels, after reduction with 2-mercaptoethanol. Under
these conditions, as shown in Fig. 3, human IgG was completely dissociated into heavy chains and light chains. Under the same conditions, the hagfish Ig fraction exhibited an unusual pattern as seen
in Fig. 3; no heavy chain is detected and the main band is in the
light chain region. The molecular weight of the main band as calculated from SDS-acrylamide electrophoresis is about 22,000 daltons.
The position and shape of this band were similar to the human 7 S
light chain that was used as a standard (Fig. 3). Other bands were
also present, a diffuse one at approximately 33,000 daltons composed
of several peptide chains, and two other very homogeneous peptide
bands weighing approximately 17,000 daltons and 18,000 daltons. At

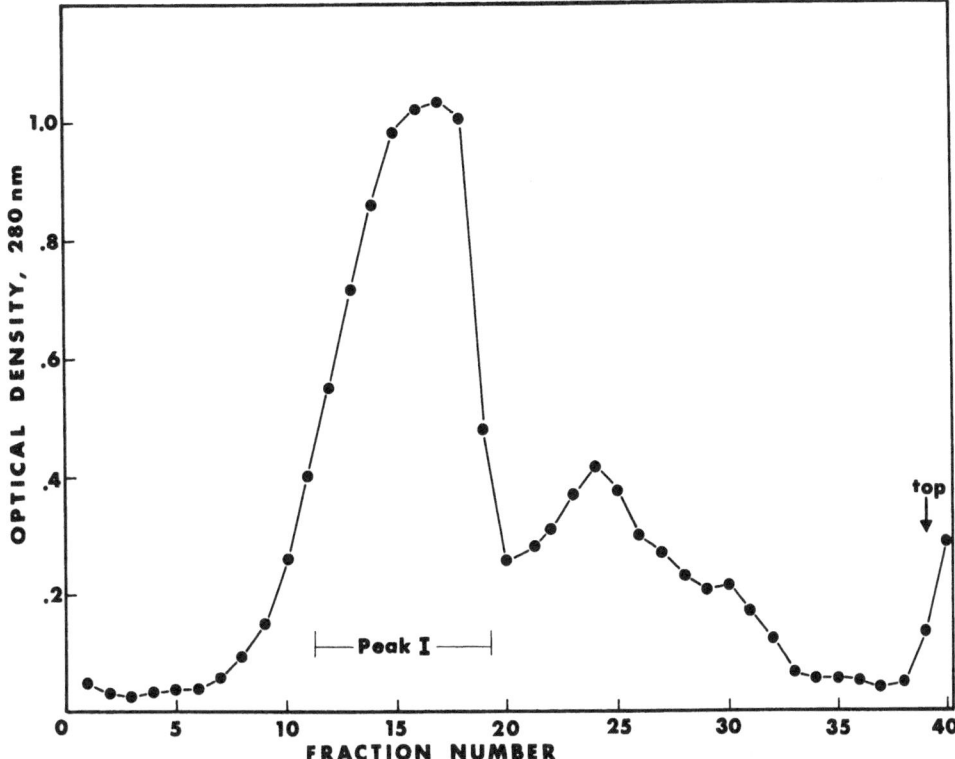

Figure 1. Sucrose gradient (10%-40%) ultracentrifugation of hagfish serum previously enriched for high molecular weight proteins by preparative ultracentrifugation. Peak 1 was reconcentrated and used for further purification and analysis.

present, experiments are underway to determine the relationship between the peptide of 22,000 daltons and the other peptides.

DISCUSSION

The unexpected observation that the pattern of hagfish macroglobulin dissociation lacked heavy chain components following SDS acrylamide electrophoresis was surprising. Possible interpretations of this finding were that (a) there was proteolytic cleavage during the purification process, (b) the immunoglobulin fraction was only a small part of the whole macroglobulin fraction or (c) the macroglobulin actually was devoid of heavy chain. Yet even when the macroglobulin fraction was analyzed by overloading the gels, the stained gel from the top to the 33,000 dalton fraction remained absolutely

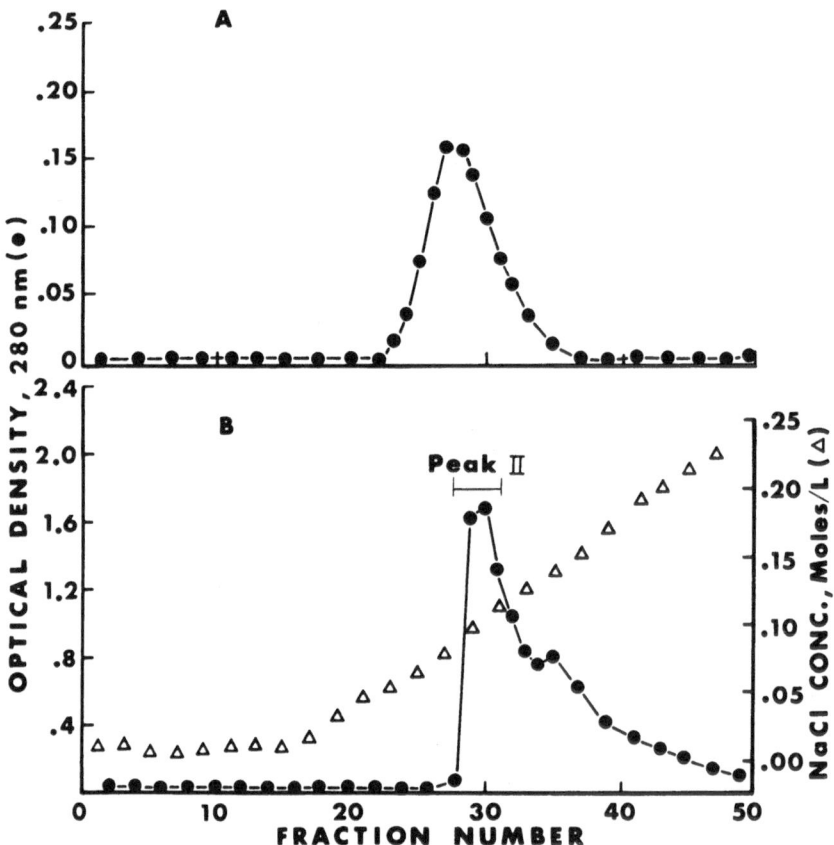

Figure 2A. Sepharose 6B gel filtration of reconcentrated "Peak II" from DE-52 ion exchange chromatography.

Figure 2B. DE-52 ion exchange chromatography of reconcentrated "Peak I" from sucrose gradient purification of the macroglobulin fraction from hagfish serum.

clear of bands. Proteolysis leading to total disappearance of possible heavy chain polypeptide appears quite unlikely, because the macroglobulin fraction after purification retained the same elution position upon Sepharose 6B gel filtration, and was intact by this

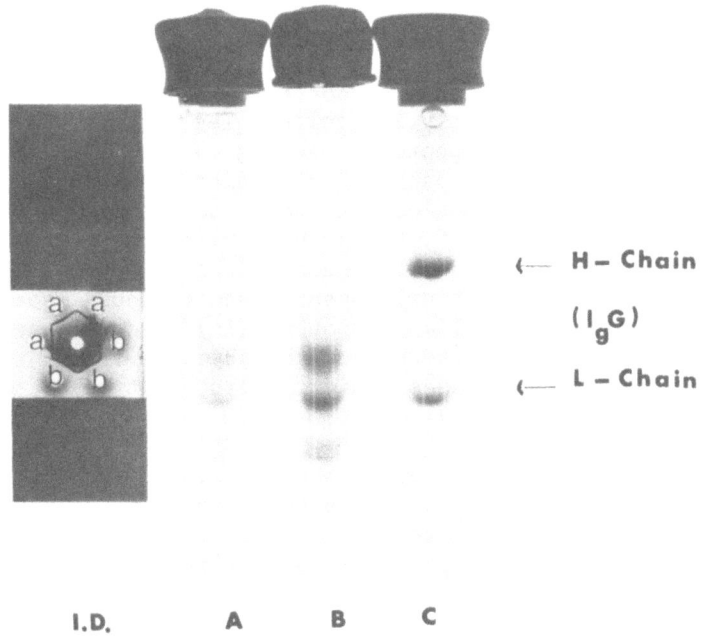

Figure 3. Immunodiffusion pattern in agarose (I.D.). Sepharose 6B
- purified fraction (peripheral wells "a") and whole hagfish serum
(peripheral wells "b") were tested against rabbit anti-whole hagfish
serum (center well). SDS-acrylamide gel electrophoresis was performed
on either differing concentrations of Sepharose 6B purified hagfish
macroglobulin (tubes A and B), or human IgG, used as a standard
marker (tube C).

criterion. Moreover, purification of hagfish immunoglobulin on
immunoadsorbant columns (14) yielded the same Ig constituents lacking
heavy chains.

     Consistent with the assumption of a multimeric light polypeptide
structure for hagfish immunoglobulin is the evidence of Clem (pers.
comm.). Under dissociating conditions of reduction and alkylation
with macroglobulin labelled by ^{3}H-iodoacetamide in 7 M guanidine-Cl,
most of the radioactivity following G-200 gel filtration in 7 M
guanidine-Cl was in the excluded fraction. However, some radioactivity was detected in the light chain region. Although Clem

could not efficiently dissociate hagfish macroglobulin under the above conditions, shark IgM was nicely dissociated into heavy and light chains under these same conditions.

The combination of SDS as a dissociating medium and acrylamide SDS electrophoresis as an analytic tool enabled us to resolve hagfish macroglobulin into polypeptides ranging in size from 33,000 to 17,000 daltons. The only band which displayed homology by molecular size to a known immunoglobulin chain was the 22,000 dalton peptide that comprises most of the macroglobulin fraction. The 33,000 dalton bands exhibited heterogeneity while the remaining two bands (17,000-18,000 daltons) appeared homogeneous. Isoelectric focusing of the light chain-like component (14) revealed the polypeptide to have a diffuse pattern over the pH range from 5 to 8. Thus, this polypeptide possesses a microheterogeneity typical of a polyclonal immunoglobulin (25).

Preliminary characterization of hagfish immunoglobulin by electron microscopy (15) suggests an asymmetric molecule with dimensions of 250 Å x 43 Å consistent with a molecular weight of about one million. Available evidence is still insufficient to propose a definitive model for hagfish antibodies. Additional information required includes (a) peptide composition and ratio of the molecular components (b) subunit structure (c) extent of disulfide bonding and (d) precise determination of molecular weights and sedimentation coefficients. At this juncture, hagfish immunoglobulin appears to be a multimer of lower molecular weight polypeptides, but consisting predominantly of a light chain-like peptide.

Several schemes of possible evolution of Ig polypeptide chain genes have recently been suggested based on studies of mammalian myeloma proteins (16, 17). Assumption of an ancestral immunoglobulin gene coding for a precursor peptide of approximately 110 amino acids with subsequent gene duplication yielding constant (C) and variable (V) region units is common to all current schemes (16-19). This V/C divergence to produce the equivalent of Ig light chains followed by interchain association of two or more units could have yielded the first antibody molecules in species antecedent to modern cyclostomes. Further gene duplication and adaptive selection to yield μ-type heavy chains with four constant region subunits may first have occurred in the progenitors of modern elasmobranchs. IgM-type antibodies are surely found in sharks and all classes of higher vertebrates. However, occurrence of the requisite H/L chain divergence in cyclostomes is now doubtful because of the apparent absence of heavy chains in hagfish.

Postulation of a model consisting mainly of light chain-like subunits in hagfish immunoglobulins appears in agreement with current theories of immunoglobulin emergence (16-19). However, the active

site on the other known immunoglobulins is believed to require collaborative interconnection of the V-region from a light chain and the
V-region from a heavy chain. Light chain dimers or light chains
alone have exhibited low affinity interaction with corresponding
haptens (22, 23). Nevertheless, one light chain dimer was reported
to possess binding activity associated with two light chains of
identical sequences but exhibiting different conformations as revealed by X-ray diffraction (20, 21, 24). From this perspective,
the combining site of the hagfish immunoglobulin could be derived
from (a) one light chain with one active site (b) collaborative
interaction of two identical light chains with one active site, or
(c) collaborative interaction of two different light chains with
differing V-regions forming an active site, reflecting the situation
found in higher vertebrates. Effective antibody function in evolving
cyclostomes as well as elasmobranchs may have been achieved by
increasing polymerization of subunits. The role of carbohydrate
components and J-chain-like or other joining units in the assemblage
and stabilization of these primordial immunolglobulins remains open
to speculation.

ACKNOWLEDGEMENTS

    We thank Ms. Birgitte Anthony for expert technical assistance
and Pacific Bio-Marine Supply Co. for excellent facilities. Dr. De
Ioannes was supported by a fellowship from the Catholic University
of Santiago, Chile. This research was supported by NIH grants
AI-07970 and CA-15788.

REFERENCES

1. Papermaster, B.W., Condie, R.M., Finstad, J. and Good, R.A.,
      J. Exp. Med. 119: 105 (1964).
2. Good, R.A. and Papermaster, B.W., Advances in Immunol. 4: 115
      (1964).
3. Linthicum, D.S. and Hildemann, W.H., J. Immunol. 105: 4 (1970).
4. Hildemann, W.H. and Thoenes, G.H., Transplantation 7: 506 (1969).
5. Thoenes, G.H. and Hildemann, W.H., In Developmental Aspects of
      Antibody Formation and Structure, Eds: J. Sterzl and I. Riha.,
      2: 711 (1969).
6. Marchalonis, J.J. and Edelman, G.M., J. Exp. Med. 127: 891 (1968).
7. Litman, G.W., Frommel, D., Finstad, J., Howell, J., Pollara, B.A.
      and Good, R.A., J. Immunol. 105: 5 (1970).
8. Litman, G.W., Rosenberg, A. and Good, R.A., Federation Proc. 29:
      774 (1970).
9. Clem, L.W. and Small, P.A., Jr., J. Exp. Med. 125: 893 (1967).
10. Hirschfeld, J., In Handbook of Immunodiffusion and Immunoelectro-
      phoresis, Ed: Ouchterlony (Ann Arbor Science Publishers,
      Ann Arbor, p.139, 1968).

11. Laemmeli, U.K. and Favre, M., J. Mol. Biol. 80: 575 (1973).
12. Laemmeli, U.K., Nature, 227: 680 (1970).
13. Atwell, J.L., The Structure and Evolution of Immunoglobulins.
        Ph.D. thesis submitted to the University of Melbourne (1974).
14. De Ioannes, A.E. and Hildemann, W.H., in preparation.
15. De Ioannes, A.E., Karp, R.D. and Hildemann, W.H., in preparation.
16. Spiegelberg, H.L., Nature 254: 723 (1975).
17. Capra, J.D., Chuang, C., Kaplan, R.D. and Kehoe, J.M., Adv. Exp.
        Med. Biol. 45: 191 (1974).
18. Hildemann, W.H., Ann. Rev. Genetics 1: 19 (1973).
19. Marchalonis, J.J., In Progress in Immunology II, vol. 2, p. 249,
        Eds: I. Brent and J. Holborow (1974).
20. Edmundson, A.B., Ely, K.R., Girling, R.L., Abola, E.E., Shiffer,
        M. and Westholm, F.A., In Progress in Immunology II, vol. 1,
        p. 103, Eds: I. Brent and J. Holborow (1974).
21. Edmundson, A.B., Ely, K.R., Girling, R.L., Abola, E.E., Shiffer,
        M., Westholm, F.A., Faush, M.D. and Doutch, H.F., Biochemistry
        13: 3817 (1974).
22. Metzger, H. and Singer, S.J., Science 142: 674 (1963).
23. Fleishman, J.B., Pain, R. and Porter, R.R., Arch. Biochem.
        Biophys. Supply. 1: 174 (1962).
24. Shiffer, M., Girling, R.L., Ely, K.R., and Edmundson, A.B.,
        Biochemistry 12: 4620 (1973).
25. Williamson, A.R., Europ. J. Immunol. 1: 390 (1971).

ANTIBODIES AGAINST SALMONELLA AND SRBC IN URODELE AMPHIBIANS:

SYNTHESIS AND CHARACTERIZATION

Annick Tournefier and Jacques Charlemagne

Université Pierre et Marie Curie, 75230 Paris, France

Laboratoire de Biologie animale 2, 9 Quai Saint Bernard

An understanding of the primitive immune responses in inverte-brates and poikilothermic vertebrates, such as fishes and amphibians, will give a better insight of the ontogeny of immune mechanisms in mammals.

Fishes and amphibians exhibit cell-mediated immune responses in rejecting allografts and tumours (1,2). The immune mechanisms implied in the allograft rejection are the same as in mammals, but with a delayed rate of response. The humoral immunity to allografts (3) and to soluble antigens exists also in these poikilothermic vertebrates. In higher vertebrates the antibody response consists of an initial 19S IgM response supplanted by a 7S IgG response, however the antibody response in fishes consists of only one immuno-globulin class (19S) (4). In some cases in dipnoi (5) and teleosts (6) a 7S IgG precursor is synthesized, but this immunoglobulin has the same antigenic determinant as the 19S IgM.

Recent data in anuran amphibians demonstrate that larvae (7,8,9) and adults (10,11,12,13) synthesize high levels of 19S IgM and 7S IgG immunoglobulins. In Xenopus laevis, one of the most primitive anurans, these two distinct IgM and IgG immunoglobulins are present and share no common antigenic determinant on their heavy chains (14). In urodele amphibians very little data concerning immunoglobulin synthesis have been published, although they may represent the phylogenetic pathway between the primitive IgM synthesis of fishes and the more sophisticated IgM and IgG synthesis of anurans and higher vertebrates. The two urodele species investigated were Ambystoma mexicanum (15,16,17) and Necturus maculosus (18).

They synthesize exclusively IgM. However, these animals are very
primitive and neotenic; and their peculiar physiological state,
more larval than adult, may influence their ability to respond to
an antigenic challenge by an IgG synthesis.

In a previous work we found in two metamorphosed Salamandridae,
Pleurodeles waltlii Michah. and Triturus alpestris Laur., humoral
antibodies against sheep red blood cells (SRBC). Fifty per cent
of the immunized animals, after a long period of immunization with
heavy doses of SRBC, were able to synthesize "incomplete" antibodies.
These incomplete antibodies seemed to be very similar to incomplete
IgM isoagglutinins in man (19). The characterization of these antibodies revealed that the only immunoglobulin synthesized is an IgM-
like protein, even after a booster injection (20).

It remained to be known if, as in anurans (21), the nature of
the immunoglobulin is dependent upon the nature of the antigen, and
also to explain the "incomplete" nature of anti-SRBC antibodies.
Using the same two species, Pleurodeles and Triturus, we determined
their antibody responses to Salmonella antigens and the classes of
immunoglobulins involved in these responses. The nature of the
"incomplete" antibodies obtained after SRBC immunization also was
investigated by indirect immunofluorescence technique.

MATERIAL AND METHODS

Immunization

The animals were adult Triturus alpestris Laur. and Pleurodeles
waltlii Michah.; some of them were thymectomized at larval stage (22).
They were bred in our laboratory, maintained at 18-20°C in tap water
and fed with hashed meat twice a week.

The first antigen used was Salmonella typhi H and O suspension
(Institut Pasteur-Paris). The animals received one intraperitoneal
injection (IP) of 5×10^8 cells in saline or Freund's complete adjuvant (FCA). A booster dose was injected 12 weeks after the initial
challenge in Pleurodeles. The second antigen was SRBC (Institut
Pasteur-Paris) in saline. A 25% SRBC suspension was injected IP at
weekly intervals (2×10^7 SRBC in 0.2 ml) in Triturus and (6×10
SRBC in 0.3 ml) in Pleurodeles. Bleeding was performed before the
first injection and every three weeks during the course of immunization. The animals were anesthetized (MS 222, Sandoz) and 50 µl
blood samples were collected from the iliac vein. The sera were
immediately tested after centrifugation for 10 minutes at 5,000
rev/minute.

Antibody titrations were carried out in microtiter plates
using two haemagglutination assays. The classic haemagglutination
assay (HA) was used with anti-Salmonella sera. Twenty-five micro-
liters of either H or O antigen were added to equal volumes of
two-fold serial dilutions of antisera. The end point of agglutination was taken for the H antigen after 1 hour at 37°C and one
night at room temperature, and for the O antigen after 2 hours at
37°C and one night at room temperature. The papainized erythrocyte
agglutination test (HAP) was performed with anti-SRBC sera inactivated 30 minutes at 56°C, as previously described (19). Controls
were made using saline and nonimmune Triturus and Pleurodeles sera.

Anti-Pleurodeles IgM sera were obtained in rabbits by one
injection of 0.5 ml of the active protein starch-gel fraction
emulsified in FCA. A booster dose in incomplete Freund's adjuvant
was injected one month later and the rabbits were bled one week
after the booster. The purity of the injected active fraction was
determined by polyacrylamide electrophoresis and immunoelectrophoresis.

Characterization of Immunoglobulin

2-Mercaptoethanol (ME) sensitivity was assayed by incubating
the sera for 2 hours at 37°C with 2-ME (0.2 M) before titrating by
the HA or the HAP test. For controls, these sera were incubated
with saline.
Sucrose density gradient centrifugation. Fractionation of
anti-Salmonella sera was carried out on a 7% to 40% sucrose gradient
as previously described (20). Each fraction collected was analysed
for agglutinating activity and absorbance measured at 660 nm.
Zone electrophoresis. Normal, immune sera, and density gradient fractions of normal and immune sera were subjected to horizontal
starch-gel and gradient polyacrylamide gel electrophoresis. Details
of these techniques were described elsewhere (23). After migration
and staining, the staining density of the different proteins were
analysed in immune and control sera using a photo-integrator densi-
tometer. Immune sera anti-Salmonella and anti-SRBC also were fractionated by micropreparative starch-gel electrophoresis by applying
0.2 ml of serum to 11% starch-gel (120 x 120 x 5 mm). At the ending
of the migration, the gel was first sliced horizontally, then 5 mm
segments from the point of insertion of the sample to the α2 macroglobulin region were cut off and eluted by centrifugation (24).
Each fraction was tested by agglutination for its antibody activity
and rerun in acrylamide gel electrophoresis to determine the exact
localization and mobility of the antibody protein.
Double diffusion in Ouchterlony plates was performed with
control and immune anti-SRBC sera against sonicated papainized SRBC
(25). Finally, purity of zone electrophoresis fractionated proteins

and specificity of the immune rabbit anti-Pleurodeles immunoglobulin sera were checked by immunoelectrophoresis (23).

Indirect Immunofluorescence

Indirect immunofluorescence was performed on normal and papainized SRBC sensitized by incubating 45 min. at 37°C with an anti-SRBC Pleurodeles serum (diluted 1:8). The sensitized SRBC were washed 6 times in saline, then incubated 20 min. at room temperature with rabbit anti-Pleurodeles IgM (diluted 1:10). After 3 washes in saline, the SRBC which had been sensitized with Pleurodeles IgM and coated with rabbit anti-Pl IgM, were incubated once again for 20 min. in an ice-bath with FITC (fluoresceine isothiocyanate) conjugated goat IgG anti-rabbit IgG (MILES). The cells were examined for their fluorescence after 3 washes in saline (for the fluorescence microscopy, see J. C. and A. T. in this volume). As controls, papainized and normal SRBC were incubated with non-immune and immunized but non-responding Pleurodeles sera.

RESULTS

Responses to Salmonella Antigens

H antigen in saline. Seven Pleurodeles waltlii which had no natural anti-H agglutinins before immunization had good antibody responses. The titers increased regularly ($\log_2$ 2-7) until the 6th week. The antibody response reached a level which remained constant until the 15th or the 18th week. A booster injection failed to increase the titers (Fig. 1). Seven normal Triturus alpestris tested with H antigen had natural agglutinins prior to immunization ($\log_2$ 1-3). As determined by HA tests all the immunized Triturus had good antibody responses ($\log_2$ 4-16). As in Pleurodeles, the antibody titers steadily increased until the 6th week, but then suddenly decreased at the 12th week. At this time, a booster resulted in a slightly enhanced response ($\log_2$ 5-6) which dropped quickly and disappeared by the 18th week. The maximum titers varied considerably (Fig. 1).

O antigen in saline. This antigen elicited a very low response ($\log_2$ 2-3) in Pleurodeles and Triturus which remained unchanged until the 18th week.

H antigen in FCA. In 12 immunized Pleurodeles the antibody titers increased exponentially during the first 6 weeks and reached maximum titers by the 6th week ($\log_2$ 7-13). The peak titers remained constant or decreased slightly after the 18th week. In 10 thymectomized Pleurodeles immunized in the same way, the antibody titers increased exponentially from the first to the third week. However, the titers increased more slowly between the third and the sixth weeks than control titers. In the thymectomized animals the maxima

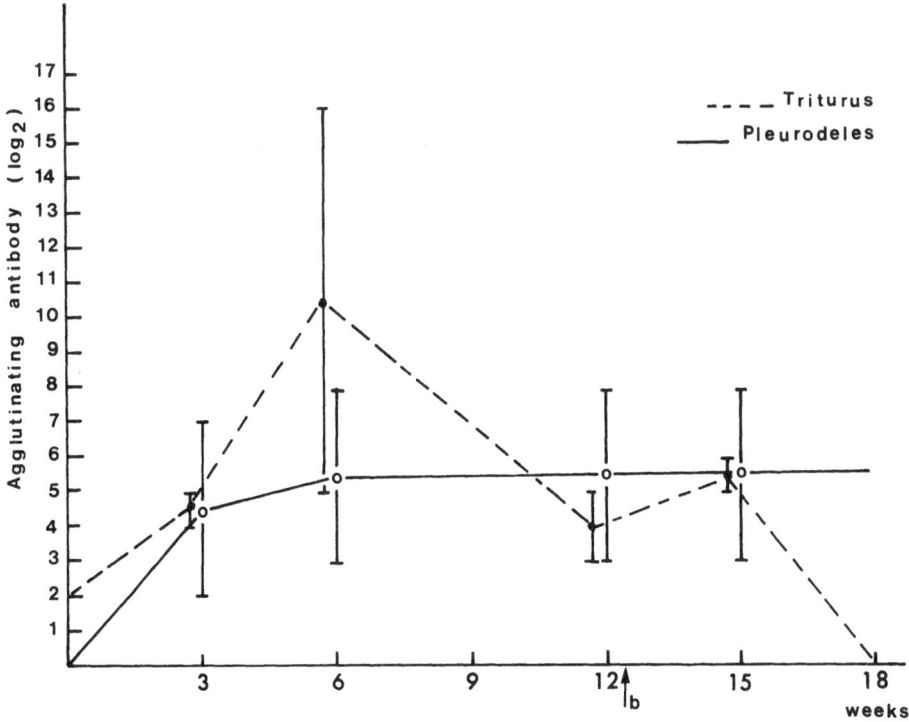

Fig. 1. Kinetics of appearance of agglutinating antibodies against Salmonella H antigen and serum titers in Pleurodeles and Triturus. Each point represents the geometric mean and the standard deviation of 7 animals.

also remained constant until the 18th week, but perceptibly lower ($\log_2$ 8-12)(Fig. 2).

O antigen in FCA. In 12 immunized Pleurodeles the agglutinating titers increased until the 18th week, followed by peak titers which remained constant ($\log_2$ 4-9). In 10 thymectomized Pleurodeles immunized with the O antigen in adjuvant the titers increased faster than in controls. The same maxima as in controls were reached in 9 or 12 weeks, then the titers decreased slightly ($\log_2$ 3-7) and remained constant (Fig. 3).

Generally, one injection of 5 x 10^8 cells of H or O Salmonella antigen in adjuvant elicited in all of the normal and thymectomized Pleurodeles good humoral antibody responses with agglutinin titers between $\log_2$ 7 and $\log_2$ 11. A booster injection at the 25th week

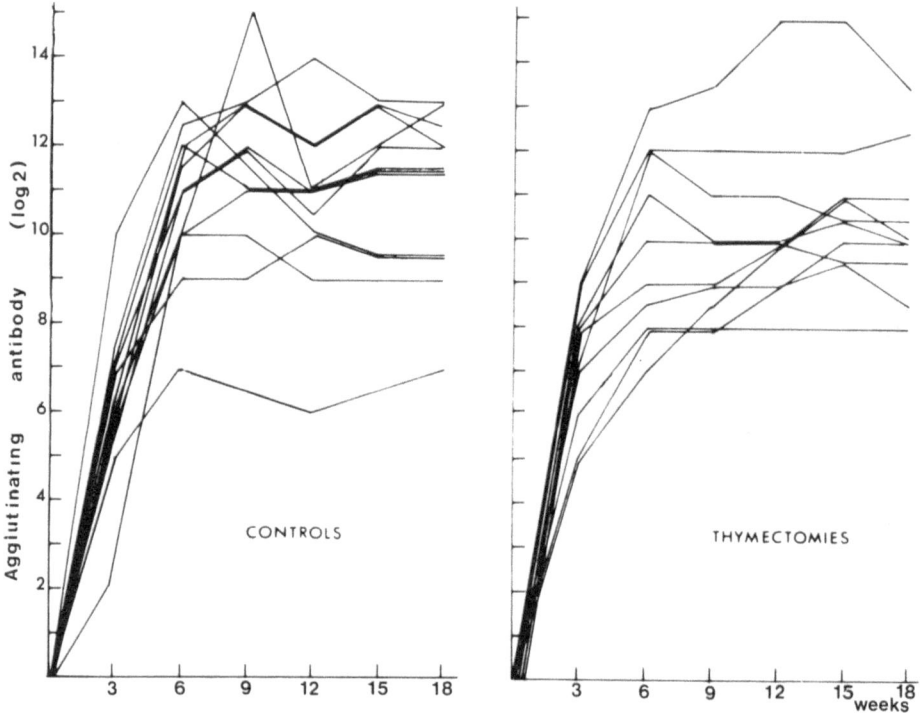

Fig. 2. Kinetics of the response of normal and thymectomized
Pleurodeles to Salmonella H antigen in adjuvant. Each curve
represents one animal.

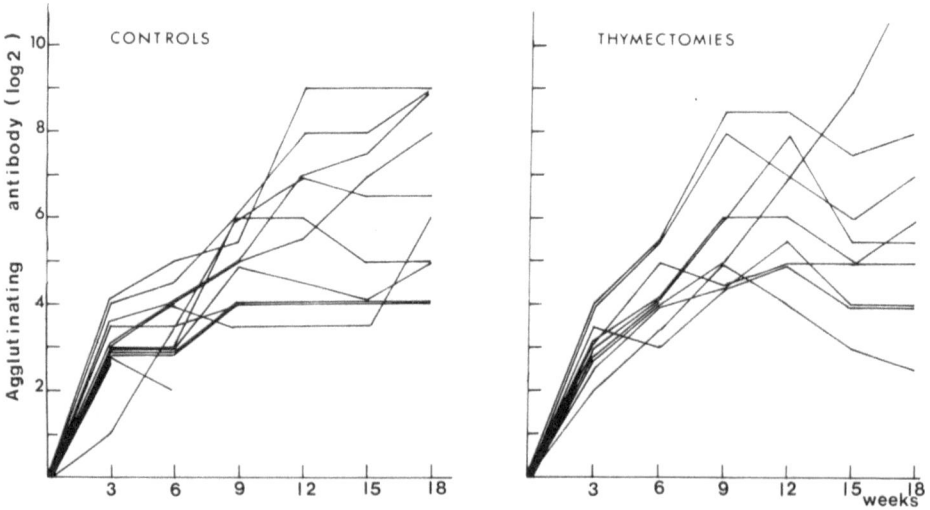

Fig. 3. Kinetics of the response of normal and thymectomized
Pleurodeles to Salmonella O antigen in adjuvant.

after the primary immunization fails to enhance the response and induces in more than 50% of the animals hypersensitivity crisis with edema and paralysis causing death in the few hours after boosting. Injection of Salmonella antigens in adjuvant elicits edema in Triturus alpestris followed by death in 3 weeks.

Responses to SRBC

With this antigen at least 3 repeated injections are necessary to elicit a humoral antibody response. "Incomplete" antibodies are detected in 45% of Triturus and 52% of Pleurodeles. In the responders, considerable individual variations were observed, but a good humoral antibody response is usually obtained ($\log_2$ 3-14). The antibody titers steadily increased up to the 8th week, and then slowly decreased until the 10th week. A booster elicits a more acute response in one third of the animals with a peak on the 6th week after boosting. The antibody titer is dependent on the number of immunizations rather than on the dose or nature of antigen (normal or papainized SRBC).

Immunoglobulin Characterization

As previously found with anti-SRBC immunoglobulins, Triturus and Pleurodeles anti-Salmonella antisera had agglutinating activity exclusively associated with the initial protein peak in Sperose density fractions. The sedimentation coefficient of anti-Salmonella immunoglobulins (18.2 S) was the same as the sedimentation coefficient of the anti-SRBC immunoglobulins.

2-ME treated immune anti-Salmonella and anti-SRBC sera did not have agglutinating activity, even in sera with high haemagglutination titers after booster injections.

Polyacrylamide gel electrophoresis and density analysis of normal and immune sera show the thickening of a slow protein in the γ zone (Fig. 4). When gradient density fractions are analyzed with the same techniques, this slow-moving protein is present only in the agglutinating fractions, but always associated with the α2 macroglobulins. The slow-moving protein isolated by starch-gel electrophoresis was found to be the only protein responsible for the antibody activity. The slow mobility is characteristic of IgM. When Pleurodeles and Triturus anti-SRBC sera were reacted with sonicated erythrocytes in Ouchterlony plates, a single precipitating arc was obtained. This indicates that Pleurodeles and Triturus have been immunized against a single type of erythrocyte antigen.

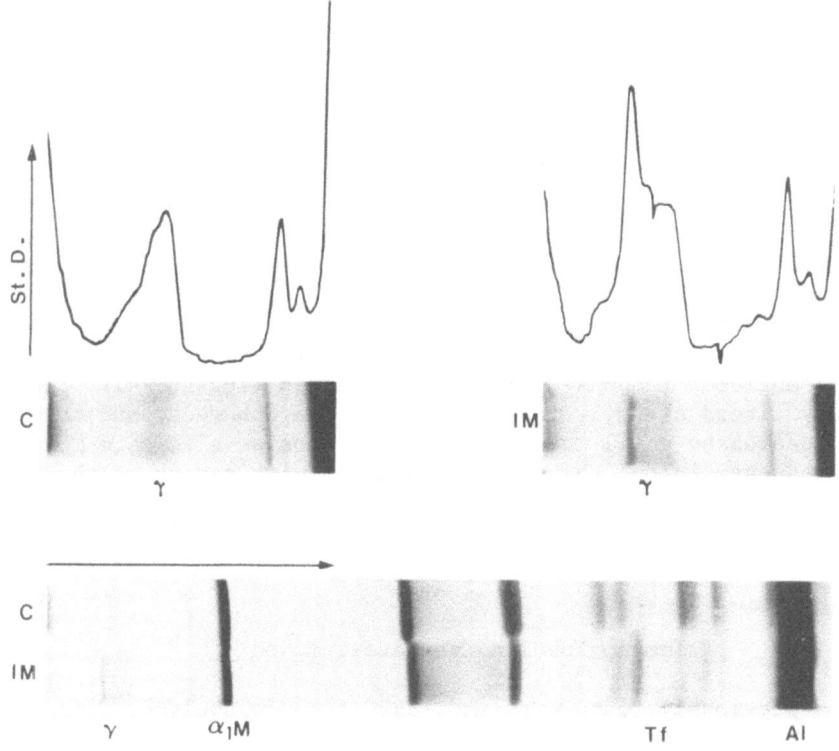

Fig. 4. Polyacrylamide gel electrophoresis of control (C) and immune (IM) anti-SRBC Triturus sera. The staining density analysis of the γ zone of these two sera shows a thickening of the slower-moving protein in the IM serum.

Indirect Immunofluorescence

The papainized erythrocytes sensitized by an anti-SRBC Pleurodeles serum, coated with a rabbit anti-Pleurodeles IgM, and then stained with fluorescent goat anti-rabbit IgG, show multiple fluorescent spots brightly patched all around their membrane. These strongly stained erythrocytes are mostly agglutinated. In this case, non-fluorescent erythrocytes are very scarce (7-14%).

In non-papainized erythrocytes treated in the same way, as controls, cells with a typical positivity are almost absent. A diffuse fluorescence in a uniform ring appearance was found in few agglutinated erythrocytes. Erythrocytes with bright fluorescent spots are very scarce, and they turned almost immediately to ghosts during the observation as if the antibody binding had weakened their membrane (Fig. 5).

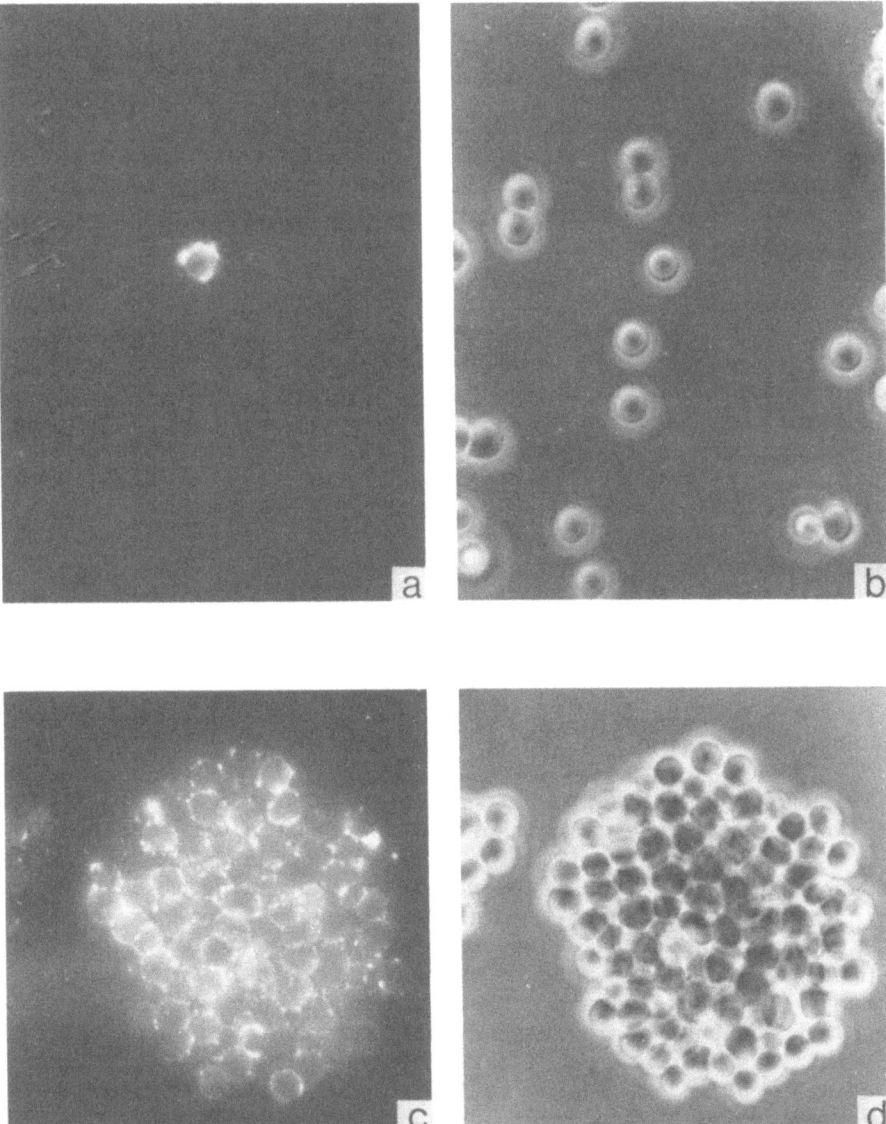

Fig. 5. a. Normal SRBC coated with Pleurodeles anti-SRBC serum
and labeled with rabbit anti-Pleurodeles IgM serum and FITC-
conjugated goat anti-rabbit IgG;
        b. The same microscopy field as a, shown in phase-
contrast light;
        c. Papainized SRBC coated and labeled as in a;
        d. The same field as c, shown in phase-contrast light.

DISCUSSION

The major finding of these experiments is that regardless of the antigen used (Salmonella or SRBC), the type of immunization (with adjuvant or not) and the dose (a single or repeated injections), the immunized Pleurodeles and Triturus synthesized only one type of immunoglobulin. The 2-ME sensitivity, the slow electrophoretic mobility and the 18.2 S sedimentation coefficient suggest that this immunoglobulin is an IgM. However, the antibody responses to Salmonella antigens and to SRBC are quite different. When Salmonella antigens are used, a single injection is sufficient to elicit a good antibody response in all of the immunized animals. Better antibody responses are obtained when Salmonella antigens are injected in FCA, especially in Pleurodeles. A slight difference is noticed in the response of normal and thymectomized Pleurodeles. With the H antigen, if the titers obtained are the same in normal and thymectomized, the response is slower in thymectomized. On the contrary, with the O antigen the thymectomized Pleurodeles are more stimulated than normal animals, especially early in the response. These results are in agreement with the data in mammals demonstrating that the H antigen is thymus-dependent and the O antigen thymus-independent. Nevertheless, thymectomized Pleurodeles elicit a good response to H and O antigens. If the presence of T lymphocytes seems to influence the kinetics of the response, their lack doesn't affect the magnitude of the response. Bacteria are common in the urodele biotype, and, as a matter of fact, urodeles have a much greater ability to respond to Salmonella antigens than to SRBC antigens.

The urodele response to SRBC antigens is very peculiar. First of all, only 50% of the immunized animals are able to elicit an immune response to this antigen. This response is dependent upon the number of immunizations rather than on the antigenic dose. Fifty per cent of the animals never respond, regardless of the number of immunizations and the dose used. In some assays we performed on allogeneic Pleurodeles chimeras, we obtained the same percentage of responders and nonresponders although these chimeras possess a permanently stimulated lymphoid system. It seems that the nonresponders do not possess the genetic equipment to recognize SRBC antigens or to synthesize anti-SRBC antibodies. Moreover, we have noticed that the good responders are numerous in aged animals (5 to 8 years old). Good antibody titers have been obtained in some thymectomized Triturus. In urodele, the antibody response to SRBC may be thymus-independent as it is in mammals when high doses of SRBC are injected. The second characteristic of this anti-SRBC response is the "incomplete" nature of the antibodies. The indirect immunofluorescence technique indicates that these antibodies are directed against a peculiar antigenic determinant of the erythrocyte membrane. The papain treatment exposes this antigenic determinant and allows these antibodies to bind and to agglutinate the erythrocytes. The double diffusion in agar of immune anti-SRBC sera against sonicated SRBC showed that only one precipitation arc is obtained. This result seems to indicate the urodele inefficiency to synthesize antibodies against the surface antigenic components of the erythrocyte membrane (26). The natural haemolytic factor always present in urodele sera, the high doses of antigen injected and the numerous immunizations may finally result in a thymus-independent antibody synthesis against a crypto-antigen of the erythrocyte membrane in a restricted lymphocyte population.

REFERENCES

1. Perey, D. V. E., Finstad, J., Pollara, B. and Good, R. A., Lab. Invest., 19: 591 (1968).
2. Du Pasquier, L., Curr. Topics Microbiology Immunology, 61: 37 (1973).
3. Badet, M. T., Chateaureynaud-Duprat, P. and Voisin, G., C. R. Acad. Sc. Paris, 278: 1297 (1974).
4. Carton, Y., Ann. Biol., 12: 139 (1973).
5. Gitlin, D., Perricelli, A. and Gitlin, J. D., Comp. Biochem. Physiol., 44B: 225 (1973).
6. Clem, L. W., J. Biol. Chem., 246: 9 (1971).
7. Geczy, C. L., Green, P. C. and Steiner, C. A., J. Immunol., 111: 261 (1973).
8. Haimovitch, J. and Du Pasquier, L., Proc. Nat. Acad. Sci. (U.S.A.), 70: 1898 (1973).
9. Moticka, E. J., Brown, B. A. and Cooper, E. L., J. Immunol., 110: 855 (1973).
10. Marchalonis, J. J., Allen, R. B. and Saarni, E. S., Comp. Biochem. Physiol., 35: 49 (1970).
11. Marchalonis, J. J., Amer. Zool., 11: 171 (1971).
12. Hadji-Azimi, I., Immunology, 21: 463 (1971).
13. Rosenquist, G. L. and Hoffman, R. Z., J. Immunol., 108: 1499 (1972).
14. Jurd, R. D. and Stevenson, G. T., Comp. Biochem. Physiol., 48B: 411 (1974).
15. Ching, Y. and Wedgwood, R. J., J. Immunol., 99: 191 (1967).
16. Ambrosius, H., Hemmerling, J., Richter, R. and Schimke, J. R., Developmental Aspects of Antibody Formation and Structure, 727 pp. (Sterzl and Riha, Academic Press, New York, 1970).
17. Houdayer, M. and Fougereau, M., Ann. Immunol. Inst. Pasteur, 123: 3 (1972).
18. Marchalonis, J. J. and Cohen, N., Immunology, 24: 395 (1973).
19. Tournefier, A., Ann. Immunol. Inst. Pasteur, 125: 637 (1974).
20. Tournefier, A., Immunology, 23 (in press) (1975).
21. Turner, R. J. and Manning M. J., Europ. J. Immunol., 4: 343 (1974).
22. Charlemagne, J., Europ. J. Immunol., 4: 390 (1974).
23. Charlemagne, J., Thèse Université Paris 6 (1972).
24. Moretti, J., Boussier, G. and Jayle, M. F., Bull. Soc. Chim. Biol., 40: 59 (1958).
25. Waterston, R. H., Immunology, 18: 431 (1970).
26. Adachi, H. and Furusawa, M., Exp. Cell. Res., 50: 490 (1968).

IMMUNOGLOBULINS IN RANID FROGS AND TADPOLES

L.A. Steiner, C.A. Mikoryak, A.D. Lopes, and C. Green

Dept. of Biology, Massachusetts Institute of Technology

77 Massachusetts Avenue, Cambridge, MA 02139

INTRODUCTION

One approach to gain insight into the evolution of the immune system is to investigate the structure of the immunoglobulins (Igs) in a variety of species. The results of such studies (reviewed in reference 1) have usually been interpreted to indicate that the diversity of the Ig classes increases in the course of evolution. Thus, most primitive vertebrates (e.g., cartilaginous and bony fish) have Igs that apparently correspond to mammalian IgM, whereas most higher vertebrates have 2 or more Ig classes. To understand how the Igs in these various groups of animals are related to one another, it is necessary to obtain detailed information regarding their structure.

In this paper, we shall summarize our work on one aspect of this general problem.[1] Our specific objective is the isolation and characterization of immunoglobulins in the anuran amphibian, Rana catesbeiana. Two major classes of Igs in these animals were first described by Marchalonis and Edelman (4). In addition to studying the structure of these proteins in adult frogs, we are investigating the nature of the immunoglobulins in the developing tadpole. A comparison of tadpole and adult Igs is of particular interest because of the numerous biochemical changes associated with amphibian metamorphosis (reviewed in reference 5).

---

[1] An account of the earlier portions of this work has appeared (2), and the more recent studies will be published in detail elsewhere (3).

IDENTIFICATION, ISOLATION AND ANTIGENIC ANALYSIS OF IMMUNOGLOBULINS

To provide a marker for serum Igs, R. catesbeiana frogs and tadpoles were immunized with the bacteriophage f_2, and the resulting antisera were fractionated by gel filtration. In the case of frog serum, some of the neutralizing activity was eluted near the front of the column and will be referred to as "high molecular weight" (HMW) Ig. The remainder of the activity was eluted in more retarded fractions, either as a single peak, with possibly a shoulder on its leading or trailing edge, or as a pair of partially resolved peaks (Fig. 1). The active material in this region will be referred to as "low molecular weight" (LMW) Ig. In the case of tadpole antiserum, most of the activity was eluted near the front of the column, but in certain samples, some activity also appeared in the more retarded fractions (Fig. 1).

The immunoglobulins containing the HMW and LMW antibodies were isolated from frog serum by standard preparative procedures (gel filtration, ion-exchange chromatography and zone electrophoresis). In our early experiments, all of the LMW Igs were isolated together (2), but recently it has been possible to prepare 2 distinct Igs (designated LMW I and LMW II) by purifying material derived from the 2 regions of the gel filtration fractionation indicated in Fig. 1 (3). In contrast to many varieties of mammalian IgG, these LMW Igs are not the most cathodal proteins of frog serum. Accordingly, they

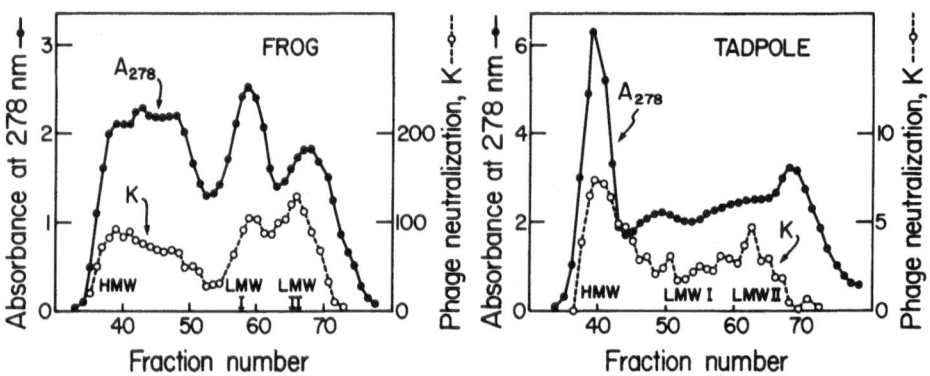

Fig. 1: Gel filtration of R. catesbeiana frog and tadpole serum proteins with Bio-Gel A 1.5 M in 0.1 M NaCl, 0.02 M Tris, 0.01 M HCl, 0.002 M NaN$_3$ (pH 8.2). Frogs were immunized with 100 μg and tadpoles with approximately 2 μg of bacteriophage f_2 emulsified in complete Freund's adjuvant. Frog: 13 ml of (NH$_4$)$_2$SO$_4$ concentrate from 23 ml of antiserum obtained from 5 frogs were applied to a 4 x 98 cm column. Tadpole: About 20 ml of antiserum obtained from 50 tadpoles (stages 28-29 (6)) were concentrated to 1.8 ml and applied to a 1.5 x 90 cm column.

are relatively difficult to isolate, and we have obtained them in
highly purified form only in very low yield. Most of our preparative work has been carried out with frog antisera, but small quantities of highly purified HMW and LMW Igs have also been isolated from
tadpole sera (2). As will be shown in a later section, R. catesbeiana tadpoles also contain both varieties of LMW Ig, and a partial
separation of these has recently been effected (3).

    Antisera were prepared in rabbits to each of the purified frog
Igs. The reactions of these antisera with frog serum and with the
individual Igs are shown in Fig. 2. As expected, each antiserum
forms a single precipitin arc with the homologous antigen. However,
because of the cross-reactivity among the Igs and their antibodies,
the reactions with frog serum are more complex. The number of distinct precipitin bands depends on the concentrations of the various
antigens and antibodies, and also on their rates of diffusion in
the agar. With the antiserum to HMW Igs, 2 major precipitin bands
were formed, one presumably containing the homologous antigen (HMW
Igs), and the other the cross-reacting LMW Igs. However, with the
antiserum to either of the LMW Igs, only 1 major precipitin band
was formed, although this band sometimes consisted of 2 partially
fused components. The failure to form a separate precipitin band
containing the cross-reacting HMW Igs can be explained in terms of
the "umbrella effect" (7): the precipitin band(s) formed by the more
rapidly migrating LMW Igs forms a barrier or "umbrella" that absorbs
all of the antibodies, cross-reacting as well as homologous.

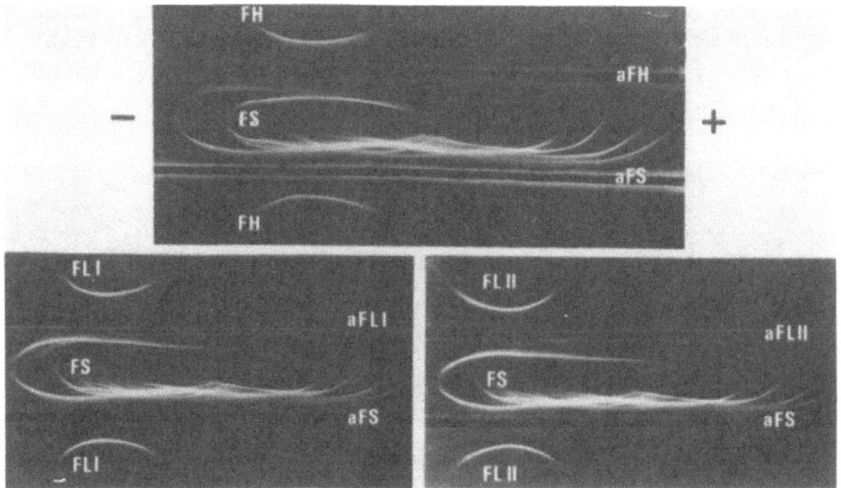

Fig. 2: Immunoelectrophoresis of R. catesbeiana Igs with their homologous antisera. FH, purified frog HMW Igs; FLI and FLII, purified
frog LMW I and II Igs; FS, frog serum; aFH, aFLI, aFLII, and aFS
are antisera prepared in rabbits to these antigens.

The specificities of these antisera and the antigenic relations among the 3 Igs were demonstrated in more detail by double diffusion. As shown in Fig. 3a, the antiserum to HMW Igs contains 2 types of antibodies: those that are specific for the HMW Igs and those that cross-react with both varieties of LMW Ig. The precipitin band formed by the LMW I Igs and the antiserum to HMW Igs fused with the band formed by the same antiserum and the LMW II Igs. Therefore, the same set of antibodies reacts with each of the 2 LMW Igs. As demonstrated, these cross-reacting antibodies can be absorbed by adding LMW Igs in excess.

The properties of antisera to the LMW I and LMW II Igs are also shown in Fig. 3. The precipitin band formed by the LMW I Igs and the homologous antiserum spurred over the band formed by the LMW II Igs and the same antiserum; this band in turn spurred over that formed by the HMW Igs (Fig. 3b). A similar set of reactions was observed with the antiserum to the LMW II Igs (Fig. 3c). Thus, each of these antisera contains antibodies of 3 different specificities: those that react with all 3 Igs, those that react with both LMW Igs, but not with the HMW Igs, and those that are specific for the immunogen. The antibodies that cross-react with the HMW Igs can be absorbed by adding this antigen in excess (Fig. 3d). As expected, the absorbed antisera still react with the LMW I and LMW II Igs (Fig. 3b, c and d).

We have not yet established the location of the relevant antigenic determinants on the Ig molecules. However, by analogy with mammalian Igs, we expect that the determinants that are shared by HMW and both LMW Igs will be primarily or exclusively on light chains, whereas the other determinants will be on heavy chains.

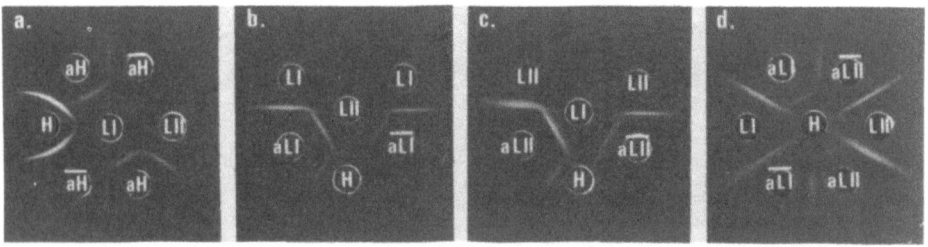

Fig. 3: Antigenic analysis of R. catesbeiana Igs by double diffusion. H, LI and LII are purified frog HMW, LMW I, and LMW II Igs, respectively. aH, aLI, and aLII are rabbit antisera to these proteins. aH is aH absorbed with excess pooled LMW Igs (as demonstrated by the line between aH and aH). aLI and aLII are aLI and aLII absorbed with excess HMW Igs. These reactions indicate that there are 3 antigenically distinguishable Igs in the serum of R. catesbeiana frogs.

Two possible sources for the heterogeneity in the LMW Igs were considered: allotypic (genetic) and isotypic variation. To distinguish between these possibilities, 22 individual R. catesbeiana frogs, obtained from geographically diverse regions of North America, were tested with the antisera to LMW I and II Igs. Sera from all of these frogs contained the specific LMW I and LMW II antigenic determinants (3). It was therefore concluded that the 2 LMW Igs are probably isotypic variants, corresponding either to Ig classes or (more likely) to subclasses.

MOLECULAR SIZE AND SUBUNIT STRUCTURE OF IMMUNOGLOBULINS

The HMW and LMW frog Igs, as well as a number of mammalian Igs, were analyzed by polyacrylamide gel electrophoresis (PAGE) in the presence of sodium dodecyl sulfate (SDS). The results, summarized in Fig. 4, demonstrate that: 1) The 3 frog Igs are each composed of 2 subunits designated, in analogy with mammalian Igs, as heavy and light chains. 2) The mobility of the light chains of frog and mammalian Igs is about the same. 3) The mobility of the heavy chain of frog HMW Igs is about the same as that of mammalian μ chain. 4) The mobility of the heavy chain of both frog LMW Igs is similar to that of human α chain, intermediate between that of mammalian γ and μ chains. 5) The LMW I and II Igs are indistinguishable no matter whether the samples were unreduced, partially reduced and alkylated (presumably only interchain S-S bonds cleaved), or extensively reduced in SDS (presumably all disulfide bonds cleaved). 6) In contrast to the mammalian Igs, the 3 frog Igs can be dissociated into 2 components by the detergent without reduction. The results are consistent with the possibility that these 2 components are free light chains and a dimeric (in the case of the LMW Igs) or higher (in the case of the HMW Igs) aggregate of heavy chains. It was considered that the dissociation could be the consequence of a disulfide exchange reaction in the detergent. However, it occurred equally well in the presence or in the absence of iodoacetamide, a thiol-binding reagent that might be expected to inhibit disulfide interchange.

The presence of 2 varieties of LMW Ig in frog serum was first suspected because some gel filtration fractions formed 2 precipitin bands with antiserum to LMW Igs (2). This possibility was strengthened when it was observed that there were sometimes 2 peaks of neutralizing activity in fractions containing LMW Igs (e.g., Fig. 1). Since some separation of the LMW I and II Igs seemed to take place upon gel filtration, it was anticipated that these 2 Igs would differ in molecular size. However, the results of SDS-PAGE suggest that there probably is no difference in the size or in the covalent aggregation of the subunits of these 2 Igs. To detect possible differences in non-covalent aggregation, the 2 purified LMW Igs, at a

concentration of approximately 0.6 mg/ml, were sedimented in the
analytical ultracentrifuge. The sedimentation rates were approximately the same (∿7S).

Finally, the 2 purified LMW Igs were again subjected to gel
filtration with Bio-Rad A 1.5 M, under conditions similar to those
used in the original fractionation of frog serum (e.g., Fig. 1),
but in a smaller column. A small amount of either the pure frog
LMW I Igs or the LMW II Igs was mixed with 2 internal markers, rabbit IgG and ε-dinitrophenyl-L-lysine. The elution position of the
antibody-containing frog Igs was determined by neutralization assays,
and that of the markers by absorbance measurements. The frog LMW II
Igs and rabbit IgG were eluted in exactly the same position, whereas
the frog LMW I Igs were slightly (∿3%) less retarded on the column
(3). However, this small difference, which would have been difficult to detect without internal markers, was considerably less than

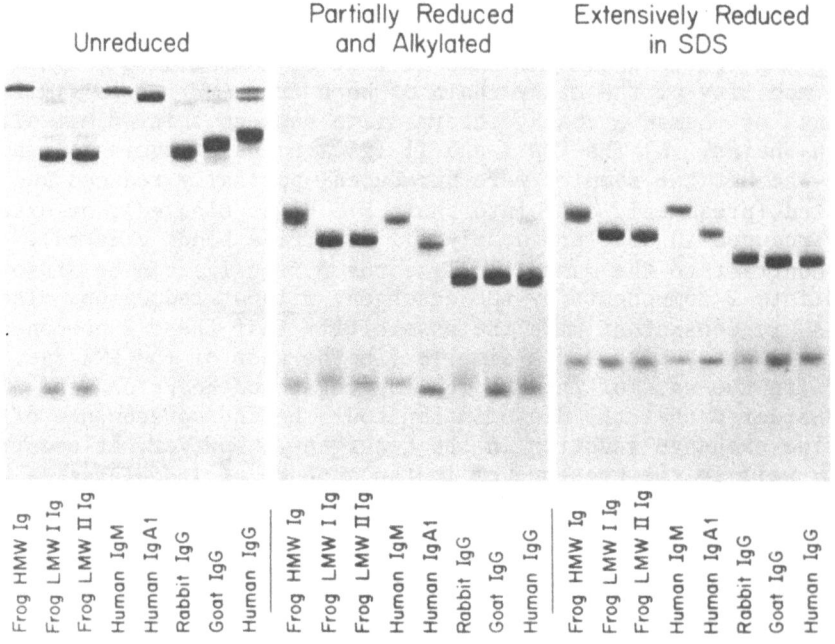

Fig. 4: Polyacrylamide gel electrophoresis in SDS. Unreduced samples
were incubated in 1% SDS, 0.075 M iodoacetamide at 100° for 1 min.
Partially reduced and alkylated samples were reduced with 0.01 M dithiothreitol, alkylated with 0.075 M iodoacetamide and then incubated
in 1% SDS at 100° for 1 min. Extensively reduced samples were incubated in 0.05 M dithiothreitol, 1% SDS at 50° for 1 hr. Human IgM
is macroglobulin Ou and human IgA1 is myeloma protein Mor. Rabbit,
goat, and human IgG were purifed by DEAE-cellulose chromatography.

the difference between the 2 LMW Ig peaks in Fig. 1. Thus, there
does not appear to be a substantial difference in the size of the
2 purified LMW Igs. Consequently, in the original fractionation
of frog serum, the LMW I Igs must have been retarded for some other
reason (e.g., a tendency to aggregate with other serum proteins).

IMMUNOGLOBULINS IN ADULTS AND TADPOLES OF 3 SPECIES OF RANID FROGS

It has been shown that R. catesbeiana tadpoles have Igs that
closely resemble, in structural and antigenic features, the corresponding Igs in frogs of this species (2). In a preliminary report,
it was also noted that sera from Rana pipiens and Rana clamitans
frogs and tadpoles contain proteins that cross-react with R. catesbeiana HMW and LMW Igs (8). However, the antisera specific for the
LMW I and II Igs were not available in these earlier studies. Accordingly, the antigenic properties of the Igs in the 3 species
have now been re-examined with the antisera characterized in
Figures 2 and 3 of the present study. As shown in Fig. 5, each of
the frog and tadpole sera precipitated with all of the absorbed
antisera, although some of the reactions were quite weak. It is
interesting to note that the patterns of cross-reactivity are different for each antiserum. For example, in the reaction with anti-
HMW Igs, the precipitin band formed by R. pipiens tadpole serum
spurred over that formed by R. clamitans frog serum (Fig. 5a),
whereas in the reaction with anti-LMW I Igs, the reverse spur was
seen (Fig. 5b).

It is also demonstrated in Fig. 5 that the precipitin band
formed by each of the absorbed antisera with R. catesbeiana tadpole
serum fused with the band formed by R. catesbeiana frog serum. Sometimes (not illustrated here), the absorbed antisera to the LMW I or
II Igs formed 2 distinct precipitin bands with R. catesbeiana frog
or tadpole sera. (Whether 1 or 2 bands appear depends on the concentrations of the cross-reacting antigens (i.e., LMW I and LMW II
Igs) and antibodies, and can be explained in terms of the "umbrella
effect" described in an earlier section.) The precipitin bands
formed by the tadpole and frog sera also fused in those cases. It
was concluded, therefore, that the Igs in R. catesbeiana tadpoles
have the 3 specific antigenic determinants (HMW, LMW I, and LMW II)
of the Igs in adult frogs of this species.

Sera from R. clamitans frogs and tadpoles also form either 1
or 2 precipitin bands with the antisera to R. catesbeiana LMW I Igs.
In Fig. 5b, the tadpole serum formed 2 bands (1 strong and 1 weak)
whereas the frog serum formed only 1 band. These bands fused with
one another, as well as with the band formed by R. catesbeiana serum.
Evidently, R. clamitans frogs and tadpoles also have 2 varieties of
LMW Igs, one of which is antigenically identical to the R. catesbeiana
LMW I Igs. In contrast, the Igs in R. clamitans sera are antigenically

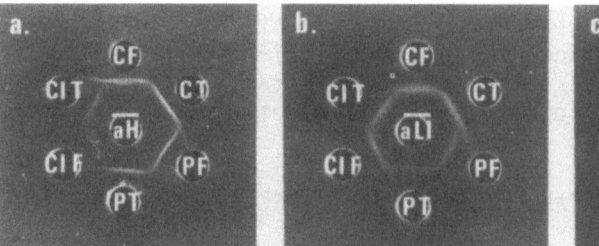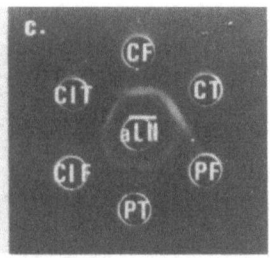

Fig. 5: Antigenic analysis of sera from frogs and tadpoles of 3 ranid species. CF and CT, PF and PT, ClF and ClT are R. catesbeiana, R. pipiens, and R. clamitans frogs and tadpoles. Serum was obtained by cardiac puncture from a single frog or pooled from at least 10 tadpoles. (Serum from tadpoles is usually diluted by some tissue fluid.) CF and ClF were obtained from the U. of Mich. Amphibian Facility (Ann Arbor, MI), PF from J.M. Hazen & Co. (Alburg, VT). CT (stage 28 (6)) and ClT (stages 26-27) were from Conn. Valley Biological Supply Co. (Southampton, MA). PT (stages 28-29) were offspring (8 weeks after fertilization) of wild-caught animals bred at the U. of Mich. Amphibian Facility. aH is a 1:4 dilution of antiserum to R. catesbeiana HMW Igs absorbed with excess LMW Igs; aLI and aLII are antisera to R. catesbeiana LMW I and II Igs, each absorbed with excess HMW Igs. The sera were used at the following concentrations, expressed relative to undiluted serum (beginning with CF and proceeding clockwise): a, 1/10, 2, 2, 12, 2, 20; b and c, 1/20, 1/4, 1/4, 12, 1/5, 10.

deficient with respect to both the LMW II Igs (Fig. 5c) and the HMW Igs (Fig. 5a). The Igs in R. pipiens frog and tadpole sera are antigenically deficient with respect to all 3 R. catesbeiana Igs. The reactions of sera from adult R. pipiens and R. clamitans with the antisera to the LMW I and II Igs will be considered in more detail elsewhere (3). Sera from adult Xenopus laevis did not react with any of the antisera to R. catesbeiana Igs.

DISCUSSION AND CONCLUSIONS

One of the major implications of these studies is that the Igs in R. catesbeiana are relatively complex. In addition to the HMW Igs and the 2 varieties of LMW Igs, it seems probable that further heterogeneity will be uncovered as these proteins are examined in more detail. In particular, the possible presence of 2 antigenic varieties of light chain must be evaluated (e.g., see (2)), as well as the existence of a secretory Ig system. Other studies (e.g., 9,10) have also indicated that the diversity of the Igs in certain poikilotherms may be greater than has been generally recognized.

Since the 2 types of LMW Ig were found in the serum of each of 22 R. catesbeiana frogs, it was concluded that these proteins are probably isotypic variants. The 2 purified Igs were found to be very similar in a number of structural properties: behavior in SDS-PAGE, sedimentation velocity, and mobility in gel filtration. One apparent difference was the behavior in gel filtration when the 2 Igs were present in crude serum fractions. Possibly, the LMW I Igs have a greater tendency to aggregate with other serum proteins and are consequently less retarded. The 2 proteins cross-reacted with antisera prepared in rabbits to either, even after these antisera had been absorbed with HMW Igs. Although the cross-reactivity may be enhanced because the antisera were prepared in a distant species, it seems likely that the 2 LMW Igs are sufficiently similar to be considered subclasses. We have reported elsewhere that fractions containing pooled LMW Igs fix guinea pig complement (11), and it will be interesting to investigate the reactivity of the LMW I and II Igs with both amphibian and mammalian complement components.

The R. catesbeiana Igs are unusual in that they dissociate in SDS without reduction, releasing subunits with the mobility of free light chains. The several mammalian Igs examined did not dissociate under these conditions. Further experiments are required to establish that the dissociation is not an artifact of the particular experimental conditions (e.g., that it occurs also in other dissociating solvents). Among mammalian Igs, molecules lacking disulfide bonds between heavy and light chains are usually confined to the IgA class (12,13). It has recently been reported that the IgA in chicken bile contains non-covalently linked, predominantly monomeric, light chains (14).

When 2 major classes of Ig were first isolated in the amphibian, R. catesbeiana, an analysis of their physical-chemical properties led to the suggestion that the HMW Igs correspond to mammalian IgM and the LMW Igs to IgG (4). However, we have observed that the heavy chains of frog LMW Igs migrate, in SDS-PAGE, to a position corresponding approximately to that of human α chains (midway between μ and γ chains). It has been reported that the mobility in these gels of the heavy chains of the LMW Igs of another anuran amphibian, Xenopus laevis, is also less than that of human γ chains (15). Such variations in mobility do not necessarily indicate differences in molecular weight, since the migration in these gels can be affected by factors such as charge (16) and carbohydrate content (17). Nevertheless, these findings do suggest that there is probably some significant structural difference between the heavy chains of the amphibian LMW Igs and mammalian γ chains. The possibility should be considered that the amphibian LMW Igs are related to the 7S Igs of reptiles and birds, proteins with heavy chains somewhat larger than mammalian γ chains (18-20). Additional studies (e.g., determination of amino acid sequence) are required to evaluate the phylogenetic relationships among these proteins.

The results presented here and elsewhere indicate that tadpoles contain Igs that are very similar in antigenic and/or structural properties to the HMW and LMW Igs in adults (2,21). In other studies, HMW Igs were found in tadpoles, but LMW Igs or antibodies were not detected (22,23). It is probable that these apparent discrepancies are related to the difficulty in detecting small quantities of Igs. The similarity in the Igs of tadpoles and adult frogs contrasts with the transition in the hemoglobins that occurs at metamorphosis in these animals. Hemoglobin in tadpoles is different from that in adults in a number of structural features, including antigenicity (5,24,25). Of course, it is still possible that there is a temporal progression in the synthesis of Igs during the earlier developmental stages of the tadpole. We are currently utilizing a sensitive radio-immunoassay to evaluate this possibility.

SUMMARY

Three distinct immunoglobulins (Igs) have been isolated from serum of Rana catesbeiana frogs. One of these is high in molecular weight and probably corresponds to the IgM-like Igs that have been isolated from a variety of vertebrate species. The other 2 Igs are lower in molecular weight (∿7S) and very similar in subunit structure. They were highly cross-reactive, although each contained unique antigenic determinants. Their relationship to other vertebrate Ig classes remains to be established. The mode of subunit linkage in all 3 Igs is unusual since the unreduced proteins were partially dissociated in detergent. Serum from R. catesbeiana tadpoles contained Igs that were antigenically identical to each of the Igs in adults of this species. Sera from R. pipiens and R. clamitans frogs and tadpoles contained Igs that cross-reacted with the R. catesbeiana high and low molecular weight Igs.

ACKNOWLEDGMENTS

We thank Drs. C.M. Richards and G.W. Nace of the Amphibian Facility, U. of Michigan, for specimens and for advice on the care of amphibians. We are indebted to Dr. S. Lowey for the ultracentrifugation, to Dr. H.F. Lodish for supplies of bacteriophage f2, to Drs. H. Metzger and A. Plaut for contributing proteins Ou and Mor, and to Ms. Pamela Evleth for expert typing of the manuscript.

REFERENCES

1. Kubo, R.T., Zimmerman, B. and Grey, H.M., in The Antigens, M. Sela, ed., Vol. I, p. 417 (Academic Press, New York, 1973).
2. Geczy, C.L., Green, P.C. and Steiner, L.A., J. Immunol., 111: 1261 (1973).

3. Green, C. and Steiner, L.A., to be published.
4. Marchalonis, J. and Edelman, G.M., J. Exp. Med., 124: 901 (1966).
5. Frieden, E., in Metamorphosis: A Problem in Developmental Biology, W. Etkin and L.I. Gilbert, eds., p. 349 (Appleton-Century-Crofts, New York, 1968).
6. Witschi, E., Development of Vertebrates, p. 78 (Saunders, Philadelphia, 1956).
7. Shore, S.L., Phillips, D.J. and Reimer, C.B., Immunochemistry, 8: 562 (1971).
8. Geczy, C.L., Green, P.C., Gaydos, K.C. and Steiner, L.A., Fed. Proc., 31: 750 (1972).
9. Ambrosius, H., Hemmerling, J., Richter, R. and Schimke, R., in Developmental Aspects of Antibody Formation and Structure, J. Sterzl and I. Ríha, eds., Vol. II, p. 727 (Academic Press, New York, 1970).
10. Gitlin, D., Perricelli, A. and Gitlin, J.D., Comp. Biochem. Physiol., 44B: 225 (1973).
11. Romano, E.L., Geczy, C.L. and Steiner, L.A., Immunochemistry, 10: 655 (1973).
12. Grey, H.M., Abel, C.A., Yount, W.J. and Kunkel, H.G., J. Exp. Med., 128: 1223 (1968).
13. Abel, C.A. and Grey, H.M., Biochemistry, 7: 2682 (1968).
14. Vaerman, J.P., Lebacq-Verheyden, A.M. and Heremans, J.F., Immunol. Comm., 3: 239 (1974).
15. Hadji-Azimi, I., Immunology, 21: 463 (1971).
16. Tung, J-S. and Knight, C.A., Biochem. Biophys. Res. Commun., 42: 1117 (1971).
17. Segrest, J.P., Jackson, R.L., Andrews, E.P. and Marchesi, V.T., Biochem. Biophys. Res. Commun., 44: 390 (1971).
18. Leslie, G.A. and Clem, L.W., J. Exp. Med., 130: 1337 (1969).
19. Zimmerman, B., Shalatin, N. and Grey, H.M., Biochemistry, 10: 482 (1971).
20. Leslie, G.A. and Clem, L.W., J. Immunol., 108: 1656 (1972).
21. Du Pasquier, L., Current Topics in Microbiology and Immunology, 61: 37 (1973).
22. Marchalonis, J.J., Develop. Biol., 25: 479 (1971).
23. Moticka, E.J., Brown, B.A. and Cooper, E.L., J. Immunol., 110: 855 (1973).
24. Aggarwal, S.J. and Riggs, A., J. Biol. Chem., 244: 2372 (1969).
25. Maniatis, G.M. and Ingram, V.M., J. Cell Biol., 49: 380 (1971).

STRUCTURAL DATA ON CHICKEN IgA AND FAILURE TO IDENTIFY THE IgA OF THE TORTOISE

J.P. Vaerman,* J. Picard,** and J.F. Heremans*

Dept. of Experimental Medicine,* Institute of Cellular
Pathology and Univ. Catholique de Louvain, Brussels,
Belgium, Lab. of Embryology, Comparative Anatomy and
Anthropology,** 5, Place de la Croix du Sud, Louvain-
La-Neuve, Belgium

1. STRUCTURAL DATA ON CHICKEN IgA

IgA from Chicken Bile

In 1972, our group had demonstrated the existence in chicken
serum, intestinal secretions and bile, of an immunoglobulin (Ig)
which was clearly physicochemically and antigenically different
from chicken IgM and IgG (1). The occurrence of this Ig at relatively high concentrations in bile, saliva, seminal plasma, lachrymal
and intestinal secretions (2), and in the majority of plasma cells
from the <u>lamina propria</u> of the intestinal mucosa (3), has allowed
us to call this Ig the chicken homologue of mammalian IgA. These
findings have since been confirmed by several groups (4-9).

More recently, we have shown that IgA purified from chicken
bile possesses light (L) chains which are non-covalently linked to
its heavy (H) chains (10). When unreduced chicken bile IgA is
submitted to gel filtration in 5 M guanidine, three protein peaks
(Fig. 1A) are eluted. Such a dissociation did not occur for
unreduced purified serum IgM and IgG. Analysis of these three
peaks by means of polyacrylamide gel electrophoresis in 8 M urea
at pH 3.5 (Fig. 1B) revealed that peaks two and three migrated in
the gel at positions compatible with L-chain dimers and monomers,
respectively, whereas peak 1 barely penetrated the gel. In
addition, immunoelectrophoreses of the three concentrated gel-
filtration peaks revealed that peak one reacted with anti-α-chain
antibodies whereas both peaks two and three precipitated with an
anti-L-chain antiserum.

185

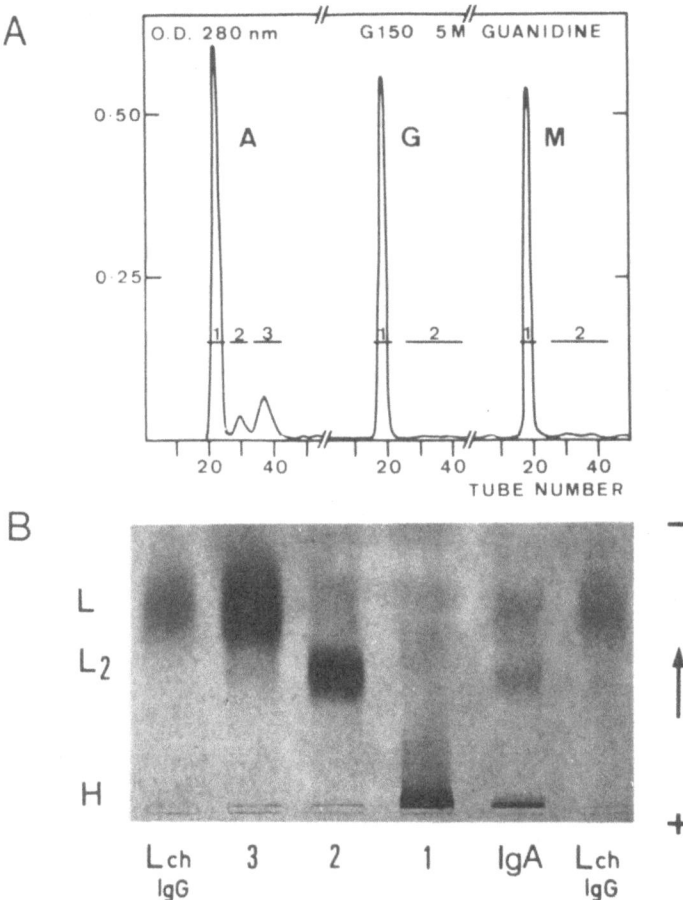

Fig. 1. Splitting of fowl biliary IgA in dissociating solvents.
A. Elution profile of chicken biliary IgA (A), serum IgG (G) and
IgM (M) from a column of Sephadex G-150 in 5 M guanidine.
B. Acid urea gel electrophoresis. Lch IgG : light chains purified
from reduced-alkylated chicken serum IgG; 3,2 and 1 are the
Sephadex-fractions of fowl biliary IgA (see A); L, L$_2$ and H :
position of L-chain monomers, -dimers and of polymeric α-chains,
respectively.

IgA from Intestinal Secretions

It was recently observed (11) that in the chicken, only the IgA from intestinal secretions, which sedimented as a 9-12S molecule, possesses the "secretory component" (SC), which is typical in mammals for the secretory IgA (SIgA) found in all exocrine secretions. Bile IgA, which sedimented as a 15-16S molecule, did not appear to have this "SC".

We have purified IgA from chicken intestinal secretions and have verified, thanks to a gift of anti-"SC"-antiserum kindly provided by Dr. K. Kobayashi, that it contained the chicken "SC". In addition, we have checked that our preparations of IgA from bile, as well as from serum and from egg-white (12), do not react with the anti-"SC"-antiserum, confirming the data of Watanabe and Kobayashi (11).

In a previous study (13), it was demonstrated that those human IgA2 molecules, which had no disulfide bridges between their H and L chains, could combine in vitro with human SC and thereby acquired an H-L disulfide bond by a disulfide interchange reaction. Since our chicken intestinal IgA was shown to have "SC" bound in its structure, it seemed of interest to verify whether or not its L chains were covalently linked. We found that chicken intestinal IgA submitted, unreduced, to acid-urea gel electrophoresis, did release light chain dimers and monomers in amounts very similar to those released by unreduced bile IgA.

Pertinence to Phylogeny

The absence of disulfide bridges between H and L chains observed for the IgA in chickens confers an archaic appearance to this immunoglobulin, since the same non-covalent H-L association occurs in the Igs of one of the most primitive vertebrates, i.e. the sea lamprey (14). One may propose additional arguments to substantiate the hypothesis that α chains are perhaps the most ancient H chains of Igs.

The secretory IgA system has been called the first line of defense of the organism against foreign invaders. It is conceivable that a protection of the internal mucosae, and particularly of the intestinal mucosa, has evolved earlier than the internal humoral defense system.

In the lamprey, the same antigenic class of Igs exists in monomeric and polymeric forms. This characteristic seems to apply at least as well to IgA as to IgM.

The mode of action of IgA antibodies, which are unable to trigger the classical pathway of complement activation or to opsonize various particles for phagocytosis, seems to be of a more direct, solitary nature : they just combine with their antigens. This again may be considered as an archaic feature.

Finally, a strong homology has been observed by Heremans (15) between the sequences of the 19 C-terminal residues (called "tails") of the human α chain and the hinge region of the human γ1 chain. He suggested an evolutionary scheme for an ancestral C region, by which the actual human γ1 hinge region would have evolved from the "tail" of the ancestral C region by the usual mechanism of crossing over between misaligned chromatids. However, the filiation between the γ1 hinge and the "tail" transpires much more clearly for the α chain "tail" than for the μ chain "tail", despite the very strong homology existing between the μ- and α chain tails; hence, the possible seniority of the α chain over the μ chain.

2. FAILURE TO IDENTIFY IgA IN THE TORTOISE

We have attempted to detect an Ig in the tortoise (Testudo hermanni Gmelin) which would differ antigenically from the three Igs which have been characterized in turtles, namely a 19S Ig, a

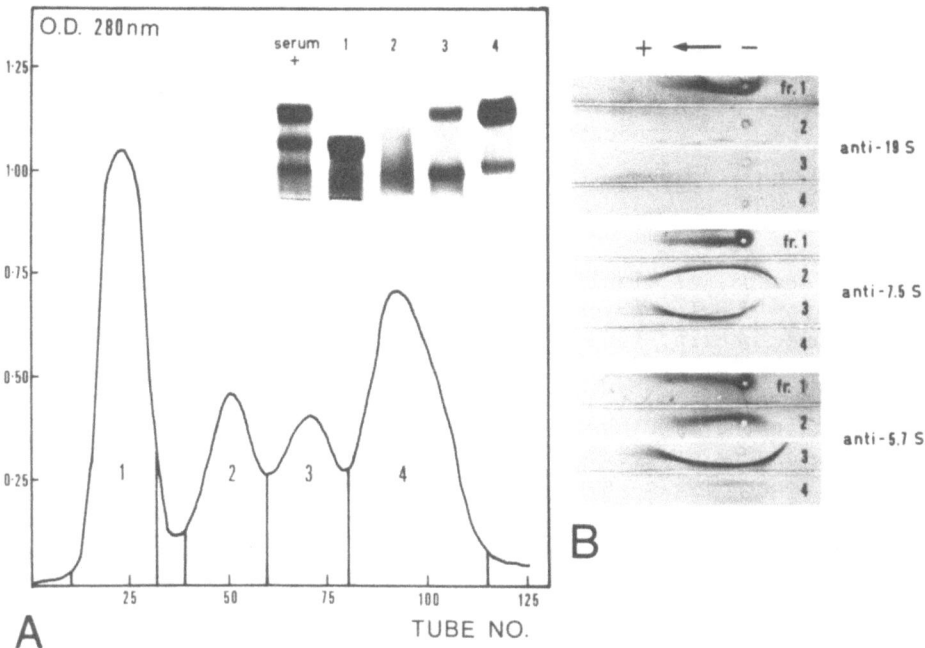

Fig. 2. Gel-filtration of tortoise serum on Sephadex G-200. Left : elution profile and agarose gel electrophoresis of the 4 fractions pooled as indicated. Right : immunoelectrophoresis of the 4 G-200 fractions of tortoise serum developed with specific antisera against the 19S-, the 7.5S- or the 5.7S-immunoglobulins, respectively.

7.5S Ig and a 5.7S Ig (16,17). We have searched for such a
distinct Ig in bile and intestinal secretions, and, by means of
immunohistology, in the immunocytes present in the lamina propria
of the intestinal mucosa.

Preparation of Specific Antisera against Tortoise Igs

Tortoise serum (80 ml) was submitted to gel-filtration on
Sephadex G-200 (Fig. 2, left). Four protein peaks were eluted and
the agarose gel electrophoresis of these 4 peaks is also
illustrated in Fig. 2. The three first peaks were each recycled
on G-200.

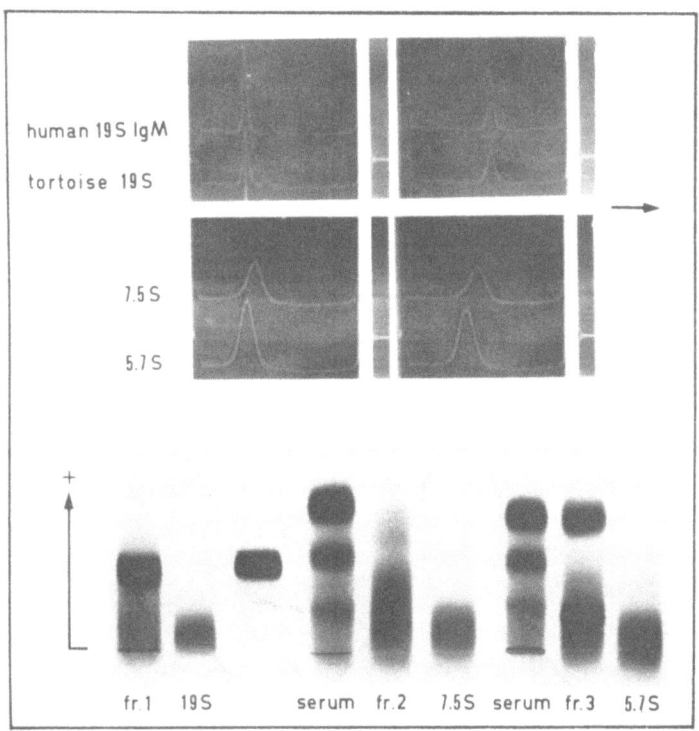

Fig. 3. Top : analytical ultracentrifugation of purified tortoise
immunoglobulins, compared to a human 19S IgM. Bottom : agarose gel
electrophoresis of tortoise serum, of the 3 purified tortoise
immunoglobulins and of the Sephadex fractions 1,2 and 3 from which
they were isolated.

The tortoise 19S Ig was purified from the first G-200 peak by
preparative electrophoresis on a Pevikon block, whereby it was
separated from a major high molecular weight component of α_2
mobility (Fig. 3, bottom left).

The recycled G-200 peaks 2 and 3 were submitted to
chromatography on DEAE-cellulose in pH 8.0, 0.02 M Tris-HCl buffer
with a linear NaCl gradient. Fractions eluted at low ionic strength
were salted-out at 35 % saturation in ammonium sulfate. The
resultant precipitates consisted in relatively pure preparations of
7.5S and 5.7S Igs, from peak 2 and 3 of the G-200 column,
respectively (Fig. 3, bottom middle and right).

The three purified Ig preparations were also submitted to
analytical ultracentrifugation, where they gave rise to essentially
symmetrical boundaries (Fig. 3, top). However, immunoelectrophoreses
of these 3 preparations, when developed with a very polyvalent rabbit
antiserum against tortoise whole serum, displayed minor impurities
in the 7.5S and 5.7S Ig samples. Therefore, these two preparations
were further purified by a small scale agarose gel electrophoresis
on glass plates. The more cathodal fractions were cut out of the
gel and used as antigens.

Rabbit antisera were raised against each of the three purified
Igs. After suitable absorption, specific antisera were obtained
for each of the three tortoise Igs. The specificity of these
antisera, as tested on the 4 gel-filtration peaks of tortoise serum,
is illustrated in Fig. 2, right.

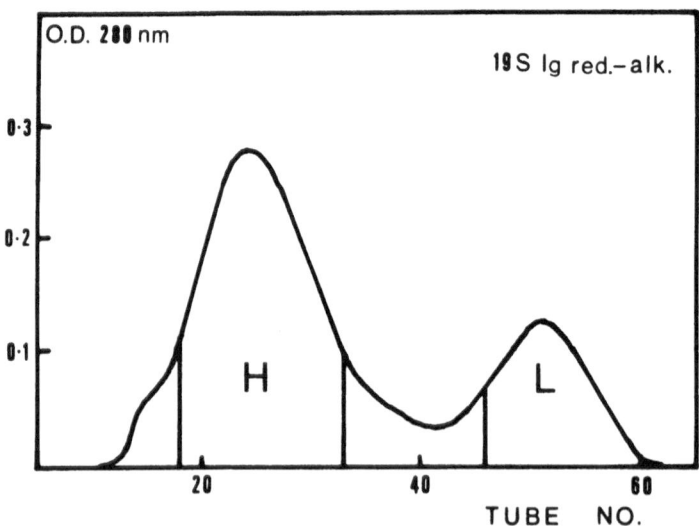

Fig. 4. Separation of H and L chains of partially reduced and
alkylated tortoise 19S Ig by means of gel-filtration in 5 M
guanidine. H: heavy chains; L: light chains.

In addition to these three antisera, an antiserum was raised
against the light chains purified from the 19S Ig. The latter
was reduced with 20 mM dithiothreitol and alkylated with excess
iodoacetamide. Heavy and light chains were separated by gel-
filtration in 5 M guanidine (Fig. 4). After several injections of
the light chains with complete Freund's adjuvant, a small amount
of rabbit antiserum was finally obtained which gave a precipitin
line of identity between the 19S, 7.5S and 5.7S Igs.

Tortoise Bile and Intestinal Secretions

Bile (12 ml) was aspirated from the gall bladder of 11
dissected tortoises. After extensive dialysis against saline, it
was concentrated four-fold and clarified by high speed centrifugation
before being submitted to gel-filtration on Sephadex G-200.

Intestinal secretions were obtained by rinsing the gut with
ice cold saline containing a protease inhibitor (Trasylol, Bayer).
After centrifugation to remove insoluble matter, intestinal
globulins were prepared by salting out at 50 % saturation in
ammonium sulfate. The precipitate was dissolved in and dialysed
against the buffer of the subsequent gel-filtration on Sephadex
G-200.

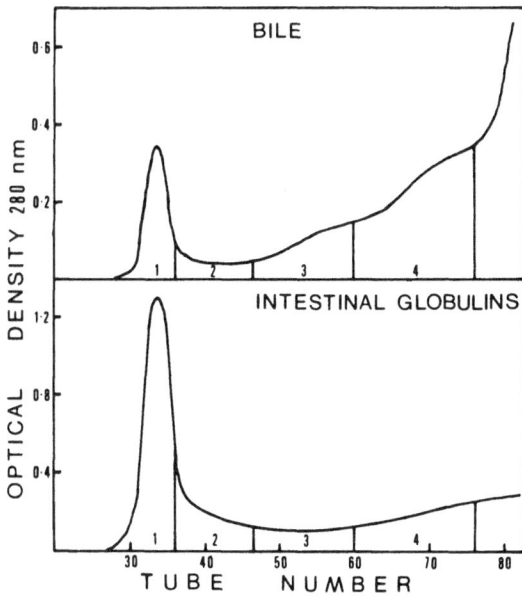

Fig. 5. Gel-filtration on Sephadex G-200 of tortoise bile and
intestinal globulins.

The elution profiles of bile and intestinal globulins, shown in Fig. 5, were divided into four fractions corresponding to the elution positions of the 4 peaks given by serum. The four fractions were concentrated to one ml and analyzed by means of immunoelectrophoresis and Ouchterlony analyses, using the antisera described above.

The anti-L chain reacted distinctly with G-200 fraction 1 of both bile and intestinal secretions. Very weak reactions were obtained with fractions 2 and 3, particularly for bile. The specific anti-19S antiserum also precipitated distinctly with fractions 1 of bile and intestinal secretions, and the morphology of the precipitin lines suggested that the same component was involved with both antisera. This was corroborated by an Ouchterlony analysis where both anti-19S and anti-L chain antisera were allowed to diffuse against fraction 1 of intestinal secretions a line of identity was observed.

Only traces of 7.5S and 5.7S Igs could be detected in G-200 fractions 2 and 3, using the specific antisera. Here, again, these lines merged with those given by the anti-L-chain antiserum.

Finally, an antiserum was also raised against the first G-200 fraction of intestinal secretions. However, this antiserum, after absorption with 5.7S Ig, appeared again to reveal only the 19S Ig both in bile and intestinal secretions.

Immunohistology on the Intestinal Mucosa

In humans, the vast majority (80-85 %) of plasma cells in the intestinal mucosa synthesizes IgA (18). Such an association between IgA and the gut plasma cells has been a reliable criterion for the identification of IgA in all mammalian species where it has been investigated (19), and has confirmed the identification of chicken IgA as well (3).

If one finds many more cells stained with a fluorescent anti-L-chain reagent than the sum of the cells staining with various fluorescent specific anti-H chain antisera, then one may suspect the existence of another H chain than those against which antisera were available. We have used such an approach for the tortoise intestinal mucosa.

Figure 6 illustrates our results. Many cells were stained with the anti-19S reagent. These cells were usually located close to the epithelial layer (Fig. 6A). The core of the intestinal villi displayed bright non-specific fluorescence, as shown in a control section (Fig. 6B) stained with fluorescein labelled anti-19S absorbed with 19S Ig. This obscures the interpretation of the results. Anti-L chain antibodies did not seem to stain many more cells (Fig. 6C) than anti-19S antibodies. The anti-7.5S and anti-5.7S reagents only revealed an occasional positive cell (Fig. 6D and E).

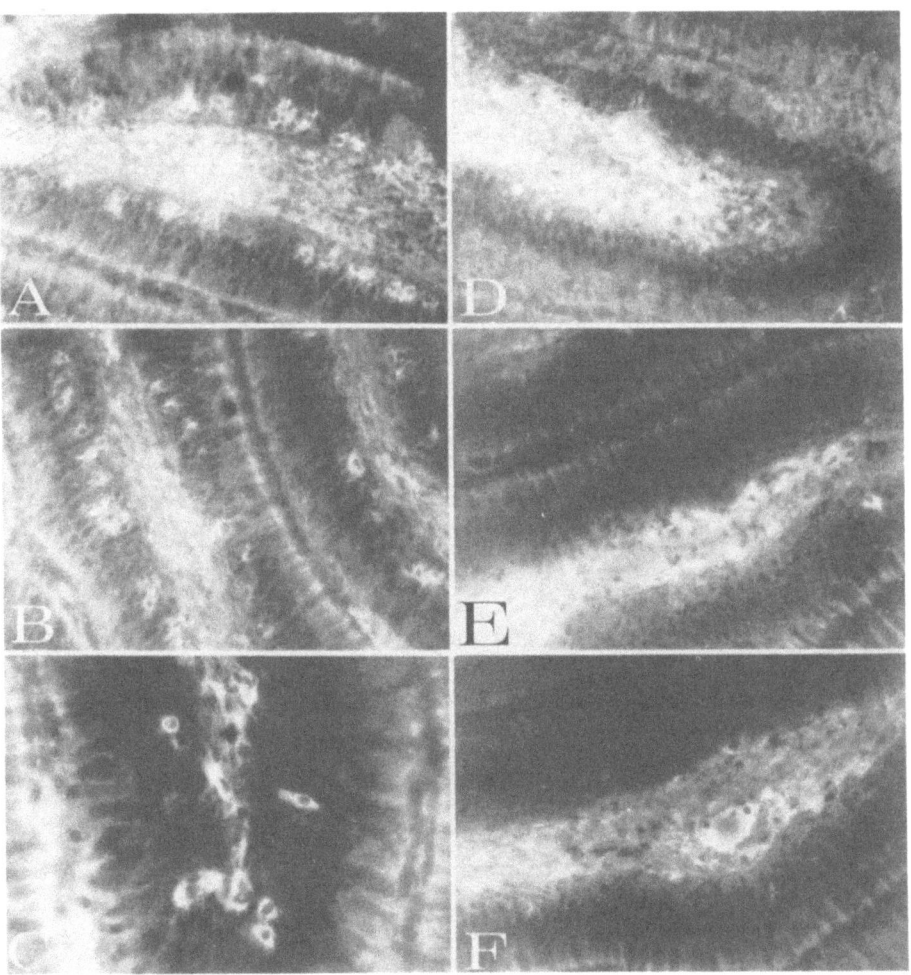

Fig. 6.   Immunohistologic studies on cryostat sections of tortoise
intestinal mucosa incubated with various fluorescein-labelled
antisera against tortoise immunoglobulins.   A: specific anti-19S Ig;
B: anti-L-chain; C: same as A; D: same as A, but absorbed with
purified 19S Ig; E: anti-5.7S Ig; F: anti-7.5S Ig.
Magnification: x 175, except in E: x 280.

Interpretation

The present data suggest that, in the tortoise, the 19S Ig is the predominant immunoglobulin occurring both in secretions and in intestinal immunocytes. However, our failure to detect an IgA-like Ig in the tortoise may be due to the very low concentration of this Ig in serum and secretions. This Ig could then have escaped detection with our anti-L chain antiserum. This also may explain why our antiserum against Sephadex fraction 1 from intestinal secretions failed to reveal the existence of another Ig. Further attempts to identify IgA in the tortoise are being undertaken on animals subjected to oral or parenteral immunization and larger amounts of secretions will be collected.

However, if one considers the evolution of reptiles, it appears that the therapsids, from which IgA-possessing mammals have evolved, and the thecodonts from which crocodiles and IgA-possessing birds have originated, are both more recent forms than the primitive stem reptiles (the cotylosaurs) from which turtles and tortoises are thought to be direct descendents. Thecodonts and therapsids are also believed to have the cotylosaurs as ancestors. It is difficult then, to admit that IgA may have evolved independently in two branches of evolution (for birds and mammals). Therefore, our personal opinion is that turtles and tortoises probably possess an IgA-like Ig and that further attempts to identify this IgA in reptiles are justified.

Acknowledgements. This work was supported by grant No. 1192 from the FRSM and grant No. 10.013 from the FRFC, Brussels, Belgium.

REFERENCES

1. Lebacq-Verheyden, A.M., Vaerman, J.P., and Heremans, J.F., Immunology, 22: 165, 1972.
2. Lebacq-Verheyden, A.M., Vaerman, J.P., and Heremans, J.F., Immunology, 27: 683, 1974.
3. Lebacq-Verheyden, A.M., Vaerman, J.P., and Heremans, J.F., J. Immunol., 109: 652, 1972.
4. Bienenstock, J., Perey, D.Y.E., Gauldie, J., and Underdown, B.J., J. Immunol., 109: 403, 1972.
5. Orlans, E., and Rose, M.E., Immunochemistry, 9: 833, 1972.
6. Leslie, G.A., and Martin, L.N., J. Immunol., 110: 1, 1973.
7. Bienenstock, J., Perey, D.Y.E., Gauldie, J., and Underdown, B.J., J. Immunol., 110: 524, 1973.
8. Leslie, G.A., and Martin, L.N., Int. Arch. Allergy, 46: 834, 1974.
9. Perey, D.Y.E., and Bienenstock, J., J. Immunol., 111: 633, 1973.

10. Vaerman, J.P., Lebacq-Verheyden, A.M., and Heremans, J.F.,
    Immunol. Comm., 3: 239, 1974.
11. Watanabe, H., and Kobayashi, K., J. Immunol., 113: 1405, 1974.
12. Rose, M.E., Orlans, E., and Buttress, N., Eur. J. Immunol., 4:
    521, 1974.
13. Jerry, L.M., Kunkel, H.G., and Adams, L., J. Immunol., 109:
    275, 1972.
14. Marchalonis, J.J., and Edelman, G.M., J. Exp. Med., 127: 891,
    1968.
15. Heremans, J.F., Behring Inst. Mitt., 54: 1, 1974.
16. Litman, G.W., Chartrand, S.L., Finstad, J., and Good, R.A.,
    Immunochemistry, 10: 323, 1973.
17. Benedict, A.A., and Pollard, L.W., Folia Microbiol., 17: 75,
    1972.
18. Crabbé, P.A., Carbonara, A.O., and Heremans, J.F., Lab. Invest.,
    14: 235, 1965.
19. Vaerman, J.P., Res. Immunochem. Immunobiol., 3: 93, 1973.

EVOLUTIONARY DIVERGENCE OF IMMUNOGLOBULIN CONSTANT
REGION GENES

J. Michael Kehoe

Department of Microbiology
Mount Sinai Medical Center of the City
    University of New York
New York, New York 10029

INTRODUCTION

The development of the humoral immune response over
evolutionary time has resulted in the occurrence of
numerous immunoglobulin gene products in animal serum.
The variable region gene products which are now known to
be responsible for providing the distinct combining specificities that are required for interacting with the mult-
itude of antigens a given individual encounters in its
lifetime (1) are of obvious importance in this regard.
Genetic complexity also exists on another level in the
humoral response, however, albeit less pronounced. This
complexity is presented at the level of constant region
genes. The precise extent of this diversity is not yet
clear, especially in any complete phylogenetic context
since extensive information concerning the question is
available at present only for higher species, particularly
mammals. While this information has provided much knowledge regarding the extent of constant region diversity
in these higher species, and may show us the highest
degree of such divergence that has yet occurred in the
biological world, the data obviously can speak only for
a limited spectrum of the animal kingdom.
    The purpose of the present article is to analyze

current information regarding constant region gene
divergence in a phylogenetic context. The analysis is
based on data available for immunoglobulin heavy chain
constant regions (Figure 1) and will show that much
information is still lacking concerning the detailed
molecular structure of immunoglobulin molecules from
lower species.

METHODS FOR ANALYSIS OF HEAVY CHAIN
CONSTANT REGION DIVERGENCE

Three main approaches, which are complementary and
not mutually exclusive, have been used to discern and
characterize immunoglobulin molecules which reflect
divergence in constant region genes. These approaches
are biophysical characterization, determination of
serological relationships, and amino acid sequence
analysis. Selected examples of the use of each approach
in the study of immunoglobulins from various species
will be given to illustrate the type of information
that can be obtained.

Physical Characterization of Isolated
Molecules

Physical measurements of immunoglobulin molecules
have been an important aspect of their analysis for many
years. This can be traced back to the early distinctions
of macroglobulins, now known to be members of the IgM
class, from other antibodies found in the gamma globulin
fraction of serum (2). Such characterizations have been
extremely useful in understanding the class and subclass
diversity that results from the divergence of heavy chain
constant region genes. The methods used include analytical
ultracentrifugation, molecular exclusion and ion-exchange
chromatography, polyacrylamide gel electrophoresis, and
amino acid composition determinations. Such analyses,
while of obvious value, have definite limitations and
pitfalls with respect to the accurate delineation of the
extent of heavy chain constant region divergence. One
example of the kind of problem that can develop is

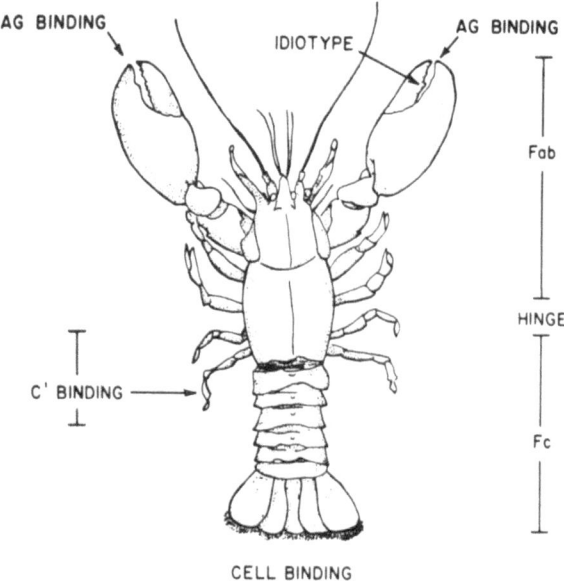

Figure 1. Representation of a prototypic lower molecular weight immunoglobulin molecule (or monomeric subunit of a polymeric molecule) illustrating features that have been observed for such molecules in numerous animal species. Constant region divergence has been studied most completely to date for the Fc portion (carboxy-terminal section of the heavy chains). The submolecular localization of various important immunoglobulin properties is indicated.

illustrated by the discovery of the human IgE class by the Ishizakas (3). Before the specific identification of this fifth class of human immunoglobulins, reaginic antibodies were found in an IgA isolate that had been prepared from whole serum by ion-exchange chromatography (3). Only the most careful observation indicated that it was not the IgA per se but representatives of an entirely different class, termed IgE by the Ishizakas, which was, in fact, responsible for the reaginic activity. Such methodological masking of certain immunoglobulin classes or subclasses is a potential danger for any analysis of the extent of constant region diversity through the examination of serum immunoglobulins. This

is particularly true for the majority of species where
no myeloma paraproteins are available.

Nonetheless, no description of an antibody protein
is complete without at least some minimal statement as
to its physical characteristics.

Determination of Serological
Relationships

After an immunoglobulin has been purified and
physically characterized at least in a preliminary way,
it is usually very useful to prepare an antiserum against
this protein to provide for the establishment of serological relationships. The production of such an antiserum requires a purified immunoglobulin initially and,
depending on the purification technics available, this
may pose a problem, especially where myeloma proteins
are not available. The successful use of such antisera
is illustrated for some of the frog immunoglobulin characterizations described in this volume (4).

Specific antisera are valuable for both intra- and
interspecies comparisons. They can be used to establish
relationships or non-relationships of immunoglobulins
isolated from the sera of members of the same species,
as has been done in great detail for the various classes
and subclasses of man (5). They can also be used for
cross species comparisons of isolated immunoglobulin
molecules. Problems inherent in such comparisons are
exemplified by the results of studies of some cat
immunoglobulins using antisera prepared against human
proteins (6). This study showed that of ten antisera
specific for human IgG proteins only one would react
with all of a panel of three cat IgG myeloma proteins.
Thus, an indication of the divergence of the genes coding
for these constant regions was detectable by a serological
approach since only one of the antisera could recognize
an antigenic determinant common to these two species,
implying that such determinants were not too common.
Similar serological studies of other relatively closely
related species have shown that under certain conditions,
this kind of immunological approach can yield useful
comparative data concerning the divergence of immunoglobulins. However, cross reactions have been obtained only

with animals that are relatively closely related and,
to date, mostly with higher mammals (e.g. cat, dog,
monkeys, man). Thus, the serological analysis of
divergent immunoglobulins can be very useful but is
subject to the limitation that it seems effective only
for limited sections of the phylogenetic spectrum. In
other terms, the evolutionary divergence of immunoglobulin heavy chain constant regions has been such that
the immunological cross relatedness is evident only for
species that are quite closely related.

Amino Acid Sequence Analysis

     Sequence analysis is the most definitive approach
to the establishment of evolutionary relationships
among immunoglobulin heavy chain constant regions, outside of the direct study of the involved genes themselves.
Sequence determinations allow the establishment of the
number of homology regions, or domains (7), that exist
in the various immunoglobulin chains, as well as providing
specific data for the establishment of the degrees of
homology among the various proteins. Such data also
provides clues as to the origins of the various classes
and subclasses. Here again, up to the present, the
information is most complete for the higher species,
especially man, since much heavy chain constant region
data has been obtainable using human myeloma proteins.
Such data has allowed specific estimates of the times of
divergence of certain constant region genes for immunoglobulins. For example, Chuang et al. (8) proposed, on
the basis of sequence analysis of the carboxyterminal
section of a human alpha chain, that the gene for this
chain had diverged from the human mu chain gene approximately two hundred million years ago, assuming that
one new amino acid per one hundred residues became incorporated into the alpha chain every four to five million
years. Such computations are, of course, dependent upon
the validity of a number of assumptions including the
exact rates of mutational change for this family of
proteins, and whether the number of amino acid replacements
seen in one section of the protein is representative of
the situation for other sections. In any case, such

estimates have proven valuable in surmising the chron-
ologic sequence of constant region gene divergence and
as guidelines for what classes and subclasses of immunoglobulins might be anticipated in particular groups of
animals (e.g. IgA in birds or reptiles). Pink et al.(9)
used such an approach to argue that the IgG subclasses
of man diverged approximately twenty five million years
ago and inferred from this that subclass divergence has
occurred subsequent to speciation. The confirmation of
this as a general principle must await more extensive
constant region sequence data from proteins isolated
from additional lower animal species.

Some heavy chain constant region sequence data
useful for interspecies comparisons have been obtained
in several laboratories. In a comparison of sequences
from a number of species (mouse, ref. 10; human IgG 1,
ref. 7; human IgG 4, ref. 9; rabbit, ref. 11; and guinea
pig, ref. 12) of the region of the IgG molecule that is
involved in complement fixation (Figure 1), Kehoe et al.
(10) showed that approximately forty percent mutational
change could occur in this region without the loss of the
complement fixing function. Thus, considerable constant
region gene divergence can occur over a moderately wide
phylogenetic spectrum and yet certain important biologic
functions (such as complement fixation) can be retained.
The basis for this is a most important aspect of the
evolutionary development of immunoglobulin proteins.

Additional analyses of such sequence patterns in a
phylogenetic context are greatly hampered currently by a
serious lack of data for proteins from lower species. The
acquisition of complete and detailed amino acid sequences
of immunoglobulins from a number of lower vertebrate
species will be most helpful in enlarging our perspective
of the patterns of divergence of immunoglobulin constant
region genes. To date, there is no question that most
of the emphasis in this area has been skewed toward the
more highly evolved species. It seems clear that questions
such as the precise identity of the lower molecular
weight immunoglobulin of certain amphibians (13) can only
be definitively resolved by accurate amino acid sequence
determinations.

INVERTEBRATE MOLECULES OF POTENTIAL
IMMUNOLOGIC SIGNIFICANCE

Considerable interest has developed recently in materials from various plant and animal sources that have agglutinating properties for a variety of cell types (14, 15). One of the best studied of these molecules is the hemagglutinin of the horseshoe crab, Limulus polyphemus (16, 17). In a further effort to characterize this material and to establish whether it might share any origins with immunoglobulin proteins, we have begun the determination of the complete covalent structure of this molecule (Kaplan, R.A., Li, S.L., and Kehoe, J.M., unpublished data). In the section of this molecule completed to date (approximately sixty amino terminal residues),no relationship to any immunoglobulin chain is discernible. On the basis of this data, no direct association between this molecule and the immuno-globulin family can be inferred. A definitive answer to this question, as well as the possible relation of the Limulus polyphemus agglutinin to other proteins, must, of course, await the determination of the complete sequence.

SUMMARY

The evolutionary divergence of immunoglobulin constant region genes can be analyzed through their immunoglobulin protein products in a number of ways. These include purely physical characterization, the determination of serological interrelationships, and amino acid sequence analysis. Of these approaches, sequence analysis can give the most detailed and specific information.

Such studies have permitted estimates of when certain immunoglobulin classes and subclasses diverged from one another in time on the basis of the extent of sequence homologies that are observed at present. Two different estimates of this type have lead to the view that the IgA class may have been derived from the IgM class approximately two hundred million years ago and that the IgG subclasses of man and certain animals have

diverged subsequent to speciation. Further analysis of
this kind is limited at the moment because of the relative paucity of sequence data for constant region gene
products in lower species.

The origins of a humoral immune response are being
searched for in invertebrate species by an examination
of the primary structure of molecules which have known
ligand binding activities. Preliminary results with
one such molecule, the hemagglutinin from the horseshoe crab, <u>Limulus polyphemus</u>, suggest that this
hemagglutinin is not related to the immunoglobulin
family, at least as this protein family is known today
in higher vertebrates.

REFERENCES

1. Edelman, G. M. and Gall, W.E., Ann. Rev. Biochem.
   38:415 (1969).

2. Kabat, E. A. and Mayer, M. M., Experimental
   Immunochemistry (Thomas, Springfield, Illinois,
   1961).

3. Ishizaka, K., Ishizaka, T., and Hornbrook, M. M.,
   J. Immunol. 97:840 (1966).

4. Steiner, L. A., et al., this volume.

5. Natvig, J. B. and Kunkel, H. G., Adv. Immunol. 16:1
   (1973).

6. Kehoe, J. M., Hurvitz, A. I., and Capra, J. D.,
   J. Immunol. 109:511 (1972).

7. Edelman, G. M., Cunningham, B. A., Gall, W. E.,
   Gottlieb, P. D., Rutishauser, U., and Waxdal, M.,
   Proc. Nat. Acad. Sci. U.S. 63:78 (1969).

8. Chuang, C., Capra, J. D., and Kehoe, J. M., Nature
   244:158 (1973).

9. Pink, J. R. L., Buttery, S. H., DeVries, G. M., and
   Milstein, C., Biochem. J. 117:33 (1970).

10. Kehoe, J. M., Bourgois, A., Capra, J. D., and Fougereau, M., Biochemistry 13:2499 (1974).

11. Hill, R. L., Delaney, R., Fellows, R. E., and Lebovitz, H. E., Proc. Nat. Acad. Sci. 55:1762 (1966).

12. Tracey, D. E. and Cebra, J. J., Biochemistry 13:4796 (1974).

13. Atwell, J. L. and Marchalonis, J. J., J. Immunogen. 1:367 (1975).

14. Cohen, E., editor, Ann. N.Y. Acad. Sci. 234:1 (1974).

15. Cohen, E., this volume.

16. Marchalonis, J. J. and Edelman, G. M., J. Mol. Biol. 32:453 (1968).

17. Finstad, C. L., Litman, G. W., Finstad, J., and Good, R. A., J. Immunol. 108:1704 (1972).

EVOLUTION OF CONFORMATIONAL FLEXIBILITY OF IMMUNOGLOBULIN M

Renata E. Cathou and David A. Holowka

Department of Biochemistry and Pharmacology
Tufts University School of Medicine
Boston, Massachusetts 02111 U.S.A.

Since the initial observations of Heidelberger and Pederson (1) of a macroglobulin antibody against pneumococcus in the horse, IgM has been recognized as a major class of immunoglobulins in mammals as well as in vertebrates as phylogenetically distant as the elasmobranchii (2). In fact, IgM appears to be the first recognizable class to have evolved. It still is the first immunoglobulin to be synthesized in a mammalian immune response.

In serum, mammalian IgM is generally found as a 900,000 dalton circular pentamer of five disulfide-linked IgMs subunits, each of which is composed of two light and two heavy (μ) chains held together by disulfide bridges and noncovalent interactions (3). One molecule of a third type of chain, J chain, is also present in the pentamer and is probably involved in its assembly from subunits (4). Functionally, IgM has ten antibody combining sites, one on each Fabμ (5). The (Fcμ)$_5$ region can bind Clq to initiate the classical complement pathway (6). The IgMs subunit also functions as the specific antigen receptor on small B lymphocytes (memory cells) (7).

The recent determination of the complete amino acid sequence of two human μ chains (8,9) as well as careful molecular weight measurements (10), has provided a basis for clearer understanding of the structure and conformation of IgM. These studies have shown that in contrast to IgG, there is an additional domain (Cμ2) situated between Fabμ and the (Fcμ)$_5$ core. (see Figure 1).

IgG has been found to exhibit a discrete mode of flexibility in the nanosecond time range (11). A flexible joint at the junction of the Fab fragments allows each Fab to rotate over a small angular range which has been estimated to about 33 degrees (11). Such a

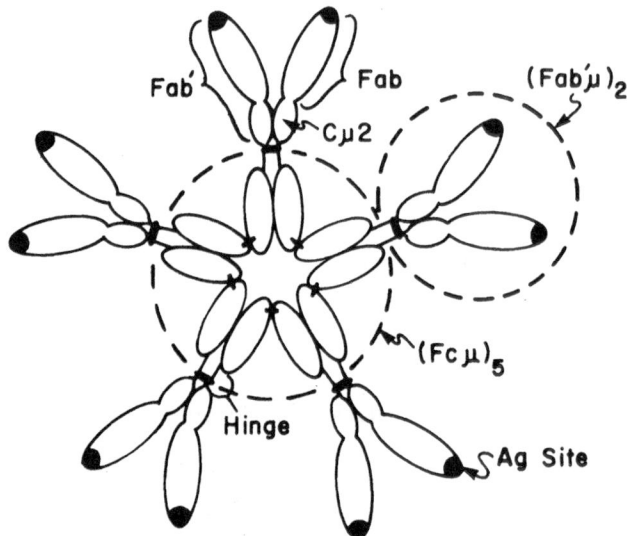

Figure 1. Structure of IgM. The locations of the fragments Fabμ,
Fab'μ, (Fab'μ)$_2$ and (Fcμ)$_5$, the Cμ2 domains, and the hinge region
are shown. The antibody combining sites for antigen or hapten
(indicated as Ag sites) are at the tips of each Fabμ (22).

flexible joint may be biologically significant in facilitating
formation of antibody-antigen complexes and may be important in
complement fixation.

     Because the μ chain contains an additional domain and the
hinge sequence is so different from that of the γ chain (12), we
asked the following questions:

1) Does IgM exhibit segmental flexibility?
2) If so, at what sites in the molecule?
3) Do IgM molecules from phylogenetically distant species differ
    in this respect?

     Flexibility is most directly studied by the technique of
fluorescence depolarization. In this method, a fluorophore on the
protein molecule is excited by plane polarized light; subsequent
depolarization of the emitted light, which is also initially plane
polarized, yields information on the rotational modes of the protein (13). There are two types of measurements that can be employed: steady-state (13) and nanosecond (14). The latter technique provides more information since fluorescence depolarization
is directly measured in the relevant time range, but because of the
specialized instrumentation required, has only been employed recently. The results that we are reporting in this paper utilize the
nanosecond approach.

A direct correlation exists between the rate of depolarization of a fluorophore rigidly bound to a protein and the rotational modes of the protein (15). However, for an unambiguous interpretation, the fluorophore should exhibit no independent rotation of its own and the rate of fluorescence emission should be comparable to the rate of rotation of the macromolecule (15).

We have satisfied these criteria by eliciting IgM antibodies to the fluorophore so that the latter will be specifically and rigidly bound in the antibody combining sites. To quantitate possible Fab flexibility, ε-dansyl-lysine (DNS-lys) is a suitable probe. For comparative measurements anti-DNS antibodies were elicited in three species: horse, pig and nurse shark (16).

RESULTS AND DISCUSSION

A. Preparation of Anti-DNS Antibodies

Immunization: In the case of the horse and sharks, the antigen employed was DNS-lys covalently coupled to streptococcus (17); in the case of the pig, the antigen was DNS conjugated to keyhole limpet hemocyanin. A horse was immunized intravenously 3 times a week for 3 weeks, boosted 3 months later with 4 injections over a period of 3 weeks, and bled the day after the last injection. Anti-DNS antibodies were initially identified by specific precipitation with the heterologous antigen DNS-human serum albumin. Three nurse sharks (20-40 lb) were immunized intraveneously with initial injections of about 40 mg of antigen and 2 months later with boosts of 60 and 100 mg on 2 successive days. The sharks were bled 2 months later. Anti-DNS antibody was found in sera from 2 of the sharks.

Antibody purification. Partially purified porcine anti-DNS was generously supplied to us by Dr. F. Franek of the Czechoslovak Academy of Science, Prague, Czeckoslovakia. These antibodies were purified by the use of a DNS-immunoadsorbent and further purified by chromatography in our laboratory on either Sephadex G-200 or Sepharose 4B. Antibodies of the IgM class were found to be pure by immunochemical, SDS-polyacrylamide gel, and sedimentation analyses (16).

Equine and shark antibodies were purified by selective adsorption to DNS-immunoadsorbent, elution with dansic acid, dialysis, and chromatography on either Sephadex G-200 or Sepharose 4B. Yields corresponding to 1.2 mg/ml serum were obtained from the horse while much lower yields, 0.15 mg/ml, were obtained from the sharks. Sedimentation velocity analysis of horse and shark antibodies showed single symmetrical boundaries and expected sedimentation constants (16). The horse preparation was immunochemically

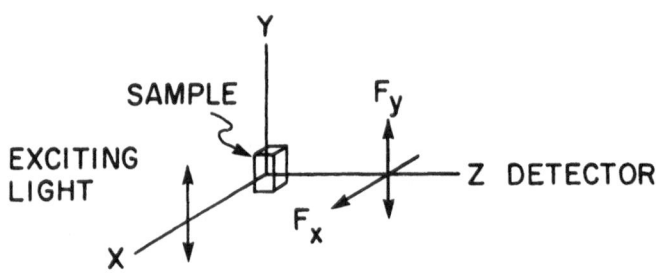

Figure 2. Coordinate axes for describing fluorescence depolarization measurements. The exciting light travels along x and is
polarized along y. The emitted light is detected along z through
a polarizer oriented either along y or x.

pure. Anti-shark antiserum was not available at the time these
experiments were done and so the shark IgM could not be analyzed
in this respect.

B.   Characterization of the Antibody Combining Sites

When DNS-lys is bound in the combining site of IgG anti-DNS,
the fluorescence emission maximum is blue-shifted and the quantum
yield is markedly enhanced (18). Similar effects were seen for
DNS-lys bound in the IgM combining sites and only small differences
were seen when antibodies from different species were compared.
In all cases, the emission maximum was in the range of 500-515 nm
and fluorescence enhancement was about 40 fold over the fluorescence
of DNS-lys in water at 500 nm.

The average binding constant for DNS-lys and anti-DNS from
the 3 species was also similar, i.e., $K_o \simeq 10^6$. This value of
K_o is higher than that expected for mammalian antibodies in the
IgM class (19); however, it should be noted that only about 30%
of the sites exhibited this value. The remainder of the obviously
heterogeneous populations had lower binding constants that could
not be measured at the concentrations employed. Measurement of
the fluorescence lifetime, τ, of bound DNS-lys, also revealed that
the horse and pig combining sites were somewhat heterogeneous.
The average value of τ was about 22 nsec and at least 2 components were seen in the fluorescence decay. In the case of the
shark antibodies, the average lifetime was about 20 nsec. Two
to three components were seen and one of these, with $\tau = 4.5$
nsec, made a significant contribution to the total fluorescence
intensity. The shark sites are therefore also heterogeneous.
Several factors could contribut to the observed spectral

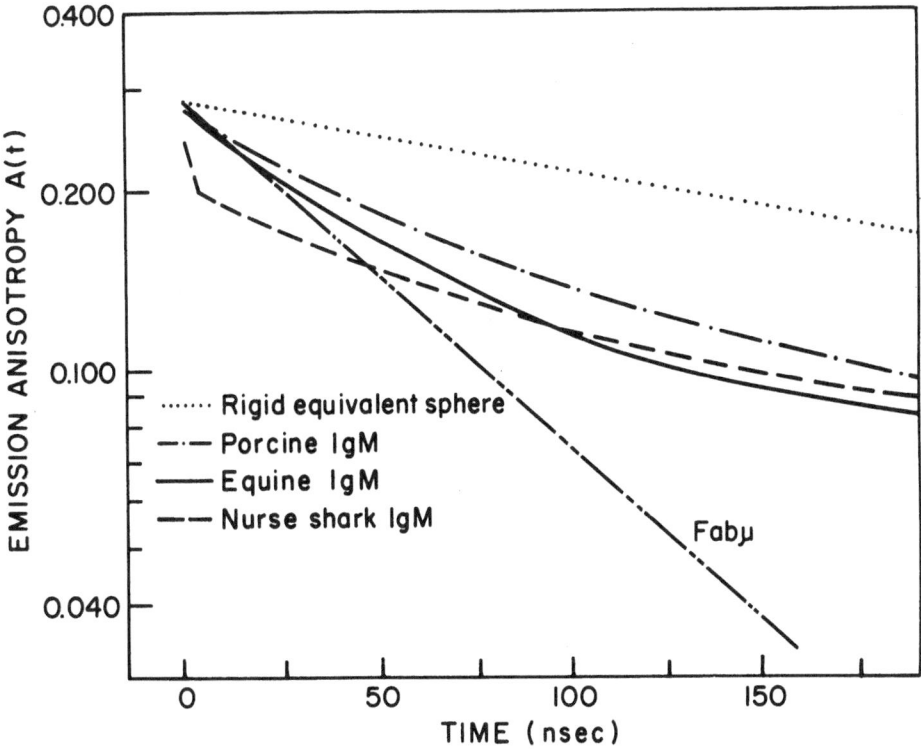

Figure 3. Time dependent emission anisotropy of DNS-lys-anti-DNS complexes of several species. The Fabμ fragment is from equine antibody. The lines are from a non-linear least squares analysis of the data and fit the equation, $A(t) = A_o[f_S e^{-t/\phi_S} + f_L e^{-t/\phi_L}]$.

TABLE I

Summary of Rotational Correlation Times of IgM of Several Species (16). See the legend to Figure 3.

Species	f_S	ϕ_S(nsec)	f_L	ϕ_L(nsec)
Horse	0.71	61	0.29	> 4000
Pig	0.57	69	0.43	568
Nurse Shark (2)	0.63	93-117	0.37	> 4000
Equine Fabμ		32		
Equine Fab'μ[a]		42		

[a] The Fab'μ fragment contains a Cμ2 domain.

characteristics of bound DNS-lys. The emission spectra suggest
hydrophobic environments in all of the combining sites. The
short lifetime component in the case of DNS-lys bound to shark
antibody, however, suggests that in some of these sites, the DNS-
lys may be more exposed to solvent. It may also be less rigidly
bound.

C. Segmental Flexibility

Nanosecond fluorescence depolarization provides direct information concerning the rotational motions of macromolecules.
Briefly, the sample is excited with a very short pulse of light
polarized in the y direction (see Figure 2). The intensities of
emission, detected at z, polarized along y, $F_y(t)$, and along a
perpendicular direction x, $F_x(t)$, are then measured as a function
of time. The most informative quantity is the emission anisotropy,
$A(t)$, which is defined by

$$A(t) = \frac{F_y(t) - F_x(t)}{F_y(t) + 2F_x(t)} \tag{1}$$

and expresses the change in orientation of the transition moment
direction between the time of excitation and emission. In the
simplest case of a rigid sphere, $A(t)$ decays exponentially and is
related to the rotational correlation time, ϕ, by:

$$A(t) = A_o e^{t/\phi} \tag{2}$$

where A_o is the initial anisotropy. The time dependent anisotropy
of particles with shapes other than rigid spheres is more complex
(15). In any case, however, it is usually possible to detect
whether the particle is rigid or flexible.

The fluorescence depolarization of DNS-lys bound in the combining sites of equine, porcine and nurse shark IgM antibodies is
shown in Figure 3. Several observations can be made. Firstly,
the equine Fabμ fragment exhibits a single value of $\phi = 32$ nsec
which is almost identical to that of Fabγ, 33 nsec (11), and indicates that Fabμ is rigid and compact. The value for porcine Fabμ
is similar. (We did not have enough shark antibody to attempt
proteolytic digestions). Thus, no sites of flexibility exist in
Fabμ. In contrast, the time dependent anisotropies of intact IgM
from the 3 species exhibit several values of ϕ, all of which are
shorter than that expected if the molecules were rigid. This can
be seen by comparing the anisotropy decays with the expected decay
for a rigid sphere of equivalent molecular weight (dotted line).
If IgM were a rigid ellipsoid, either prolate or oblate, the
shortest ϕ that would be seen would be 0.95 of ϕ of the rigid sphere
(15). Clearly, the observed values of ϕ are much shorter than

this and IgM displays flexibility. It is also clear that the decays of IgM from the 3 species are different. This observation suggests that the sites of flexibility and/or the relative amplitudes of motion are different. The horse and pig IgM, although not identical, are more similar to each other than to the IgM from shark. It is somewhat surprising that IgM from two species such as horse and pig which are reasonably close to each other on an evolutionary time scale would display any observable differences at all. These differences may be due somewhat to different purification procedures; the horse anti-DNS was eluted from immunoadsorbent with hapten, whereas the porcine antibody was eluted with acetic acid and immediately neutralized. However, differences in horse and pig IgM are also seen in the effects of proteotytic digestion and partial reduction and alkylation (16,20).

A summary of the results of analyses of the anisotropy decays is given in Table I. Interpretation of these results suggests at least two possible modes of flexibility in the IgM molecule:

1) Wagging or twisting of each Fab'μ, and 2) bending of (Fab'μ)$_2$ as a unit, out of the plane of (Fcμ)$_5$. These modes of flexibility are illustrated in Figure 4. The motions may be more complex than this but further analysis is limited by the precision of the data. The value of ϕ_s of shark IgM is too long to be due solely to Fab'μ motion (40 nsec) and is more likely due primarily to bending of the (Fab'μ)$_2$. as a unit. This result is consistent with the observation that enzymatic digestion of shark IgM yields only (Fab'μ)$_2$ and no Fabμ (23). Thus, the μ chain above or in the Cμ2 domain is not susceptible to enzymatic attack, probably because the critical bond is not exposed. The values of ϕ_s of equine and porcine IgM are intermediate between those expected for simple flexibility of Fab'μ and that of (Fab'μ)$_2$; they can be ascribed to either hindered Fab'μ rotation, due to association between adjacent Cμ2 regions, or the combined effects of some Fab'μ flexibility and some (Fab'μ)$_2$ bending. These 2 possibilities could be distinguished by measurement of the anisotropy decay of the isolated (Fab'μ)$_2$ fragment; these studies are in progress. Some association between Cμ2 regions probably exists: exposure of equine IgM to acid changes the conformation of Cμ2 and frees the Fab'μ sufficiently to result in lowering of the value of ϕ_s from 61 to about 40 nsec. ϕ_L is probably due to the global motion of the IgM. Unfortunately, because of the relatively short lifetime of DNS-lys, ϕ_L cannot be accurately measured. Values of ϕ_L are best obtained with a longer lifetime fluorophore such as pyrene-butyrate ($\tau \simeq$ 130 nsec when bound in the combining site of anti-pyrene (21).

What is most striking is that the relative motions of Fab'μ and (Fab'μ)$_2$ in horse, pig and nurse shark IgM are clearly

SIDE VIEW

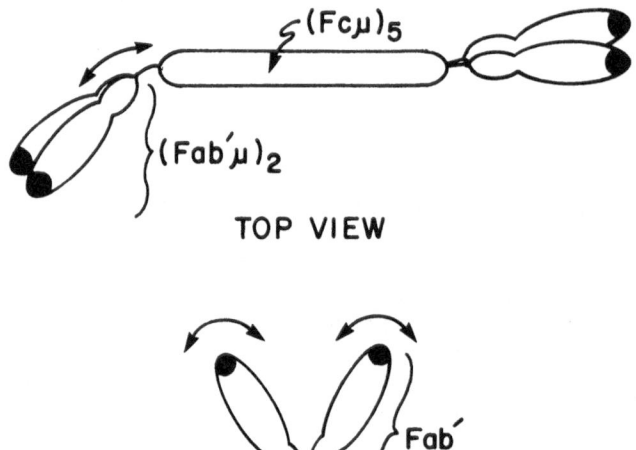

TOP VIEW

Figure 4. Modes of flexibility of IgM. Two possible motions,
consistent with the depolarization data, are illustrated. For
simplicity, only 2 of the 5 $(Fab'\mu)_2$ regions are shown in the side
view.

different. These differences probably arise from different
energies of interaction between domains as well as different
hinge regions. One can predict, therefore, that the amino acid
sequences from the end of the $C\mu1$ domain through the hinge will
show corresponding differences among these species.

Acknowledgements

    We gratefully thank Dr. William Clem of the University of
Florida for immunization and collection of sera from the sharks
and Dr. F. Franek of the Institute of Organic Chemistry and
Biochemistry, Czechoslovak Academy of Science, for the porcine
anti-DNS. This research was supported by grants from the NIH and
the American Heart Association. R.E. Cathou is a Senior Investigator of the Arthritis Foundation.

References

1. Heidelberger, M. and Pederson, K.O. (1937). J. Exp. Med. 65,
    393.
2. Marchalonis, J. and Edelman, G.M. (1965). J. Exp. Med. 122, 601.

3. Metzger, H. (1970). Adv. in Immunol. 12, 57.
4. Koshland, M.E. (1975). Adv. in Immunol. 20, 41.
5. Kim, Y.D. and Karush, F. (1973). Immunochemistry, 10, 365.
6. Plaut, A.G., Cohen, S. and Tomasi, T.B., Jr. (1972). Science 176, 55.
7. Pierce, C.W., Asofsky, R. and Solliday, S.M. (1973). Federation Proceedings, 32, 41.
8. Putnam, F.W., Florent, G., Paul, C., Shinoda, T., Shimizu, A. (1973). Science 182, 287.
9. Watanabe, S., Barnikol, H.V., Horn, J. and Hilschmann, N. (1973). Hoppe-Seyler's Z. Physiol. Chem. 354, 1505.
10. Dorrington, K.J. and Mihaesco, C. (1970). Immunochemistry 7, 651.
11. Yguerabide, J., Epstein, H.F. and Stryer, L. (1970). J. Mol. Biol. 51, 573.
12. Putnam, F.W. (1974), in Prog. in Immunol. II, ed. L. Brent and J. Holborow, volume 1, 25.
13. Weber, G. (1953). Adv. in Portein Chem. 8, 415.
14. Stryer, L. (1968). Science 162, 526.
15. Yguerabide, J. (1972), in Methods in Enzymology, Volume 26, Part C, ed. C. H. W. Hirs and S. N. Timasheff, Academic Press, N. Y. p. 498.
16. Holowka, D.A. and Cathou, R.E. Manuscript in preparation.
17. Holowka, D.A. and Cathou, R.E. (1974). Federation Proceedings 33, 1320.
18. Parker, C.W., Yoo, J.J., Johnson, M.C. and Godt, S.M. (1967). Biochemistry 6, 3408.
19. Kim, Y.D. and Karush, F. (1974). Immunochemistry 11, 147.
20. Beale, D. (1974). FEBS Letters. 44, 236.
21. Lovejoy, C., Holowka, D.A. and Cathou, R.E. (1975). Manuscript in preparation.
22. Feinstein, A. and Munn, E.A. (1969). Nature 224, 1307.
23. Klapper, D.G., Clem, L.W., and Small, P.A., Jr. (1971). Biochemistry 10, 645.

RELATIONSHIP BETWEEN STRUCTURE AND FUNCTION OF LOWER VERTEBRATE

IMMUNOGLOBULINS

G.W. Litman

Sloan-Kettering Institute for Cancer Research

New York, New York 10021

INTRODUCTION

In order to elucidate both macromolecular and genetic bases for the functional diversity expressed by immunoglobulins, extensive studies of their primary, secondary, tertiary and quaternary structure have been undertaken (1-3). Early in the course of these investigations, it became apparent that antibody function was associated with a heterogeneous group of multimeric glycoproteins and that more than one gene controlled the synthesis of individual immunoglobulin subunits. The mechanism whereby the separate gene products are generated (somatic mutation or germ line accumulation) and ultimately integrated are not fully understood (4,5). As biologic processes such as antibody formation may have become more complex during the passage of evolutionary time, one major direction in the investigation of adaptive humoral immunity has been to evaluate the immune response and antibody structure in phylogenetic perspective. Although the characterization of lower vertebrate immunoglobulins is not as complete as that of the mammalian counterparts, sufficient detail of their structure is known to permit meaningful phylogenetic comparisons. This presentation will first outline the central structural features of mammalian IgM and IgG, compare the structures of lower and higher vertebrate forms of immunoglobulins, relate immunoglobulin structure to active site formation and expression and discuss the origins of non-immunoglobulin mediated "immune-like" recognition in invertebrate and vertebrate species.

IMMUNOGLOBULIN STRUCTURE AND THE EVOLUTION OF IMMUNOGLOBULINS RESEMBLING MAMMALIAN IgM

Viewing the schematic representation of human IgM and IgG

(Fig 1), it is evident that 1) each form is comprised of equal numbers of disulfide bonded heavy and light chains; in addition, IgM
possesses a system of intersubunit disulfide bridges, 2) intrachain
disulfide linkages occur in a repetitive, periodic fashion in both
heavy and light chains and are the dominant features of structurally
homologous regions (domains) (3) of ~ 110-120 amino acids, 3) while
the light chains of both classes are of equal mass, the heavy chains
of IgM contain an additional domain. The shaded area at the amino
terminus of the heavy and light chains of both IgM and IgG indicates
intermolecular variability in amino acid sequence. This region of
the molecule accounts for the idiotypic character of homogeneous
immunoglobulin and contains the antigen combining site (8). Not indicated in this figure but nevertheless essential for our discussion
are the following: 1) immunoglobulin class is determined by the heavy
chain and not by the light chain, 2) IgM and IgG, in addition to
differing in one additional heavy chain domain, possess different C
region (class determinant) amino acid sequences, 3) IgM and IgG differ
in the content and attachment sites of carbohydrate, 4) an additional
polypeptide chain, J chain, is located in the C terminal regions of
certain mammalian IgM molecules and their homologs isolated from lower
vertebrate species (9), 5) the degree of subpopulation heterogeneity
associated with IgM, IgG and other immunoglobulin classes (2) exceeds
that described to date for any other class of plasma protein.

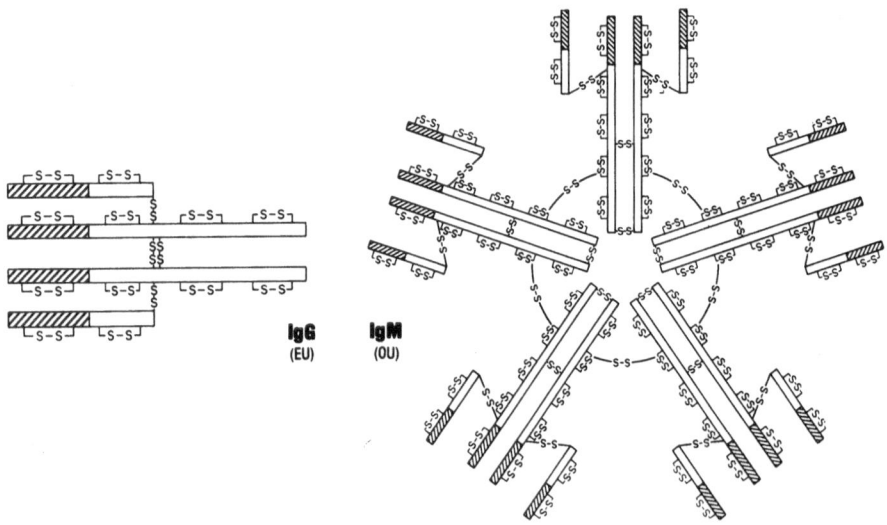

FIG. I. Schematic representation of IgM and IgG. OU (IgM, κ) and EU
(IgG$_1$, κ) are drawn from data contained in (6) and (7) respectively.
Variable regions of heavy or light chains are indicated by shading.

Immunoglobulins from a sufficient number of representative
Chondrichthyes and Actinopterygii fishes have been biochemically
characterized and, in part, substantiate the assertion that these
macromolecules resemble mammalian IgM in terms of heavy chain mass,
interchain disulfide bonding, amino acid and carbohydrate compositions
and solution conformation (10-12). Figure 2 illustrates the occurrence and polymer composition of HMW and LMW IgM-like immunoglobulins in vertebrates derived from the primitive Placoderms. While
most of the polymer configurations were proposed on the basis of biochemical estimation of subunit size and disulfide content, some of
the arrangements actually have been confirmed by direct electron
photomicrographic examination of negatively stained immunoglobulin
preparations (13). Of the vertebrate species thus far examined,
some possess both HMW and LMW forms of the IgM-like immunoglobulin
(10,14), others possess the HMW and not the LMW form (15) and some
vertebrate species which emerged after the appearance of distinct
immunoglobulin classes possess only the HMW IgM-like immunoglobulin

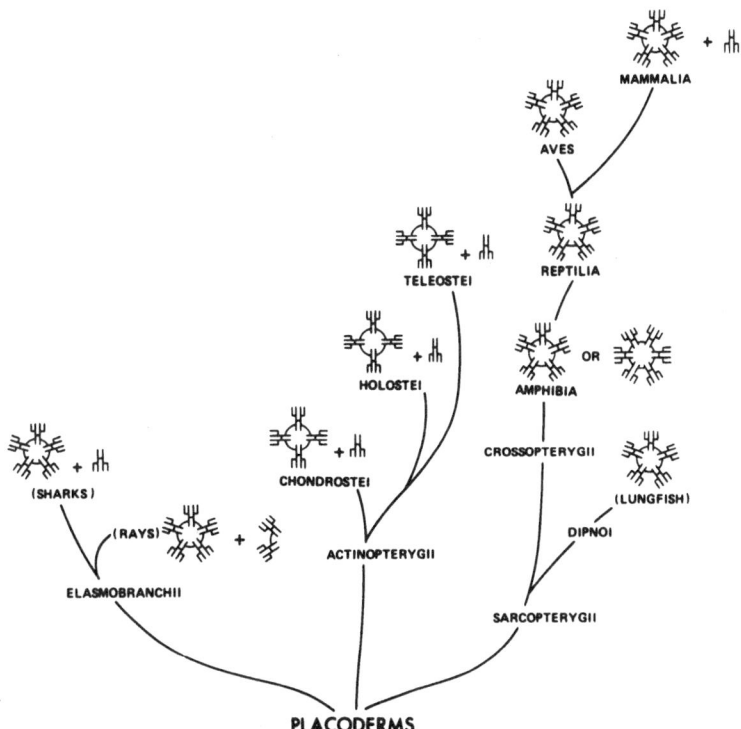

FIG. 2. Evolution of IgM-like immunoglobulins. No provision is made
for the apparent restrictions of certain Teleost and Holostean species
to a single HMW immunoglobulin class. The length of the heavy chain
is not intended to indicate heavy chain mass; deleted "μ-like" heavy
chains have been detected in several species.

(11,12). One possible fault with the above statements is that
several of the IgM-like proteins possess heavy chains of atypical
mass (less than the ~70,000 MW characteristic of the μ heavy chains)
(17,18). As immunoglobulin chains evolved by end-to-end duplication
of an ~ 330 nucleotide precursor gene (19), it is not difficult to
imagine that regular deviations in μ heavy chain length occurred and
should not be construed as class determinant events.

The evolution of the IgM-like immunoglobulins was marked by
considerable variation in the polymeric arrangements of a basic ~ 7S,
180,000 MW monomer. It is not possible to ascribe a single category
of functional significance to these structural rearrangements, however, the following provide some of the possible adaptive advantages
which could be realized: 1) variation in polymer composition would
directly affect extravascular distribution of antibody, 2) variation
in polymer composition may affect the interaction of immunoglobulin
with other secondary mediators of immune function, e.g. complement,
3) polymer composition may alter net, effective antibody affinity
and valence (20). While recent studies based on fluorescence polari-
zation have clearly indicated that antibody became progressively more
flexible in the course of vertebrate evolution, there is no apparent
relationship between segmental or rotational flexibility and polymer
composition (21). It seems more likely that polymer composition
influences the manner in which antibody is oriented on particulate
antigens, an important factor in the ultimate disposition of heavy
chain complement binding regions.

Remarkable structural similarity exists between the IgM-like
immunoglobulins found in lower and higher vertebrate species. While
it is tempting to speculate that the molecule represents a highly
conserved structure, it must be remembered that amino acid sequence
homology in class determinant regions must be demonstrated. Little
data of this type exists for lower vertebrate immunoglobulin and has
prompted us to initiate sequence analysis of the blocked heavy chains
of immunoglobulins from several species including the horned shark
(Heterodontus franciscii). To date, it has been possible to identify
eight CNBr fragments and analysis of their amino acid sequence is in
progress (Litman, G.W., Kehoe, J.M., unpublished). Such studies will
enable us to calculate rates of evolutionary divergence of individual
domains, establish the heavy chain class of lower vertebrate immunoglobulin and interpret the critical genetic events in the divergence
of immunoglobulin classes.

IMMUNOGLOBULIN CLASS DIVERGENCE

The emergence of a second, distinct immunoglobulin class occurred
at the level of phylogenetic development of the Crossopterygii. In
two species of Dipnoi fishes, the Australian lungfish, (Neoceratodus
forsteri) (22), and African lungfish (Protopterus aethiopicus) (23),

a LMW ~ 120,000 MW immunoglobulin, comprised of equal numbers of heavy ~ 38,000 MW and light ~ 22,500 MW chains and antigenically distinct from the pentameric HMW immunoglobulin also found in these species, has been partially characterized. Further evidence for class distinction between HMW and LMW lungfish immunoglobulin has arisen from analysis of amino acid composition, carbohydrate content and comparative peptide mapping of enzymatic digests of heavy chains. In addition to the HMW and LMW classes, lesser quantities of an antigenically distinct ~ 170,000 MW immunoglobulin (IMW) have been isolated from the serum of the African lungfish and detected in immunoelectrophoretic patterns of Australian lungfish serum. As will be noted below, molecules resembling the lungfish LMW immunoglobulin are found in the phylogenetically more recent deviations, the reptilia and aves. The genetic mechanism whereby these abbreviated heavy chains arose (deletion of μ chain C regions followed by mutation, independent gene duplication, etc.) is of considerable importance and may reflect a general mechanism in immunoglobulin heavy chain class expansion.

An immunoglobulin class distinct from IgM also has been detected in several amphibian species. The bullfrog *(Rana catesbiana)* (24) as well as the marine toad *(Bufo marinus)* (25) and clawed toad *(Xenopus laevis)* (26) possess a LMW immunoglobulin with a heavy chain of ~ 53,000 MW. The LMW immunoglobulin is considered to be homologous to the heavy chain of IgG in terms of mass, amino acid and carbohydrate composition[1]. As mentioned above, one species of Urodele amphibian, the mudpuppy *(Necturus maculosus)*, does not express a low molecular weight immunoglobulin and only synthesizes an IgM-like protein (16).

Examples of reptilian and avian species possessing as many as three distinct immunoglobulin classes have been described. A LMW molecule remarkably similar to the LMW immunoglobulin of the lungfish has been detected in two species of turtle *(Chelydra serpentina, Pseudamys scripta)* (27,28) and the duck *(Chordapa aves)* (29). Unlike the African lungfish immunoglobulin, the turtle and duck immunoglobulins were markedly deficient in carbohydrate (0.6-0.9% by weight) which led to the postulate that the latter two LMW proteins lacked a heavy chain region equivalent to the CH_2 domain of the γ type heavy chain (30). Although deficient in both length (110-120 residues in reference to a γ type chain) and carbohydrate, the turtle LMW immunoglobulin fixes both homologous and heterologous complement (27). It is interesting to note that species both more and less phylogenetically advanced than the amphibians possess remarkably similar immunoglobulin profiles but lack an equivalent of the LMW, IgG-like molecule thus far described in three amphibian species. The selective pressures bringing about this unusual distribution in immunoglobulin classes would be interesting to consider in terms of adaptive advantages associated with the LMW forms of immunoglobulin.

No major qualitative differences in secondary structure have been detected between the LMW, IMW immunoglobulins and the corresponding HMW immunoglobulins found in any of the species thus far analyzed (31). There is some indication, however, that one component of immunoglobulin conformation, segmental flexibility, increased in the course of evolution of the LMW and IMW immunoglobulins (21). The most apparent structural variation in the evolution of these non IgM-like immunoglobulins has been the variations in mass (length) of the heavy chains. Some of the possible functional consequences of such structural rearrangements would be: 1) broadened physiologic distribution, 2) altered (less stearically hindered) reactivity with certain classes of complex antigens, and 3) unique interaction of the molecules with secondary mediators of immune function such as fixation of complement and 4) passage to the egg or through the placenta.

While the evolution of IgM-like immunoglobulins was marked by rearrangements in polymer composition, the evolution of at least three distinct immunoglobulin classes found in Dipnoi, amphibian, reptilian and avian species, involved significant mass alteration rearrangements in the heavy chain subunit of 120,000 - 170,000 MW monomer. One possible exception, however, involves a polymer form of secretory immunoglobulins found in an avian species (32) and resembling mammalian IgA.

ACTIVE SITES OF LOWER VERTEBRATE ANTIBODY

The range of specific interactions mediated by the antigen combining site of antibody is several orders of magnitude greater than that displayed by any well characterized, polymorphic group of enzymes, carrier proteins or polypeptide hormones. The structural basis for recognition of diverse antigenic structures involves limited amino acid substitution in restricted regions of heavy and light chains which contact and form a crevice at the N terminal end of the Fab fragment (1-3). The folding of the polypeptide chains in the Fab as well as hydrogen, hydrophobic and electrostatic bonding forces are involved with specific ligand recognition. In order to achieve functional diversity within the constraints of limited amounts of DNA while still invoking established patterns of transcription and translation, macromolecules the size of immunoglobulins must possess unique structural organization. As active site heterogeneity most likely expanded during the passage of evolutionary time in response to a broadening antigenic environment, considerable interest has been generated for examining active sites of lower vertebrate antibody directed at well defined hapten structures.

When careful consideration is made of antigen dose, route of administration and physical condition of the species under study, it is evident that lower vertebrate species are capable of responding to most conventional antigens. The specificity of the induced antibody has not yet been scrutinized in a definitive fashion; it is apparent, however, that the most primitive of vertebrate species are capable of discriminating substructures on surfaces of antigens as complex as erythrocytes and bacteriophage. The capacity of lower vertebrates to respond to hapten groups such as 2,4-dinitrophenol has permitted isolation of specific antibody and characterization of active site geometry and microenvironment. Comparison of tumbling rates (correlation times), Tc, determined by electron paramagnetic resonance spectroscopy of hapten spin labels of 8-17.4Å internal molecular lengths, has been utilized to probe the depth of the rainbow trout *(Salmo gairdneri)* antibody to the dinitrophenol ligand (33). A sharp discontinuity in plots of Tc vs ℓ at 10-12 Å indicates that the depth of the active site of trout antibody is ~ 10-12Å; a similar value is obtained for rabbit antibody to the same ligand. The affinity label MNBDF has been utilized to probe the active sites of rabbit, duck and turtle LMW antibody to 2,4-dinitrophenol (34,35). Although minor differences exist in terms of the relative ratio of heavy and light chain labeling, it is evident that both the heavy and light chains participate in formation of the active sites, all of which contain tyrosine (Table 1). It would be of interest to examine affinity labeling characteristics of chicken IgY (36) antibody to 2,4-dinitrophenol, as this antibody class exhibits weak interchain non-covalent bonding (37). Spectral shift experiments which estimate

TABLE 1. Affinity labeling characteristics of reptilian, avian, and mammalian antibody to 2,4-dinitrophenol. (a) data contained in (35); LMW Ig, low molecular weight immunoglobulin; (b) data contained in (34); (c) meta-nitrobenzenediazonium fluoroborate.

	Turtle LMW Ig[a]	Duck LMW Ig[a]	Rabbit IgG[b]
Molecular weight	120,000	118,000	150,000
Combining sites/molecule	1.7 ± 0.1	1.5 ± 0.1	2.0 ± 0.1
Combining sites/molecule lost MNBDF[c] modification	0.5	0.2	0.5
Moles MNBDF incorporated/mole of antibody	0.4	0.3	0.6
Residue modified	tyrosine/histidine (5:1)	tyrosine	tyrosine
Labeling ratio heavy/light chain	2.7 : 1	1.4 : 1	2 : 1

the relative hydrophobicity of antibody active sites directed at certain colored haptens have suggested that tryptophan is a principal
active site component of shark, turtle and duck antibody to dinitrophenol (35,38). Taken together, these studies suggest a common
molecular basis for hapten recognition by antibody from phylogenetically diverse species.

If antibody is to express a range in molecular specificity, it
is necessary for primary structure heterogeneity to exist. Acrylamide
gel electrophoresis (14,39) and analytical isoelectrofocusing (unpublished) of lower vertebrate immunoglobulin heavy and light chains
have revealed a degree of microheterogeneity equivalent to that associated with mammalian immunoglobulin. N terminal amino acid sequences
of heavy and light chains from species as phylogenetically diverse
as shark (39), paddlefish (40), African lungfish (23) and several
avians (41,42) have established varying degrees of homology with mammalian immunoglobulin κ and λ chains and demonstrated the existence
and evolutionary conservation of V region subgroups. Recently a sequence of nurse shark *(Ginglymostoma cirratum)* heavy and light chains
has been reported (43). The sequence extended almost 1/4 the length
of the variable portion of the light chain and suggested the occurrence of a hypervariable region at an equivalent position to the first
hypervariable region of mammalian light chains. In the nurse shark
immunoglobulin the boundaries of the first light chain hypervariable
region and the occurrence of other light and heavy chain hypervariable
regions have not been definitively established; however, its existence
when considered along with the basic features of the combining site
microenvironment and location elucidated in the biophysical studies,
is consistent with the early evolutionary origin of a limited, specialized molecular region involved in active site function.

IMMUNOGLOBULINS IN OSTRACHODERM DERIVED VERTEBRATES AND OTHER CLASSES
OF RECOGNITION MACROMOLECULES IN VERTEBRATES AND INVERTEBRATES

From the above discussion, it is apparent that the lower and
higher vertebrate species which are descendents of the Placoderms
respond to antigenic challenge by production of antibody with a basic
structural organization (chain arrangements, active site location
and active site composition) that was conserved during the course of
evolution. The more phylogenetically primitive Ostrachoderm derived
vertebrates, the lampreys and hagfishes, respond to immunization with
bacteria, erythrocytes, protein or bacteriophage by production of a
structurally distinct, specific antibody. Sea lamprey *(Petromyzon
marinus)* antibody to f-2 bacteriophage has been characterized as an
~ 188,000 MW protein consisting of two heavy chains and two light
chains (44); the heavy chain is similar in amino acid composition to
the μ type heavy chains of higher vertebrate immunoglobulin (45).
Unlike other lower vertebrate immunoglobulins, however, the subunits
are not disulfide linked and associated functional activity is labile

under routine storage and chromatography conditions. When the same
species is immunized with either erythrocytes or gram negative bacteria, antibody activity is associated with an ~300,000 MW protein
comprised of 75,000 MW noncovalently bonded subunits (46). No evidence for a typical light chain structure was found and the molecule's
secondary structure contained significant (~ 45%) amounts of α helix
not detectable in other vertebrate immunoglobulins (31). The different lamprey immunoglobulins may reflect an alternate, antigen-dependent
class of humoral immune responsiveness. The ~ 24S antibody formed
in the Pacific hagfish (Eptatretus stoutii) in response to immunization with protein and cellular antigens appears to resemble the lamprey immunoglobulins in terms of characteristic lability and dissociation tendencies (47).

Although the hagfish (48) and several species of invertebrates
have been shown to respond to injection of bacteria with production
of bactericidins, there is little indication that these macromolecules resemble immunoglobulin (11). In addition to the bactericidins,
structurally diverse agglutinins have been isolated from the coelomic
fluids of phylogenetically critical invertebrate species (49-51).
These molecules, usually in combination with divalent cations, effect
highly specific interactions with the surface carbohydrate (glycoprotein) of erythrocytes and lymphocytes. Attempts at relating
agglutinins from various species using criteria of primary structure
have not proven successful. Furthermore, the N-terminal amino acid
sequence of the agglutinin isolated from the horseshoe crab (Limulus
polyphemus) showed no structural homology to immunoglobulin or the
functionally related plant lectins (50). The evolutionary fate of
the invertebrate agglutinins is not clear. It has been suggested
(46), however, that the 300,000 MW, inducible lamprey immunoglobulin
and some of the other both inducible and non-inducible carbohydrate
binding proteins (52), e.g. nurse shark fructosan specific protein
(53), eel (Anguilla rostrata) human blood group O hemagglutinin (54)
and inducible C reactive protein (55) may resemble these molecules.

While the evolutionary appearance of immunoglobulin with characteristic interchain bonding patterns and variable region subgroups
could be interpreted as a rather abrupt event occurring in the ancestral placoderms, it is important to remember that the emergence of
cell mediated immunity occurred far earlier in evolution (56). In
light of recent evidence for structural homology between various T
cell structures including histocompatibility antigens and immunoglobulin subunits, it has been suggested that the ancestral genes
of the immunoglobulin heavy and light chains were first expressed
(56-59) as functional surface components of primitive "T-like" cells.
Changes in these cells' biosynthetic (protein secreting) apparatus
and/or in the proteins themselves may have resulted in their secretion or shedding into extracellular space. Thus, the origins of
immunoglobulin-mediated humoral recognition may reside in species

phylogenetically distal to the vertebrates. Characterization of
cell surface associated immunoglobulin and immunoglobulin substructures in lower vertebrates and, perhaps, in invertebrate species
will aid in our interpretation of the relative roles of cell-associa-
ted vs humoral-mediated recognition in adaptive immunity.

[1] A recently published study (Atwell, J.L. and Marchalonis, J.J.,
J. Immunogen., 1: 367 (1975)) presented a revised molecular weight
estimate of 61,400 for the LMW immunoglobulin heavy chains of *(Bufo
marinus)* and *(Xenopus laevis)*. The two amphibian immunoglobulin
heavy chains were similar in mass and carbohydrate composition to
the heavy chains of the LMW chicken immunoglobulin. The dissimilar
amino acid compositions of the amphibian and chicken immunoglobulin
heavy chains, however, did not permit grouping of these immunoglobulins in a single class. In light of these findings, earlier
classifications of LMW amphibian immunoglobulins as IgG-like may
require revision.

Abbreviations: HMW, high molecular weight; IMW, intermediate molecular weight (used to designate immunoglobulin classes in Dipnoi,
amphibian, reptilian and avian species (12)); MNBDF, meta-nitrobenzenediazonium fluoroborate; MW, molecular weight.

Acknowledgments: supported by NCI CA-08748, CA-17404 and CA-16889.

REFERENCES
1. Milstein, C. and Pink, J.R.L., in Progress in Biophysics and
    Molecular Biology, Butler, J.A.V. and Noble, D., eds., (Pergamon
    Press, Oxford & New York, 1970), p. 209.
2. Edelman, G.M. and Gall, W.E., Ann. Rev. Biochem., 38: 415 (1969).
3. Poljak, R.J., Amzel, L.M., Chen, B.L., Phizackerlay, R.P. and
    Saul, F., Proc. Nat. Acad. Sci., 71: 3440 (1974).
4. Hood, L.E., Fed. Proc., 31: 177 (1972).
5. Hood, L. and Ein, D., Nature, 220: 764 (1968).
6. Putnam, F.W., Florent, G., Paul, C., Shinoda, T. and Shimizu, A.,
    Science, 182: 287 (1973).
7. Edelman, G.M., Cunningham, B.A., Gall, W.E., Gottlieb, P.D.,
    Rutishauser, U. and Waxdal, M.J., Proc. Nat. Acad. Sci., 63: 78
    (1969).
8. Capra, J.D. and Kehoe, J.M., Adv. Immunol., 20: 1 (1975).
9. Koshland, M.E., Adv. Immunol., 20: 41 (1975).
10. Marchalonis, J. and Edelman, G.M., Science, 154: 1567 (1966).
11. Marchalonis, J.J. and Cone, R.E., Aust. J. Exp. Biol. Med. Sci.,
    51: 461 (1973).
12. Litman, G.W., in Comparative Immunology, Marchalonis, J.J., ed.,
    (Blackwell Press, Oxford, Great Britain, in press).
13. Acton, R.T., Weinheimer, P.F., Hall, S.J., Niedermeier, W.,
    Shelton, E. and Bennett, J.C., Proc. Nat. Acad. Sci. 68: 107
    (1971).
14. Clem, L.W. and Small, P.A., J. Exp. Med., 125: 893 (1967).

15. Bradshaw, C.M., Clem, L.W. and Sigel, M.M., J. Immunol., 106: 1480 (1971).
16. Marchalonis, J.J. and Cohen, N., Immunol., 24: 395 (1973).
17. Clem, L.W., J. Biol. Chem., 246 (1971).
18. Litman, G.W., Frommel, D., Finstad, J. and Good, R.A., J. Immunol., 107: 881 (1971).
19. Hill, R.L., Delaney, R., Fellows, R.E., Jr. and Lebovitz, H.E., Proc. Nat. Acad. Sci., 56: 1762 (1966).
20. Hornick, C.L. and Karush, F., Immunochem., 9: 325 (1972).
21. Zagyansky, Y.A., Arch. Biochem. Biophys., 166: 371 (1975).
22. Marchalonis, J.J., Aust. J. Exp. Biol. Med. Sci., 47: 405 (1969).
23. Litman, G.W., Wang, A.C., Fudenberg, H.H. and Good, R.A., Proc. Nat. Acad. Sci., 68: 2321 (1971).
24. Marchalonis, J. and Edelman, G.M., J. Exp. Med., 124: 901 (1966).
25. Acton, R.T., Evans, E.E., Weinheimer, P.F., Niedermeier, W. and Bennett, J.C., Biochem., 11: 2751 (1972).
26. Marchalonis, J.J., Allen, R.B. and Saarni, E.S., Comp. Biochem. Physiol., 35: 49 (1970).
27. Chartrand, S.L., Litman, G.W., Lapointe, N., Good, R.A. and Frommel, D., J. Immunol. 107: 1 (1971).
28. Leslie, G.A. and Clem, L.W., J. Immunol. 108: 1656 (1972).
29. Zimmerman, B., Shalatin, N. and Grey, H.M., Biochem., 10: 482 (1971).
30. Litman, G.W., Frommel, D., Chartrand, S., Finstad, J. and Good, R.A., Immunochem., 8: 345 (1971).
31. Litman, G.W., Frommel, D., Rosenberg, A. and Good, R.A., Biochem. Biophys. Acta, 36: 647 (1971).
32. Bienenstock, J., Perey, D.Y.E., Gauldie, J. and Underdown, B.J., J. Immunol., 110: 524 (1973).
33. Roubal, W.T., Etlinger, H.M. and Hodgins, H.O., J. Immunol., 113: 309 (1974).
34. Good, A.H., Traylor, P.S. and Singer, S.J., Biochem., 6: 873 (1967).
35. Litman, G.W., Chartrand, S., Finstad, C. and Good, R.A., Immunochem., 10: 323 (1973).
36. Leslie, G.A. and Clem, L.W., J. Exp. Med., 130: 1337 (1969).
37. Dreesman, G.R. and Benedict, A.A., Proc. Nat. Acad. Sci., 54: 822 (1965).
38. Voss, E.W., Russell, W.J. and Sigel, M.M., Biochem., 8: 4866 (1969).
39. Suran, A.A. and Papermaster, B.W., Proc. Nat. Acad. Sci., 58: 1619 (1967).
40. Pollara, B., Suran, A., Finstad, J. and Good, R.A., Proc. Nat. Acad. Sci., 59: 1307 (1968).
41. Kubo, R.T., Rosenblum, I.Y. and Benedict, A.A., J. Immunol., 107: 1781 (1971).
42. Grant, J.A., Sanders, B. and Hood, L., Biochem., 10: 3123 (1971).
43. Sledge, C., Clem, L.W. and Hood, L., J. Immunol., 112: 941 (1974).
44. Marchalonis, J.J. and Edelman, G.M., J. Exp. Med., 127: 891 (1968).

45. Marchalonis, J.J., Nature, 236: 84 (1972).
46. Litman, G.W., Frommel, D., Finstad, J., Howell, J., Pollara,
     B.W. and Good, R.A., J. Immunol., 105: 1278 (1970).
47. Linthicum, D.S. and Hildemann, W.H., J. Immunol. 105: 912 (1970).
48. Acton, R.T., Weinheimer, P.F., Hildemann, W.H. and Evans, E.E.,
     J. Bact., 99: 626 (1966).
49. Marchalonis, J.J. and Edelman, G.M., J. Mol. Biol., 32: 453
     (1968).
50. Finstad, C.L., Good, R.A. and Litman, G.W., Ann. N.Y. Acad. Sci.,
     234: 170 (1974).
51. Hammarström, S., Ann. N.Y. Acad. Sci., 234: 183 (1974).
52. Sigel, M.M., Ann. N.Y. Acad. Sci., 234: 198 (1974).
53. Harisdangkul, V., Kabat, E.A., McDonough, R.J. and Sigel, M.M.,
     J. Immunol., 108: 1259 (1972).
54. Bezkorovainy, A., Springer, G.F. and Desai, P.R., Biochem.,
     10: 3761 (1971).
55. Baldo, B.A. and Fletcher, T.C., Nature, 246: 145 (1973).
56. Hildemann, W.H., Nature, 250: 116 (1974).
57. Gally, J.A. and Edelman, G.M., Ann. Rev. Genet., 6: 1 (1972).
58. Peterson, P.A., Rask, L., Sege, K., Klareskog, L., Anundi, H.
     and Ostberg, L., Proc. Nat. Acad. Sci., 72: 1612 (1975).
59. Dayhoff, M.O., McLaughlin, P.J., Barker, W.C. and Hunt, L.T.,
     Naturwissenschaften, 62: 154 (1975).

VERTEBRATE IMMUNOLOGY

Evolution of Lymphoid
and Immunocyte Systems

QUANTITATIVE AND QUALITATIVE ASPECTS OF THE ANTIBODY LIBRARY OF SHARKS

L. William Clem, W. Edsel McLean, and Vincent Shankey

Department of Immunology and Medical Microbiology
College of Medicine, University of Florida
Gainesville, Florida 32610

INTRODUCTION

At the present time there are sufficient data available to allow two rather basic generalizations regarding the humoral immune response of sharks. The first is that sharks can respond with the production of circulating antibodies to a wide variety of antigens and thus are not necessarily primitive in an immunologic sense. The second generalization is that these antibodies belong to an immunoglobulin class whose gross architecture resembles 19S IgM of mammals, i.e. a pentamer of disulfide-linked monomers each composed of 2 μ–like and 2 L chains (reviewed 1,2,3). Similar types of studies indicate the presence of a 7S immunoglobulin that resembles a monomer of IgM; no molecules homologous to mammalian IgG have been found in sharks.

In considering the antibody response of sharks, one misconception has apparently arisen, namely that sharks are innately poor antibody producers in a quantitative sense. A portion of this paper is devoted to data indicating this is not always the case. Another area of considerable importance in understanding immunologic phylogeny involves the question of the combining site "library" in animals such as sharks. A priori one cannot necessarily predict whether a) antibodies to a defined antigenic determinant from a single shark would be homogeneous or heterogeneous, b) the nature of the antibody site(s) to a defined antigenic determinant would differ from shark to shark within the species and c) these antibody sites are stable or alternatively change (mature) with respect to time of immunization in a single shark. The second portion of this paper discusses data dealing with these questions.

EXPERIMENTAL RESULTS

Quantitative Aspects of Shark Antibody Responses

Previous studies on the production of antibodies by sharks
usually involved the usage of soluble antigens incorporated into
adjuvants, viruses, or bacterial vaccines administered in relatively small amounts (reviewed 3). The results obtained from
such studies indicated that antibody titers were usually rather
low—hence the idea that sharks are innately poor responders.
Therefore, in light of the success obtained in rabbits, mice, and
more recently birds, using intravenous hyperimmunization with
streptococcal and pneumococcal vaccines (4,5) similar studies
were undertaken with the nurse shark Ginglymostoma cirratum.
Initial efforts in this direction were quite successful in that
as previously reported (6), 2 of 3 nurse sharks immunized with
heat killed, pepsinized streptococcal A-variant vaccine responded
with the production of > 7 mg ab/ml to the group specific A-
variant carbohydrate between 72–116 days after initial immunization. These studies have now been extended to include 14 nurse
sharks immunized with A-variant streptococcal cells; 10 of these
animals have responded with > 5 mg ab/ml to the group specific
carbohydrate. Some of these results are presented in Table I.
Also included here are some representative results obtained with
group A streptococcal vaccine. It can be seen that this immunogen appears to preferentially elicit the production of antibodies
reactive with the A-variant carbohydrate and not the A carbohydrate. One probable explanation for this observation may be
that sharks have an enzyme capable of hydrolysing terminal amino
sugars from the group A carbohydrate. Hence the effective immunogen may in reality be the underlying A-variant streptococcal
backbone. In either case, these results should leave little
doubt that streptococcal vaccines are reasonably potent immunogens in sharks.

In attempting to extend this range of bacterial cell "superimmunogenicity" in nurse sharks, four animals were immunized with
Type III pneumococcal vaccine under a similar protocol as
employed with the streptococci. While each of these animals produced detectable precipitating antibody to the SSS, none made in
excess of 0.4 mg/ml over an 8 month period. However each of four
other sharks immunized with Type VIII pneumococcal cells made in
excess of 2 mg ab/ml to the Type VIII SSS between 2–12 months of
immunization. Surprisingly two of these animals also made at
least 1.5 mg ab/ml reactive with the type III polysaccharide in
addition to antibodies reactive with the homologous antigen in-
spite of never having been immunized with Type III vaccine.

TABLE I

IMMUNIZATION SCHEDULES AND SERUM ANTIBODY LEVELS IN
NURSE SHARKS IMMUNIZED WITH STREPTOCOCCAL VACCINES

Shark Number	Immunogen	Immunization	Bleeding	Antibody Concentration(mg/ml) A-Variant	A
225	A-variant	1, 2, 3, 5	38	2.3	----
		39	72	10.0	----
		76	116	9.1	0.3
226	A-variant	1, 2, 3, 5	38	<0.25	----
		39	72	5.7	----
		76	116	7.4	1.0
1919	A-variant	1, 2	33	<0.25	----
		35,37,39	76	7.7	0.5
			140	3.5	
			220	0.4	
239	A-variant	1, 2, 3, 4, 5	49	7.4	0.6
Frances	A-variant	1, 2	90	2.0	0.8
		93	140	6.4	3.0
		143	190	7.7	4.0
261	A	1, 2, 3, 4	70	<0.25	<0.25
		74	110	2.0	0.6
		113	145	2.5	0.5
		148	175	1.5	0.3
263	A	1, 2, 3, 4	70	0.5	<0.25
		74	110	2.2	1.1
		113	145	2.5	0.7
		148	175	1.4	0.25

Purification of shark antibodies to streptococcal and pneumococcal polysaccharides was readily accomplished by affinity
chromatography (7). These experiments resulted in recovery of
> 75% of the precipitating antibody present in the serum and
indicated that > 95% of the recovered material was 19S immunoglobulin. Some of these sharks were immunized for over 2 years
without yielding significant amounts of 7S antibody.

The high degree of success in eliciting the production of
large amounts of relatively homogenous antibody in mammals (and
sharks as discussed below) with streptococcal vaccines, suggested
an adjuvant effect somehow involving the "monotonous" carbohydrate
surface of the cells employed as vaccine. In spite of uncer-
tainties as to the mechanism of this "superimmunogenicity", it was
decided to continue such studies by immunizing animals with the
same vaccines containing "monotonous" surfaces of our choosing.
Preliminary experiments with rabbits involved immunization with
group A streptococcal cells containing ε-2,4-dinitrophenyl lysine
coupled covalently (by the CNBr reaction) to the bacterial cell
surface carbohydrate at a concentration of $\sim 0.2~\mu M$ DNP lysine/mg
cell suspension. Rabbit antibody responses to the DNP moity were
quite variable (as is also true for the anticarbohydrate response
in our hands) although most animals (6 of 8) responded after 2-4
courses of immunization with the production of 5-10 mg IgG ab/ml
(Yocum and Clem. in preparation). In some cases these antibodies
exhibited considerably restricted heterogeneity, i.e. Sips heterogeneity indices of 1.0 and isoelectric focusing patterns reminiscent of myeloma proteins.

In light of this success in rabbits, a series of nurse sharks
(totaling 8) were immunized with the DNP-lysine-streptococcal
vaccine. While none of these animals appeared to synthesize sufficient amounts of antibody for quantitative precipitin analysis,
all animals made anti-DNP antibodies as indicated by neutralization
of DNP-T_4 phage. Isolation of these antibodies was accomplished
by affinity chromatography using ε-TNP-lysine-sepharose. Hapten
elution (0.1 M DNP-OH) indicated yields of 50-400 μg ab/ml from
about 40 days of immunization through 2 1/2 years with intermittent boosting. Analytical ultracentrifugation indicated each
shark anti-DNP preparation (with one exception discussed below)
to be at least 90% 19S Ig. As mentioned previously for anticarbohydrate antibodies, there was no significant synthesis of
7S antibodies in six sharks studied in detail over the 2 1/2 year
period. The one exception (designated nurse shark #29) yielded
between 30-40% of the isolated anti-DNP antibody as 7S Ig between
30 days and 2 1/2 years of study.

Regarding the ability of shark 19S anti-DNP antibodies to
form immune precipitates, each of the isolated preparations was

>80% (and >90% in many cases) precipitable with DNP_{10}-BSA. On
the other hand shark 7S antibodies to DNP (obtained naturally
from shark #29 or by mild reduction of 19S molecules to subunits)
were not capable of immune precipitation although binding to
affinity columns was quite efficient. This latter point (binding to affinity columns) in conjunction with good recoveries by
the elution techniques employed, supports the argument that such
7S molecules were not missed in the original purification
schemes.

Molecular Heterogeneity of Shark Antibodies

The initial approach employed to assess the heterogeneity of
nurse shark 19S antibodies specifically purified by affinity
chromatography involved cellulose acetate electrophoresis. Some
of the results with antibodies to streptotoccal A-variant carbohydrate are depicted in Figure 1 and illustrate the following
points. The electrophoretic heterogeneity varies considerably
from one shark to another and ranges from being quite restricted
to being indistinguishable from a pool of normal shark 19S Ig.
There is no apparent correlation between electrophoretic hetero-
genetiy and high antibody levels. Another feature discernable
by this method is an apparent stability with time of immunization
of the electrophoretic patterns of antibodies from individual
aniamls. Several animals (such as Frances, not depicted) have
yielded similar patterns from bleedings obtained over a 3 year
period with intermittent (2-4 month intervals) immunization with
A-variant streptococcal vaccine. In fact the only exception yet
observed to this rule involved shark 225 wherein antibodies
obtained at 38 days exhibited a somewhat faster mobility than
observed with antibodies from later bleedings. The anti-group A
streptococcal carbohydrate, the anti-pneumococcal polysaccharide,
and the anti-DNP antibodies also exhibited considerable variability between animals but were quite similar on repeated
samples (with time) from individuals. This admittedly rather
crude approach does not permit any predictions regarding the
antibody homogeneity of any individual shark but it is consistent with the idea that what ever population of antibody(s)
is made early in immunization continues to be present for a
long period of time.

Alkaline urea gel electrophoresis of L chains isolated from
shark antibodies to the A-variant streptococcal carbohydrate has
served to verify the above mentioned points, i.e. there is considerable variability between animals but a marked stability within individual animals with time. Peptide maps of tryptic digests
of antibody L chains were also revealing in that all chains ex-

hibited some common peptides (these peptides were also evident
in an L chain preparation obtained from a pool of normal 19S
Ig) and each antibody L chain preparation appeared to have some
unique peptides. Thus there seems to be little room for doubt
that the concept of constant and variable regions observed in
antibodies from higher animals (reviewed 8) should also be
extended to sharks. In fact, the observation that several of
these L chains in addition to normal L chains have been subjected to automatic amino acid sequence analysis (9) for the
amino terminal 20 or so residues and found to be nearly identical,
implies that the variability revealed by the peptide maps is
likely reflecting different hypervariable regions and not
subgroups of L chains.

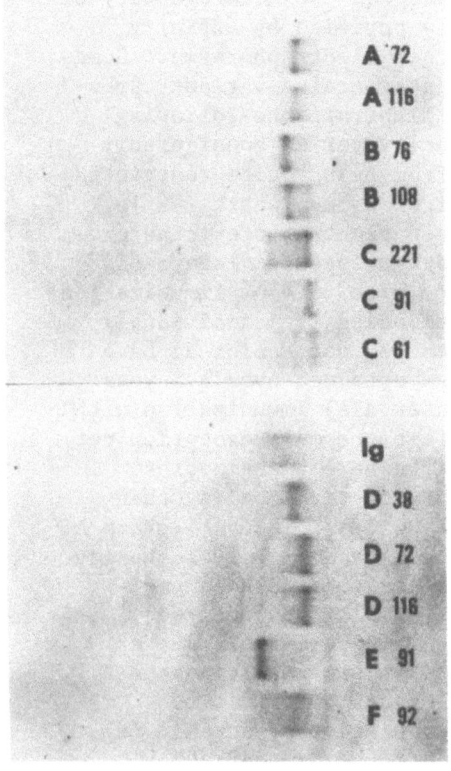

Figure 1. Cellulose acetate
electrophoretic patterns of
purified nurse shark 19S
immunoglobulin and anti-
bodies against A-variant
streptococcal carbohydrate.
The capital letters designate
antibodies from individual
sharks (A = shark 226, B =
1919, C = 1904, D = 225,
E = 1903, F = 239, Ig =
pooled immunoglobulin). The
accompanying numbers indicate
the day of bleeding.

     One approach that has proven useful in the detection of
antibody combining site differences in higher animals has involved the usage of idiotypic antibodies, i.e. antibodies directed
to the combining sites of other antibodies (10). Thus, con-

sidering the availability of relatively large amounts of restricted heterogeneity shark antibodies to the A-variant streptococcal carbohydrate, attempts at developing anti-idiotypes
for shark antibodies were undertaken. The basic protocol involved tolerization of guinea pigs to shark immunoglobulin
determinants (by intravenous injections of large amounts of
ultracentrifuged monomeric shark 7S Ig) coupled with intra-
muscular injections of shark 19S antibody emulsified in adjuvant.
As depicted in Figure 2, for a representative guinea pig antiserum, two different populations of guinea pig antibodies were
evident. One of these involved precipitation with all shark
sera studied and was readily absorbed with normal nurse shark
19S Ig (but not 7S) and was thus considered to be pentamer
specific - They do not appear to react with isolated nurse
shark J chain. The other population of guinea pig antibodies
was not absorbed with nurse shark 19S or 7S Ig, reacted only with
homologous anti A-variant streptococcal antibodies from the
shark used to elicit their production and, as illustrated by
inhibitition of precipitin reactions in gels, this homologous
reaction involved a site(s) on the shark Fab fragment. For
these reasons it seems appropriate to refer to such absorbed
guinea pig antisera as being anti-idiotypic with the implication
(without any supporting data) that the reactive site on the shark
Fab involves the antibody combining site.

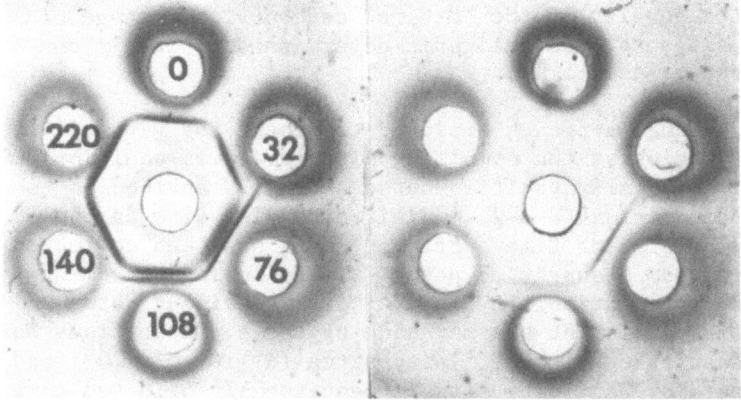

Figure 2. Immunodiffusion patterns of a guinea pig anti-idiotypic antiserum reacting with sera from nurse shark 1919. The center well on the left panel contains guinea pig antiserum to specifically purified antibody from nurse shark 1919. The outer
wells contain serum from nurse shark 1919 obtained at the indicated days after initial immunization. The right panel depicts
the same arrangement except that the guinea pig serum has been
absorbed with pooled nurse shark 19S immunoglobulin.

At the present time guinea pig anti-idiotypic sera have been
prepared against A-variant streptococcal carbohydrate antibodies
from each of 4 nurse sharks (of 8 reasonably restricted antibodies tried). Each of these guinea pig antisera appears
specific in that precipitin reactions in gels are observed only
with homologous antibodies. Quantification of homologous binding has been assessed with an indirect precipitation system
wherein radioiodinated homologous (or in some cases heterologous)
shark antibodies are bound by the appropriate guinea pig anti-
idiotype which is in turn precipitated at equivalence by rabbit
antisera to guinea pig gamma globulin (11). Inhibition of homologous binding in this system by unlabeled homologous or heterologous proteins thus permits an assessment of cross reactivity.
Each of the homologous systems thus far studied in detail (Nurse
sharks 225, 1919, 1904 and Frances) have proved to be quite
specific with binding of radioactivity ranging from about 40%
for shark 225 to about 75% for shark 1919 as compared to <4%
binding for normal shark 19S Ig. Each of these homologous
systems has proved to be uninhibited by unlabeled heterologous
(of 12 tried) shark anti-A-variant streptococcal antibodies at
1000 times the effective concentration of unlabeled homologous
inhibitor. Hence one could readily argue that the "library" of
nurse shark antibody sites for the A-variant streptococcal
carbohydrate (consisting for the most part of polyrhamnose,
12) is at least 5, i.e. one site for each of the four idiotypes
plus "others". In all liklihood, considering the electrophoretic heterogeneity of the "others" category, the range of
nurse shark sites to this antigenic determinant is likely considerably greater than 5.

One additional approach employed to assess the variability
of shark antibodies at the combining site level was equilibrium
dialysis. Specifically purified nurse shark 19S antibodies to
DNP were studied using ^{3}H-ε-2, 4-dinitrophenyl-lysine as the
hapten. At the present time sufficient data has been collected
on antibodies from 6 sharks to permit the following statements.
While considerable variability in affinity is evident between
antibodies from different sharks, each of these preparations has
5 readily measurable "high" affinity sites ($K_o \sim 10^5$-5 x 10^6) and
at least some "low" affinity sites (unequivocally 5 in two cases);
the "low" affinity sites are about two orders of magnitude less
than the "high" affinity sites. None of these shark 19S anti-
DNP preparations were homogeneous and therefore the conceptual
problem created by the failure to obtain binding of 10 sites
per each antibody molecule remains (13). Hopefully ongoing
studies with preparative isoelectric focusing will resolve this
issue, i.e. is the observed heterogeneity an intra-or intermolecular phenomenon?

In contrast to the results reported for one shark by others

(14), none of the animals studied here have exhibited significant changes in affinity for periods of time involving up to two
years of immunization. The isolated 19S and 7S anti-DNP antibodies from shark number 29 have also been studied in this
respect. The 7S molecules from this animal did not precipitate
with DNP_{10}-BSA and exhibited only one readily measurable binding
site per molecule. The K_o of this site was quite similar to
that of the 5 "high" K_o sites on the 19S molecule. Here again,
no maturation of either antibody population was evident over a
two year period of time.

In conclusion it would appear from the data discussed in this
section that the "library" of nurse shark antibodies (presumably
combining sites) for certain defined antigenic determinants is
quite large. The observed range of heterogeneity of antibodies
from individual animals implies that this "library" can also be
rather extensive within an individual. Thus while the studies
discussed here unfortunately do not permit a differentiation between germ line and somatic theories (see 15) to explain the
origin of antibody diversity, they do suggest that such diversity
had its inception in what might be called ancient animals.

Supported by NSF Grant GB29095 and an ACS Institutional Grant to
the University of Florida (70-4).

REFERENCES

1. Grey, H., Adv. Immunol., 10:51(1969).
2. Clem, L.W., and Leslie, G.A., Developmental Immunology, 26
        pp. (Spastics Society, London, 1969).
3. Carton, Y., Ann. Biol., 12:139(1973).
4. Krause, R., Fed. Proc., 29:59(1970).
5. Haber, E., Fed. Proc., 29:66(1970).
6. Clem, L.W., and Leslie, G.A., Proc. Nat. Acad. Sci., U.S.,
        68:139(1971).
7. Eichman, K., and Greenblatt, J., J. Exp. Med., 133:424(1971).
8. Gally, J., and Edelman, G., Ann. Rev. Genet., 7:1(1972).
9. Sledge, C., Clem, L.W., and Hood, L., J. Immunol., 112:
        941(1974).
10. Brient, B., and Nisonoff, A., J. Exp. Med., 132:951(1970).
11. Eichman, K., J. Exp. Med., 137:603(1973).
12. Krause, R., Adv. Immunol., 12:1(1970).
13. Voss, E.W., Russell, W., and Sigel, M.M., Biochem., 8:
        4886(1969).
14. Voss, E.W., and Sigel, M.M., J. Immunol. 109:665(1972).
15. Cohn, M., Blomberg, B., Geckeler, W., Raschke, W., Riblet, R.
        and Weigert, M., The Immune System: Genes, Receptors,
        Signals, 28pp. (Academic Press, N.Y., 1974).

ULTRASTRUCTURE OF HAGFISH BLOOD LEUCOCYTES

D. Scott Linthicum

Department of Biology, UC San Diego

La Jolla, California   92037

INTRODUCTION

Ostracoderms were the first fishes to emerge from the primordial ooze during the Devonian and Silurian periods of the Paleozoic era, over 400 million years ago. These ancient armoured fishes are now extinct, but their direct decendents, hagfishes and lampreys, still persist throughout much of the aquatic world. Hagfishes are Agnathan cyclostomes and possess numerous primitive physiologic and morphologic traits. Phylogenetically they are considered to be the lowest living vertebrate. Because of their pre-historic lineage and primitive characteristics, hagfishes probably represent an important stage in the early evolution of advanced fishes and higher vertebrates. An evaluation of their immunologic repertoire may elucidate the early development of immune responsiveness of higher vertebrates. Futhermore, hagfishes which are notochordates represent an important transition between the protochrodates and the true vertebrates may possess immunologic mechanisms common to both groups.

Early attempts by Papermaster and co-workers (1) to demonstrate specifically induced immunity in hagfishes were unsuccessful. However, later studies by Hildemann and Thoenes (2) clearly demonstrated that hagfish had the capacity to recognize and reject skin allografts. A sequalae of specific inflammatory reactions, consisting of lymphocyte infiltration, capillary hemorrhage and pigment cell destruction, was observed in rejecting allografts. Chronic rejection was characteristic, but accelerated second-set or repeat allograft rejection revealed the persistance of specific immunologic memory. With ·appropriate antigens, long-term experiments and warm water temperatures (18°C) hagfish can be stimulated to produce specific serum

antibodies to both soluble and cellular antigens.   High titers of macroglobulin
antibodies were evoked against key-hole limpet hemocyanin as demonstrated
by immunodiffusion and passive hemagglutination (3).   Repeated immunizations
against sheep erythrocytes induced high titers of specific hemagglutinating
serum antibodies (4).   Immunoelectrophoretic and chromatographic analyses
of the antisera suggested that the antibodies belonged to the slow-γ or IgM
class.   An elegant account of recent investigations on the structure of hagfish
immunoglobulin is presented by De Ioannes and Hildemann elsewhere in this
volume.

Since hagfish clearly possess the capacity to reject foreign skin grafts and
produce serum antibodies to soluble and cellular antigens, much interest in
the development of the lymphoid cells responsible for these reactions has been
generated. It has generally been considered that hagfish do not possess a
thymus gland, but Riviere et al (5) have discovered phagocytic and antigen-
reactive cells associated with the pharyngeal muscles. They postulate that
these cells may represent a protothymus or precursor of a thymus in higher
vertebrates.

Hagfish lack bone marrow and a discrete spleen, but they have specialized
hemocytopoietic tissue in the submucosa of the gut tract which appears to
carry out both myeloid and lymphoid cell development. Diffuse perivascular
islets are comprised of myeloblasts, lymphohemoblasts and megakaryoblasts.
Jordan and Speidel (6) examined hagfish blood with the light microscope
and found that hagfish, unlike higher vertebrates, have circulating hemoblasts
which differentiate into several blood cell types. In addition, several types
of leucocytes were described on the basis of their light microscopic appearance
and staining characteristics. Hitherto, the electron microscopic morphologies
of the blood leucocytes have not been described and in this paper some ultrastructural aspects of blood granulocytes, monocytes and lymphocytes of the
Pacific hagfish, Eptatretus stoutii, are presented.

GRANULOCYTES

Granulocytes (7-9 μm in diameter) make up the majority (50%) of the blood
leucocyte population. In the buffy-coat there are a variety of granular cell
morphologies which probably represent various stages of maturation. These
cells appear to be analogous with the myeloid series described in mammals.

Immature granulocytes or promyelocytes appear to have a central nucleus
which lacks distinct lobes (Fig.1). These cells probably develop from the
myeloblasts in the hemocytopoietic tissues (7). Their nuclear chromatin
pattern is a mixture of heterochromatin and loose euchromatin, but the latter

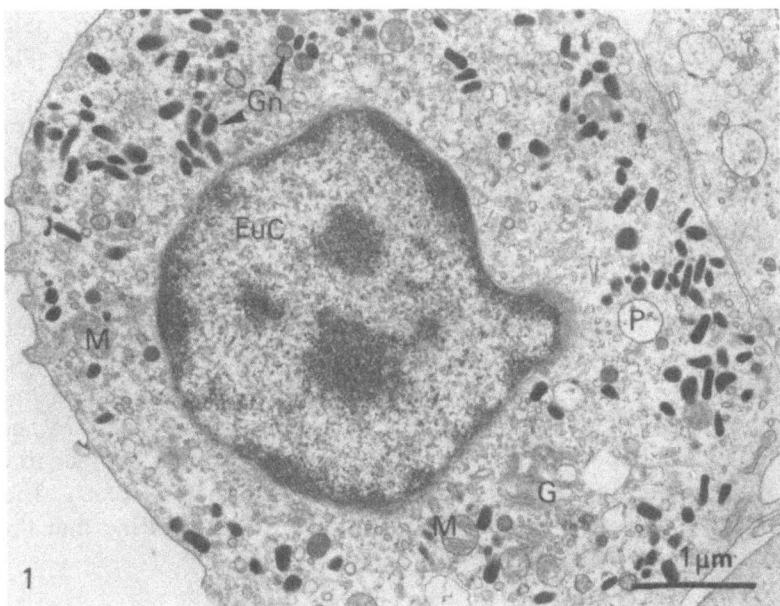

Fig. 1   Immature granulocytes have a non-segmented nucleus in which euchromatin (EuC) predominates. Extensive mitocohondria (M), golgi vesicles (G),
phagocytic vacuoles (P) and polymorphic granules (Gn) are prominant.

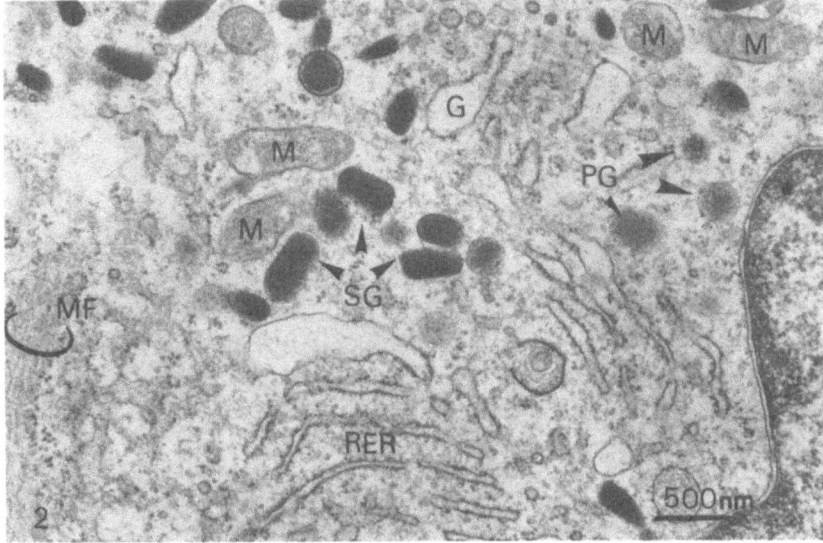

Fig. 2   In the cytosol of the immature granulocytes primary granules (PG)
and secondary granules (SG) are numerous. Rough endoplasmic reticulum (RER),
golgi vesicles (G), mitochodria (M) and microfilaments (MF) are also visible.

predominates, suggesting that there is much nuclear activity. The cytoplasm of these cells is filled with a variety of organelles. Mitochondria, golgi vesicles, and cisterna of rough endoplasmic reticulum are abundant (Fig.2). The most conspicious feature is the presence of osmiphilic granules which are generally contained within a limiting membrane. Several stages of granule development are evident. Primary granules tend to be large and round, while secondary granules are much denser and cylindrical or rod-shaped; some 2° granules present with a dumb-bell shaped configuration. In addition, phago-cytic vacuoles and secondary lysosomal or residual bodies are also present.

The metamyelocytes and granulocytes undergo final maturation in the blood. The nucleus takes on a lobed or kidney shape and occupies an excentric position in the cytoplasm. As the cells reach maturity the lobing of the nucleus becomes more complex. Nuclei with two or three lobes are common and more bizzare shapes are rare. In the granulocytes, the nuclear to cyto-plasmic ratio is greatly decreased compared to the immature forms. The heterochromatin pattern becomes much denser (Fig 3) suggesting that there is less nuclear activity.

Within the cytoplasm of the granulocytes, the once abundant organelles observed in the precursors become scarce. Few mitochondria, golgi vesicles and segments of rough endoplasmic reticulum are observed. The secondary granules increase in number and become the predominate feature. Futher differentiation of this cell type is not observed. Cells with coarse granular or crystalline-filled granules, exemplified by basophilic and eosinophilic granulocytes respectively, are not observed in these preparations. All of the granulocytes observed have the general morphology which is consistant with the neutrophilic granulocyte series of higher vertebrates.

MONOCYTES

By far the most unusual cells among the hagfish leucocytes are those which appear to be monocytes or blood macrophages. These cells, usually 6-9 μm in diameter, have a bi-lobed or W-shaped nucleus (Fig. 4). The nuclear pattern is generally heterochromatic, but areas of euchromatin and nuclear pores are readily visible. The golgi apparatus is well developed in these cells. The cytoplasm contains small numbers of mitochondria and cisterna of rough endoplasmic reticulum.

The distinctive feature of the monocyte cytoplasm is the presence of azur-philic granules. Most of these vesicles appear to be primary lysosomes, which on contact with phagocytic vacuoles probably form secondary lysosomal bodies.

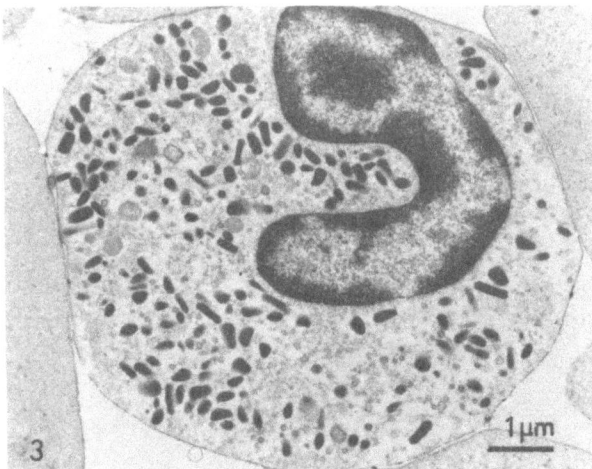

Fig.3   In mature granulocytes the nucleus takes on a lobed or segmented
appearance and the cytoplasm is almost exclusively filled with granules.

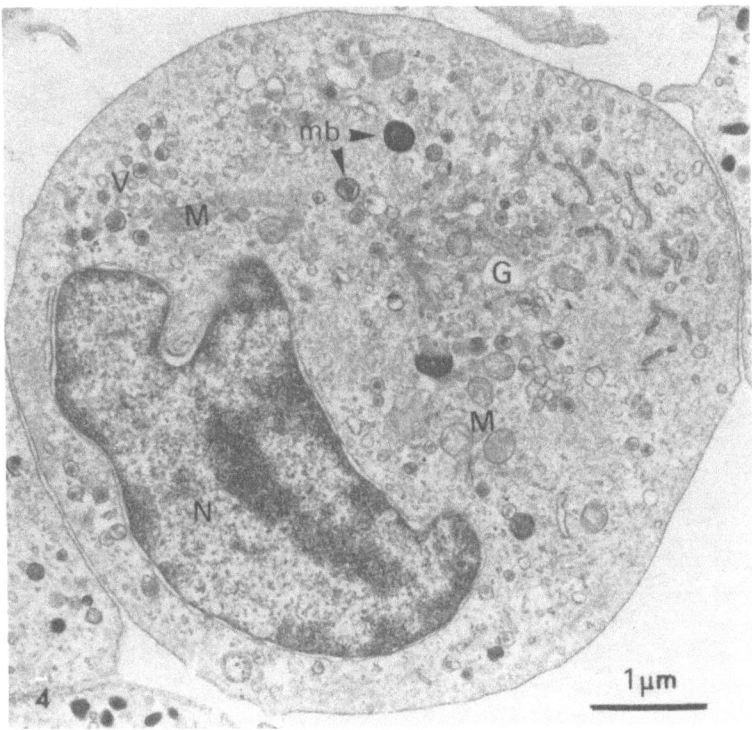

Fig. 4   Monocytes generally have a bilobed or W–shaped nucleus (N). In
addition to numerous lysosomal vesicles (V) , myelin bodies (mb) are most
conspicious. A well developed golgi (G) and mitochondria (M) are visible.

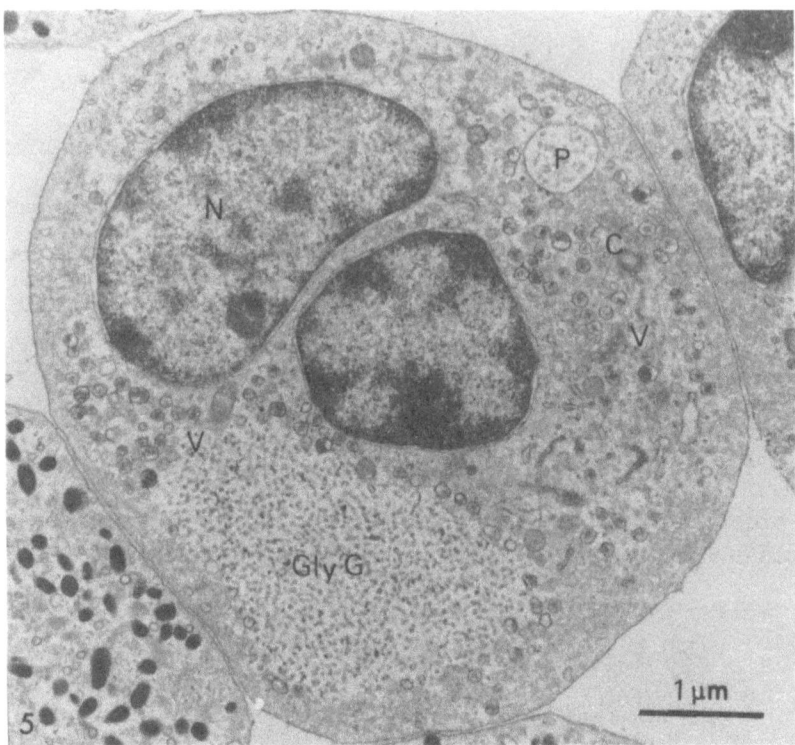

Fig. 5   Some monocytes have numerous glycogen granules (GlyG) localized
in the cytoplasm.   These may be a product of the phagocytic vacuoles (P) and
the secondary lysosomal vesicles (V).   A centriole (C) is visible in this cell.

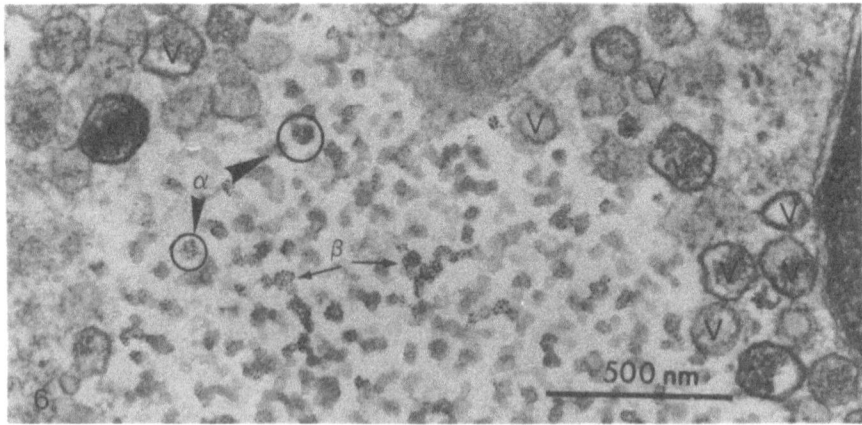

Fig. 6   The glygogen granules in the cytoplasm of the monocyte appear to
be the exudate of the lysosomal vesicles (V).   Large α particles (arrow-circle)
are made up of smaller β subunits (small arrows).

The secondary lysosomes which are membrane limited, appear as vesicles which are completely or partially filled with a dark-granular material. In some cells a good portion of the cytoplasm is occupied by a loose clustering of small (50nm) granules (Fig.5). The granules are free within the cytoplasm and are not encapsulated by an intracytoplasmic membrane. The granules appear to be the exudate of the secondary lysosomes. At high magnifications (Fig.6) these granules have the appearance of a glycogen particles (500 $\overset{\circ}{A}$) which are aggregates of smaller β particles (100 $\overset{\circ}{A}$).

LYMPHOCYTES

Some cells in the blood have the general morphological characteristics of the mammalian small lymphocytes. These cells are usually 5-6 μm in diameter and comprise approximately 15% of the buffy-coat. They are characterized by a large central nucleus (Fig.7). In some cells a nuclear cleft (Fig.8) or invagination is visible. The nucleus is generally stippled with clumps of heterochromatin; a general display of heterochromatin dominates the circumference of the nucleus, but small channels of euchromatin and nuclear pores are distinct. Often a dark staining nucleolus is visible but two nucleoli are rarely observed.

The cytoplasm of the small lymphocytes are typical of those observed in higher forms in that it is essentially devoid of extensive ogranelles. There are few mitochondria, polyribosomes or golgi vesicles; monoribosomes appear in great abundance. Some cells have several short segments of rough endoplasmic reticulum. Pinocytoic vesicles appear in the cytoplasm of most cells, but larger phagocytic vacuoles and secondary lysosomes are not visible.

Large lymphocytes, proplasmablasts and mature plasma cells were not identified in these preparations. There are some large lymphoid-like hemocytoblasts present in the blood, but these believed to be erythroblast precursors and have little resemblance to the lymphoblasts observed in higher vertebrates (6).

FINAL COMMENTS

From a phylogenetic viewpoint, hagfishes represent the lowest group in which specialized blood forming tissues are present. In the cephalochorda (amphioxus) no erythrocytes are found. Hagfish have scattered islets of hemocytopoietic tissue which carry out blood cell development; lampreys have aggregates of hemopoietic tissue localized at the spiral valve. In higher fishes, such as the African lungfish (Dipnoi) the spleen is distinctly segregated

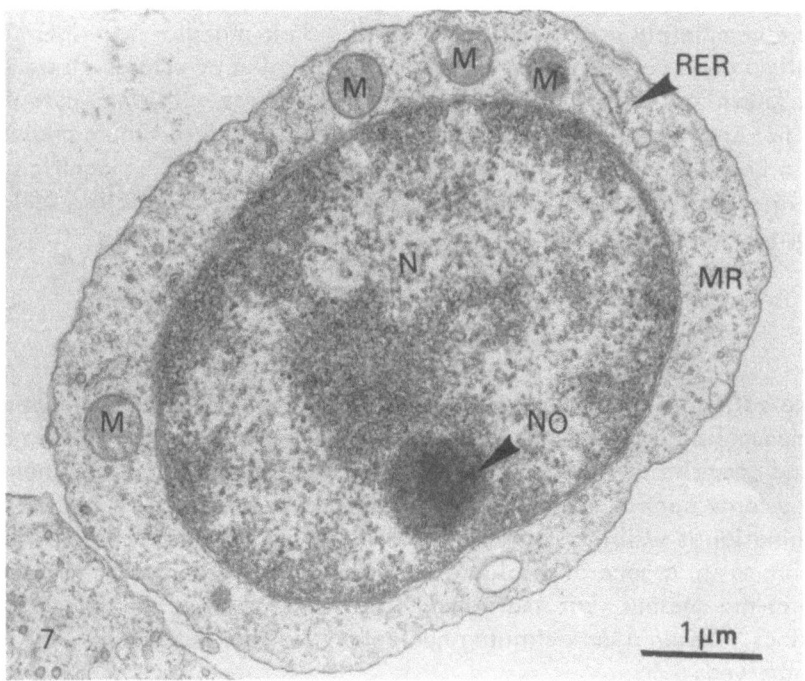

Fig. 7   Small lymphocytes are devoid of elaborate organelles. In the cytoplasm, mitochondria (M), monoribosomes (MR) and short cisterna of rough
endoplasmic reticulum (RER) are the major features. The nucleus (N) contains
much heterochromatin and sometimes distinct nucleoli (NO) are visible.

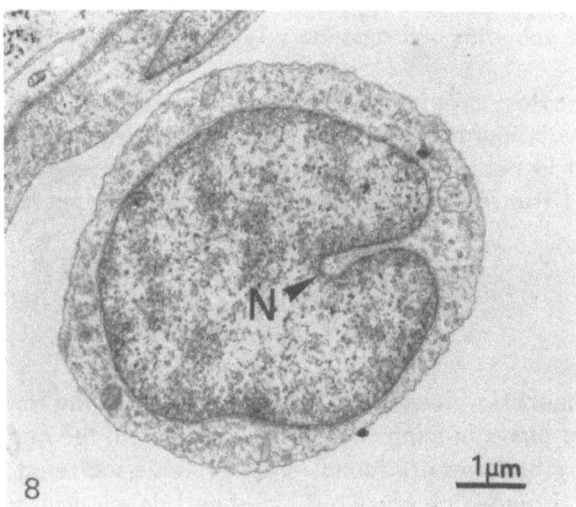

Fig. 8   Some small lymphocytes display a nuclear cleft (N, arrow).

in the stomach wall. Finally, in the sharks (Elasmobranchii) the spleen leaves
the gut tract and becomes a separate organ in the peritoneal vault. Along
with this apparent organ specialization, cellular specialization has also been
accomplished.

In hagfish blood there are a variety of complex and specialized cells.
Among these are several types of leucocytes which appear to be, at the very
least, prototypes for more advanced and sophisticated forms in higher vertebrates. Hagfish have numerous granulocytes which appear to be morphologically consistant with the neutrophilic granulocyte series of mammals. These
cells stem from the myeloid tissue of the gut tract (7). Most of the granulocytes lack extensive nuclear lobing or segmentation seen in mammalian
analogs. Extensive diversification of granulocyte granules such as those
seen in eosinophils or basophils are not observed in this species. However,
eosinophils have been reported for higher fishes (8). These granulocytes
probably represent a primitive neutrophil series.

With regard to phagocytes, hagfish have well differentiated blood monocytes or macrophages. These cells appear similar to those observed in mammals
but generally lack the extensive organelles. The presence of numerous cyto-
plasmic inclusions suggests that these cells are very active with respect to
phagocytosis. The presence of glycogen granules as lysosomal or digestive
by-products are observed in the phagocytes of many species. Even in
molluscan granulocytes, intracytoplasmic glycogen granules are the results
of bacterial phagocytosis and digestion (9).

Hagfish blood contains small lymphocytes which are very similar to
mammalian small lymphocytes. The origin of these cells is unknown, but they
probably stem from the small lymphoblasts in the gut tract or from the pronephros which has been reported to be lymphopoietic (10). Futhermore, the
fate or futher differentiation of these small lymphocytes is not clear. It may
be that these cells are an end-stage. Perhaps differentiated lymphoid forms
such as plasma cells are not observed in the blood because they are removed
from the blood and home to special tissues, the locations of which are unknown.
But the apparent absence of plasma cells is not surprising in that hagfish appear
to make only one type of immunoglobulin (IgM?) and this response tends to
be rather sluggish. In lampreys, which are also capable of making specific
immunoglobulin, plasma cells have not been found (8). Only in the higher
fishes which give vigorous responses, such as the paddlefish (Chondrostei)
are plasma cells detectable (8). However, this may be of little significance
in view of the fact that in teleosts a wide spectrum of mammalian-like cell
types, some of which are not morphologically consistant with the plasma cell,
are clearly capable of producing antibodies to sheep erythrocytes (11).
Perhaps well differentiated plasma cells are not required by these primitive

fishes. Along with a system of highly developed effector cells (monocytes and granulocytes) small lymphocytes capable of producing antibody by secretion and/or shedding may be sufficient to mediate immunocompetence at this level. The possibilities of surface immunoglobulin and/or specific antigen receptors on the surface of these small lymphocytes invite futher studies.

The author is deeply grateful to Mrs. Dianne Bass for technical assistance, Dr. L. Reddy (UCLA) for additional tissue specimens and Dr. C. Hubbs for providing marine aquaria (SIO). The author also thanks Drs. S. Sell and J. Mendelsohn for reviewing the manuscript. Special thanks goes to Dr. W. H. Hildemann for continious support, encouragment and contagious enthusiasm. This work was supported by a NSF grant (AI-11780) and the author is supported by USPHS Predoctoral Training grant AI-00453-03.

REFERENCES

(1) Papermaster, B.W., Condie, R.M., Finstad, J. and Good, R. A., J. Exp. Med., 119:105 (1964)

(2) Hildemann, W.H., and Thoenes, G.H., Transplantation, 7:506 (1969)

(3) Thoenes, G.H. and Hildemann, W.H., in Developmental Aspects of Antibody Formation and Structure, Czechoslavakian Academy of Sci, 170 (1969)

(4) Linthicum, D.S. and Hildemann, W.H., J. Immunol., 105:912 (1970)

(5) Riviere, H.B., Cooper, E.L., Reddy, A.L. and Hildemann, W.H., Am. Zool. 15:39 (1975)

(6) Jordan, H.E. and Speidel, C.C., Am.J. Anat., 46:355 (1930)

(7) Linthicum, D.S., ms in preparation

(8) Finstad, J., Papermaster, B.W., and Good, R.A., Lab Invest., 13:490 (1964)

(9) Cheng, T.C. and Cali, A., In (E. Cooper ed.) Contemporary Topics in Immunobiology, Vol 4 (Invertebrate Immunol.) p 25, Plenum Press, N.Y. (1974)

(10) Willmer, E.N., Cytology and Evolution, Academic Press, N.Y. (1960)

(11) Chiller, J.M., Hodgins, H.O., Chambers, V.C. and Weiser, R.S., J. Immunol. 102:1193 (1969)

CELL SURFACE IMMUNOGLOBULINS OF THYMUS AND SPLEEN LYMPHOCYTES

IN URODELE AMPHIBIAN PLEURODELES WALTLII (SALAMANDRIDAE)

Jacques Charlemagne and Annick Tournefier

Université Pierre et Marie Curie, 75230 Paris, France

Laboratoire de Biologie animale 2, 9 Quai Saint Bernard

Immunoglobulins associated with the surface of lymphocytes were first described in mammals (1,2,3) and then extensively studied. These membrane immunoglobulins are of special importance for the search for recognition mechanisms and cellular cooperation during the immune response. Mammalian B lymphocytes are known to carry membrane Ig; on the other hand, these molecules are not detected on T lymphocytes using classic immunofluorescence techniques except in some cases (4). More sophisticated techniques have to be used in this case, and the data are still conflicting (5,6). Nevertheless, the presence of Ig-like molecules on mammalian thymocytes seems to have been confirmed (7,8).

In an anuran amphibian, Xenopus laevis (9) and a teleostean fish, Cyprinus carpio (10), membrane-associated Ig have been described on thymocytes by indirect immunofluorescence (IF) techniques. The urodele amphibian Pleurodeles waltlii immunized with sheep red blood cells and Salmonella antigens synthesizes an 18.2 S mercaptoethanol-sensitive antibody which is an IgM-like Ig (11,12). In this work we studied membrane-associated IgM on Pleurodeles splenocytes and thymocytes.

MATERIAL AND METHODS

Animals. Pleurodeles of the A and B histocompatible strains (13) bred as previously described (12) were used. Stage 55a (14) larvae and 4 month-old metamorphosed juveniles were checked for their membrane Ig both on their thymus and splenic cells, and splenic cells only were used for adults.

Cells. Spleens and thymuses were taken from anesthesized
animals (MS 222 SANDOZ), manually dispersed in cold BSA-PBS (amphibian phosphate buffer saline with 1% Bovine Serum Albumin), and
washed 3 times by centrifugation in cold BSA-BPS.

Sera. A pure Pleurodeles IgM fraction was obtained by preparative starch-gel electrophoresis of the crude serum. Anti-Pleurodeles
IgM (anti-Pl IgM) was raised in two rabbits by injections of this
starch-gel fraction and by immunoelectrophoresis. Only one precipitating arc against crude Pleurodeles serum was formed. Before use,
these anti-Pl IgM sera were heat-inactivated and absorbed 1 hour
(v/v) with washed packed Pleurodeles erythrocytes and diluted 1:10
or 1:1000. Goat anti-rabbit FITC (fluorescein isothiocyanate)
conjugated serum (MILES: IgG FITC-conjugated goat anti-rabbit IgG)
was heat-inactivated and absorbed with Pleurodeles erythrocytes
before use in a 1:5 to 1:20 dilution.

Indirect immunofluorescence. Incubations were always performed
in the cold. Cells first were incubated 20 min. with anti-Pl IgM.
They were washed 3 times in BSA-PBS, incubated 20 min. with FITC-
conjugated serum, and washed 3 times in BSA-PBS. Cell suspensions
were observed in a Leitz microscope (Orthoplan) with an Osram HBO-200
mercury arc lamp and a Leitz vertical illuminator. FITC fluorescence
was detected with the appropriate filter combination. The percentage
of Ig-positive lymphocytes was determined by alternately examining
the same fields in specific illumination and in phase-contrast light.
Microphotographs were taken with an Orthomat camera and Kodak Tri-X
films using 2 min. exposure times. Four sets of controls were made:
(1) incubation with anti-Pl IgM omitted; (2) anti-Pl IgM substituted
by normal rabbit serum or rabbit anti-BSA serum (Difco); (3) lymphoid
cells substituted by brain cells; (4) inhibition of fluorescence by
incubating the cells in unconjugated anti-rabbit Ig serum and then
in FITC-conjugated serum.

RESULTS

Spleen Cells

With the 1:1000 diluted rabbit anti-Pl IgM, 65 ± 5% of the
splenic lymphocytes exhibited membrane fluorescence, and 35 ± 5%
were unlabeled. Morphologically, fluorescent-positive cells appeared
to possess variable shaped nuclei and a spread cytoplasm with at
least one elongated uropod at the end of which an active capping
occurred. On the other hand, the great majority of fluorescent-
negative cells were still round, spherical, with unspread cytoplasms
and no uropods. With a less diluted (1:10) rabbit anti-Pl IgM, 65%
of the spleen cells were still highly positive and it was then
possible to notice a discrete patchy fluorescence on 20% of the
previously unlabeled round lymphocytes. Nevertheless, 8 to 10% of
the splenic lymphocytes remained negative in this case.

Thrombocytes and small lymphocytes had approximately the same aspect and were difficult to discriminate in unfixed preparations. In IF, the thrombocytes were easily discriminated from the lymphocytes population by a non-specific, diffuse and general autofluorescence always present in their cytoplasms and nuclei.

Thymus Cells

With the 1:1000 anti-Pl IgM dilution, a slight patchy membrane fluorescence was seen in almost 98% of the cells. With the 1:10 dilution, some differences were observed in fluorescence intensity and repartition related to the three morphological types of lympho-cytes: small, medium and large (Figs. 1 and 2).

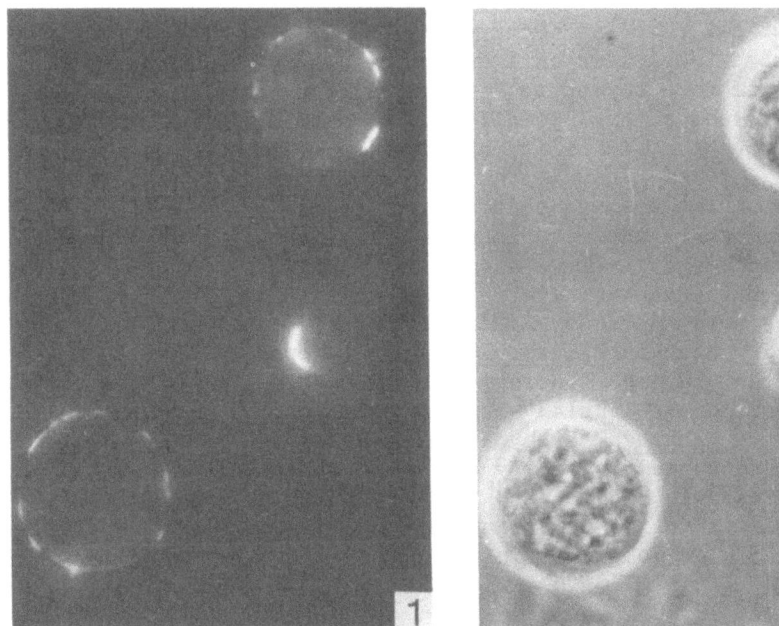

Fig. 1. Thymus lymphocytes labeled with rabbit anti-Pl IgM serum diluted 1:10 and FITC-conjugated goat anti-rabbit IgG.

Fig. 2. Same field as Fig. 1 observed in phase-contrast illumination.

The small lymphocytes (60%) exhibited a strong membrane IF
gathered in large and numerous spots turning to a bright cap at one
pole of the cell. The medium lymphocytes (30%) showed few large
spots and a slight patchy membrane IF. The large lymphocytes (10%)
exhibited few spots or not, and a slight uniform patchy fluorescence.
When these three types of lymphocytes were incubated 10 min. at 37°C,
capping occurred only on small and medium lymphocytes.

DISCUSSION

A "classical" and high percentage of membrane fluorescent
lymphocytes was found in larvae, juveniles and adults splenic
Pleurodeles lymphocytes. The use of two different dilutions (1:10
and 1:1000) of rabbit anti-Pl IgM allowed us to notice two distinct
populations: a lymphocyte population with widely spread cytoplasm
and uropod brightly labeled and another lymphocyte population with
round spherical nucleus and cytoplasm slightly labeled by patched
spots looking very much like thymic lympocytes.

A slight membrane fluorescence was also noticed on the whole
thymic population. Capping occurred in small and medium thymic
lymphocytes with the lowest anti-Pl IgM dilution. In mammals,
detection of membrane thymocyte Ig by this IF technique (4) needs
special filters and a very low dilution of anti-Ig serum of strong
titers to improve the visibility of labeling.

It is important to note that Pleurodeles lymphocytes are larger
than mammalian ones: their surface is approximately 10-fold larger
than mouse lymphocytes. If we assume that Ig molecules have approximately the same surface density on thymic cells in these two species,
they should be more numerous and easily detected in Pleurodeles
thymocytes. In fact, in Pleurodeles as in Xenopus (9) thymus
lymphocytes are much less fluorescent than spleen lymphocytes but
nevertheless obviously labeled with the classical IF technique.
The fact that in Pleurodeles thymic lymphocytes are much less
fluorescent than splenic ones may be due to the embedding of the
antigenic Ig molecule determinant in the thymocyte membrane and its
poor accessibility to the rabbit antibodies or because there are
fewer immunoglobulin molecules in thymocytes than there are in
splenocytes.

Actually various tests are performed on thymectomized Pleurodeles
to determine the thymic dependence of the spherical lymphocytes
slightly labeled in the spleen. If such is the case, the presence
of B and T lymphocytes in urodele spleen, as in mammals, may be
confirmed.

REFERENCES

1. Pernis, B., Forni, L. and Amante, L., J. Exp. Med., 132:
   1001 (1970).

2. Raff, M. C., Stenberg, M. and Taylor, R. B., Nature,
   225: 553 (1970).

3. Greaves, M. F., Transplant Rev., 5: 45 (1970).

4. Santana, V., Wedderburn, N. and Turk, J. L., Immunology,
   27: 65 (1974).

5. Marchalonis, J. J., Cone, R. E. and Atwell, J. L.,
   J. Exp. Med., 135: 956 (1972).

6. Vitteta, E. S., Bianco, C., Nussenzweig, V. and Uhr, J. W.,
   J. Exp. Med., 136: 81 (1972).

7. Roelants, G. E., Rydén, A., Hagg, L. B. and Loor, F.,
   Nature, 274: 106 (1974).

8. Moroz, C. and Hahn, Y., Proc. Nat. Acad. Sci. (Wach.),
   70: 3716 (1973).

9. Du Pasquier, L., Weiss, N. and Loor, F., Europ. J. Immunol.,
   2: 366 (1972).

10. Emmrich, F., Richter, R. F. and Ambrosius, H., Europ. J.
    Immunol., 5: 76 (1972).

11. Tournefier, A., Ann. Immunol. (Inst. Pasteur), 125C:
    637 (1974).

12. Tournefier, A., Immunology, 28 (1975), in press.

13. Charlemagne, J. and Tournefier, A., J. Immunogenet. 1:
    125 (1974).

14. Gallien, L. and Durocher, M., Bull. Biol. France et Belgique,
    91: 97 (1957).

STRUCTURE AND IMMUNOLOGICAL FUNCTION OF LYMPHOMYELOID

ORGANS IN THE BULLFROG, RANA CATESBEIANA*§

Y. Minagawa,** K. Ohnishi, and S. Murakawa

Department of Biology, Faculty of Science,

Niigata University, Niigata, 950-21, Japan

Anuran amphibians have long been known to have unique lymphoid organs in the branchial region, such as jugular body (ventraler Kiemenrest)(JB), propericardial body (corpus properi-cardiale)(PPCB) and procoracoid body (corpus procoracoideum)(PCB) (1,2). Recently, antibody-producing cells and/or plasma cells have been demonstrated in these unique organs, thymus, and bone marrow, as well as in the spleen and kidney (3-10). Accordingly, the respective role of anuran lymphomyeloid (LM) organs in the immune response seems to be considerably different from that of mammalian counterparts. The present report deals with histological structure and immunological function of bullfrog LM organs with special reference to antibody-producing sites and lymphocyte-proliferating sites.

MATERIALS AND METHODS

Animals. For histological research, both sexes of adult bull-frogs, Rana catesbeiana, weighing 200 to 500 g, were collected from Osaka or Niigata district of Japan in January or October, respectively. They were maintained in running water at 15 to 17°C, fed with pig kidneys, and used for experiments after acclimated to 25°C for one week or longer. Animals, weighing 250 to 350 g, for the study

* Communications should be addressed to K. O.
§ This work was partly carried out by K.O. at Lab. of Developmental Biology, Dept. of Zoology, Faculty of Science, University of Kyoto, Kyoto, Japan.
** Present address: Dept. of Oral Pathology (Prof. M. Katagiri), Nippon Dental College, Niigata, 951, Japan.

Table I   PFC response in bullfrog LM organs

No. of SRBC injected	Day	LM organs*	Cells per plate (X 10^5)	PFC per plate	PFC per 10^6 cells
None	--	JB	50.5	0, 0, 0	0.0
"	--	**(JB	4.1	0, 0	0.0
		{BM	2.3	0, 0	0.0
		(Spl	7.3	0, 0	0.0
4 X 10^9	3.5	(JB	4.1	1, 1, 0	1.5
		(BM	1.4	2, 0, 0	4.8
"	6	(JB	3.0	18, 16, 30	71.0
		(BM	6.6	3, 0, 3, 5	5.6
"	6	(JB	3.55	115, 91, 70	108
		(BM	1.0	8, 6, 8, 4	18
2 X 10^{10}	22	JB	1.1	6, 5	50
4 X 10^{10}	14	(JB	1.46	5	34
		{BM	0.62	3, 8, 1	65
		(Thy	0.5	3	60
4 X 10^9 day 0 & 37	40	(JB	6.8	107, 137, 111	174
		(BM	1.2	0, 1, 0	2.5
"	44	(JB	7.2	8, 6, 8, 7	10
		{BM	4.6	2, 2, 1, 4	4.9
		(Spl	3.56	0, 0, 0, 0	0.0
"	44	(JB	4.2	43, 42, 30	91
		{BM	5.1	34, 33, 48	75
		(Spl	4.1	2, 2, 1, 3	4.9
4 X 10^9, at day 0, 11, & 44	67	(JB	0.65	0, 3, 3	31
		{BM	2.3	4, 4, 3	16
		{Spl	4.5	0, 0	0
		(Thy	0.28	2, 0, 1	36

*   JB: jugular body,   BM: bone marrow,   Spl: spleen,   Thy: thymus.
** Organs grouped by bracket(s) were obtained from the same individual.

of plaque forming cells (PFC), were collected from Osaka district in various seasons. Animals were maintained at 25°C during all experiments.

    Plaque technique. Jerne's technique (11) was employed with the omission of bottom agar layer. For suspending lymphoid cells, Eagle's MEM, diluted to 55% in distilled water, and added with heat-inactivated (52°C for 30 min) bullfrog serum at 5% final concentration, was used. After plating cell suspension, plates were incubated at 25°C for 1 hr, then flooded with 1:5 diluted fresh bullfrog serum, further incubated at 25°C for 30 min, and fixed in 10% formalin-PBS. Plaques with an antibody-forming cell in the center were counted. They were stained with methylgreen and pyronin (MP).

Histological methods. LM organs were fixed in Susa solution
for haematoxylin and eosin (HE) stain, in Helly's solution for MP
stain, and in Bouin's solution for Dominici's staining method. They
were embedded in paraffin and sectioned at 6 μ. For examining hyperimmunized frogs,each animal had weekly received an i.p. injection of 1 ml of 20% SRBC (8 X 10^8 cells) per 60 g body wt for 4 to
10 wks, and was killed 7 days after the last injection. Haemolytic
and haemagglutinating titers of antisera in these immunized animals
detected by Sever's technique (12)(Microtiter: Tominaga Works Ltd.,
Tokyo) at 25°C were 1:32 to 1:256 and 1:8 to 1:32, respectively.
RE system was studied by injecting 0.2 ml of india ink (Merk) per
60 g body wt into dorsal lymph sac 16 or 24 hours before sacrifice.
    Mitotic index (MI). MI was defined as an average number of
mitotic figures per 1,000 nucleated cells other than red cells and
fully matured erythroblasts. To obtain the MI for each organ or
tissue, 3,000 to 66,000 cells were counted in each animal under the
microscope. Preparations stained with HE were used. The results
were statistically analyzed by Youden and Beal's t test (1934) and
by Cochran's t test (1964)(13).

RESULTS

    PFC. The distribution of PFC in the LM organs is shown in
Table I. A marked increase in PFC was seen in both the JB and bone
marrow (femur) one week after SRBC injection, but no marked increase
occurred after the second and third injection. It seemed that PFC
are abundant in the thymus as well as in the JB and bone marrow,
while they are scarce in the spleen. MP stain revealed that PFC are
composed of plasma cells and various types of lymphocytes.
    Histological structure of LM organs. The thymus consists of
cortex and medulla. In the peripheral region of the cortex, large
lymphocytes and mitotic figures are more abundantly found than in
the central cortex (Figs. 1-2). The JB is composed of numerous
lobules of lymphocytes separated by sinusoids lined with reticuloendothelial cells (Figs. 4-6). In the peripheral region of this
body, sinusoids are more or less expanded. Smaller lymphocytes
seems to be more abundant in the inner region than in the peripheral
region. Carbon particles were mainly distributed in the inner region
of the JB, and not or scarcely incorporated in the peripheral region. Therefore, the peripheral region might be tentatively named,
the 'cortical region(CR)' of the JB, and the inner region, the
'medullary region(MR)'. In the inner region, the lymphocytes have a
tendency to crowd more densely arround the arteries, and carbon
particles tend to be more sparsely located in this densely crowded
area than in other areas of the MR (Fig. 6). The MR can be, therefore, further distinguished into the two regions; the true 'medulla'
and the area of periarteriolar lymphoid accumulations. Mitotic
figures were more abundantly found in the CR than in the MR, and

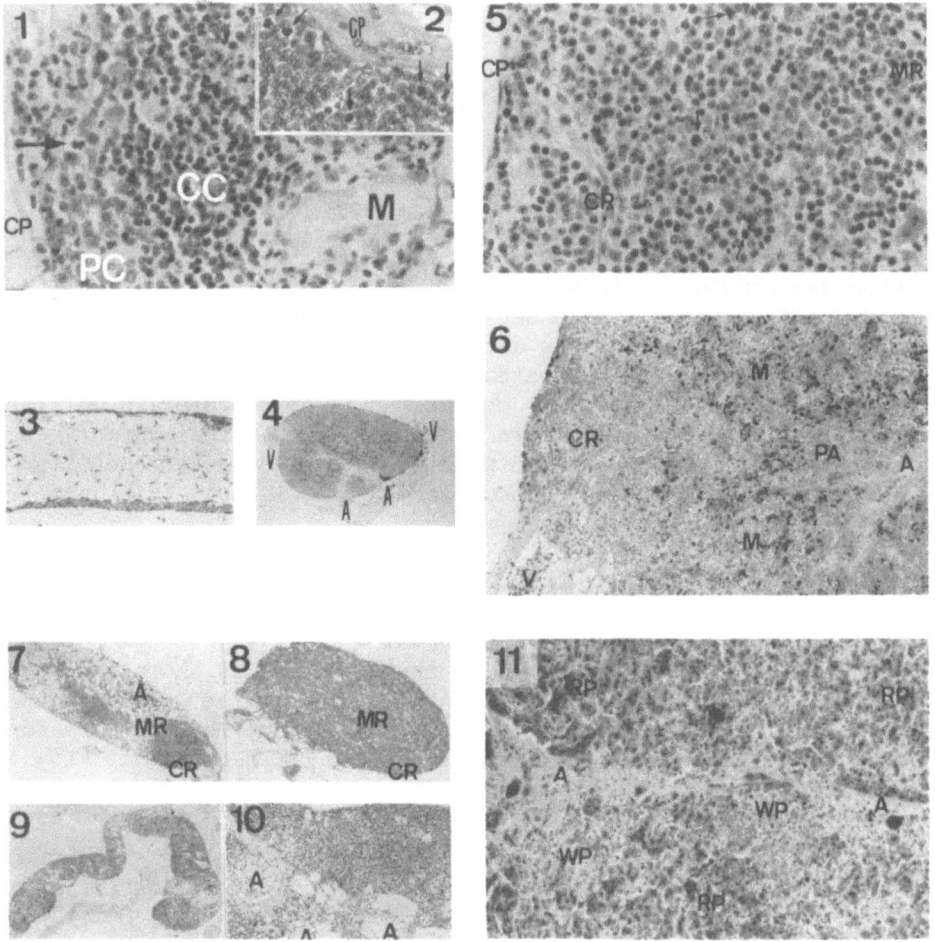

Plate I. Normal structure of bullfrog lymphomyeloid organs

Arrows show mitotic figures. See text for details.
Abbrevations: A=artery, CC=central cortex, CP=capsule, CR=cortical
region, M=medulla, MR=medullary region, PA=periarteriolar lymphoid
accumulation, PC=peripheral cortex, RP=red pulp, V=vein, WP=white
pulp.

Fig.1 Thymic cortex(HE) Fig.2 Thymic peripheral cortex;higher
magnification(HE) Fig.3 Bone marrow(HE) Fig.4 Jugular body;24hrs
after india ink injection(Dominici's stain) Fig.5 Jugular body;
higher magnification(HE) Fig.6 Jugular body;carbon particles
distributed in medulla(Dominici's stain) Figs.7-8 Propericardial
bodies(HE) Fig.9 Procoracoid body(HE) Fig.10 Procoracoid body;
higher magnification(HE) Fig.11 Spleen(Dominici's stain)

further, in the periarteriolar lymphoid accumulations than in the
true 'medulla'. The PPCB is very similar to the JB, except that
adipose tissue is more or less highly developed, especially in the
region corresponding to the MR of the JB (Figs. 7-8). The PCB is
a paired organ situated in the cavity surrounded by the coracoid
and procoracoid, and occupied by lymphoid tissues more or less
accumulated along and **around** arteria coracoclavicularis (Figs. 9-
10). This organ mainly consists of lymphoid tissues resembling
the CR of the JB (Fig. 10). The splenic white pulp is poorly developed, and the spleen is mostly occupied by the red pulp (Fig. 11).
In the bone marrow of the femur, the lymphocytes, granulocytes, and
other types of hemopoietic cells are seen crowded towards the periphery, and the inner area is occupied by adipose tissue (Fig. 3).
Colloidal carbon was incorporated into the spleen and branchial LM
organs, but not into the thymus.

Mitotic indices (MI'es). The MI'es of various LM organs are
summarized in Table II, and the results of statistical tests are
shown in Tables III-IV. To determine the MI'es of the peripheral
and central cortices in the thymus, the cells up to 20 μ deep, and
the cells deeper than 25 μ, respectively, from the surrounding capsules or trabecula of well-developed cortices, were counted. Furthermore, MI'es of the CR and MR of the JB were estimated by counting the cells up to 250 μ deep, and the cells deeper than 500 μ,
respectively, from the capsule covering this organ. Tables II-III
show high lymphocyte-proliferating activity in the thymic cortex,
especially in its peripheral region where the MI was 4.17. An
appreciable difference was demonstrated between MI'es of the CR and
MR in JB; the mitotic activity was higher in the CR than in the MR.
On the other hand, the mitotic activity of the PCB and that of the CR
of the PPCB were very similar to those of the CR in JB. The spleen
showed low mitotic activities in both white and red pulp, and also
in transitional region, whereas the bone marrow showed high activity,
indicating active hemopoiesis. Table IV shows hyperimmunization
significantly increased the MI'es of the JB, whereas no increase was
detected in the spleen and marrow. The mitotic activities in the JB
and thymus were greatly stimulated by india ink-injection.

Pyroninophilic cells. Pyroninophilic cells in various LM
organs consisted of typical plasma cells, large pyroninophilic lymphoid cells with a well-developed nucleolus (PLC) and various types
of lymphocytes. These pyroninophils occurred in both normal and
hyperimmunized states. In the thymic cortex, especially in the
peripheral cortex and in the capsular and trabecular connective
tissues adjacent to the periphery of the cortex, plasma cells and
PLC were contained in a moderate number, while in immunized animals,
a considerable increase in plasma cells were brought about (Fig. 12).
In the CR of JB, there was a marked increase in plasma cells by
immunization, while both plasma cells and PLC were abundant in unimmunized animals (Fig. 13). On the other hand, a considerable number
of PLC and a relatively small number of plasma cells occurred in the

Table II Mitotic indices* of lympho-myeloid organs of normal,
hyperimmunized and colloidal carbon-injected bullfrogs

treatment		Normal	Hyper-immunized[+]	Carbon-injected[++]
No. of animals		8	6	4
Thymus :	Cortex	1.63 ± 1.12** (7-25)***	3.17 ± 1.84 (4-20)	8.30 ± 1.79 (7- 8)
	Peripheral cortex	4.17 ± 3.11 (3-10)	5.50 ± 2.63 (3- 7)	n.d.[+++]
	Central cortex	0.70 ± 0.46 (5-15)	1.48 ± 0.93 (6-14)	n.d.
	Medulla	0.81 ± 0.82 (4-14)	0.68 ± 0.45 (3- 7)	n.d.
Jugular. body :	Total	0.93 ± 0.46 (15-56)	2.36 ± 1.07 (38-66)	2.50 ± 0.46 (10-12)
	Cortical region	1.84 ± 1.01 (6-20)	4.61 ± 3.11 (8-20)	n.d.
	Medullary region	0.54 ± 0.32 (13-30)	1.45 ± 0.47 (20-42)	n.d.
Propericardial body (Cortical region)		1.68 ± 1.16 (9-20)	3.51 ± 1.80 (6-30)	n.d.
Procoracoid body		1.68 ± 1.16 (8-26)	3.51 ± 1.80 (5-11)	n.d.
Bone marrow		3.78 ± 1.58 (6-13)	4.24 ± 2.56 (5-70)	5.36 ± 2.22 (10-15)
Spleen :	Total	0.51 ± 0.29 (23-36)	0.51 ± 0.29 (28-41)	0.51 ± 0.32 (9-16)
	Red pulp	0.44 ± 0.29 (10-18)	0.40 ± 0.37 (12-23)	n.d.
	Transitional region	0.51 ± 0.26 (11-24)	0.48 ± 0.24 (11-22)	n.d.
	White pulp	0.59 ± 0.37 (10-35)	0.96 ± 0.37 (7-20)	n.d.

*   No. of mitotic figures per 1000 cells except red cells.
**   Mean ± sample standard deviation of mitotic indices.
***   Range of the number of cells excluding red cells counted in
      each animal (X 10^3).
[+]   Each animal had weekly received an i.p. injection of 0.2 ml of
      20 % SRBC per 60 g body weight for 4 to 10 weeks, and were
      sacrificed 7 days after the last injection.
[++] Animals were sacrificed 15 or 24 hours after injection of
      0.2 ml of colloidal carbon per 60 g body weight.
[+++] Not done.

Table III Statistical analysis of mitotic indices in Table II
by Youden and Beale's t-test (13): Comparison of LM organs

LM organs compared	P values	
	Normal group	Immunized group*
Thymus : Cortex - Medulla	< 0.0025	< 0.00125
Thymus : Peripheral - Central	< 0.005	< 0.005
Jugular body :		
Cortical region - Medullary region	< 0.025	< 0.025
Thymic cortex - Jugular body	(< 0.10)**	N.S.***
Bone marrow - Thymic cortex	< 0.025	(< 0.10)
Jugular body - Spleen	(< 0.10)	< 0.0125

*   Hyperimmunized against SRBC.   ** Doubtfully significant.
*** Not significant (P > 0.1).

Table IV Statistical analysis of mitotic indices in Table II
by Cochran's t-test (13): Effect of hyperimmunization or
colloidal carbon-injection

LM organs	Comparison	
	A*	B**
Thymus :		
Cortex	(< 0.10)+	< 0.05
Peripheral cortex	N.S.++	n.d.+++
Central cortex	(< 0.10)	n.d.
Jugular body :		
Total	< 0.0025	< 0.0025
Cortical region	< 0.05	n.d.
Medullary region	< 0.01	n.d.
Propericardial body :		
Cortical region	N.S.	n.d.
Procoracoid body	(< 0.10)	n.d.
Bone marrow	N.S.	N.S.
Spleen	N.S.	N.S.

*   A : Effect of hyperimmunization: Comparison of hyperimmunized
    group with normal one.
** B : Effect of colloidal carbon-injection: Comparison of
    Carbon-injected group with normal one.
+ P values: Doubtfully significant cases are parenthesized.
++ Not significant (P > 0.1).   +++ Not done.

MR of JB, but any remarkable change was not produced after repeated
injections of SRBC (Fig. 15). The changes in pyroninophilia of the
PPCB and PCB were nearly identical to those of the JB and the CR of
JB, respectively (Figs. 16-17). However, only occasional occurrence

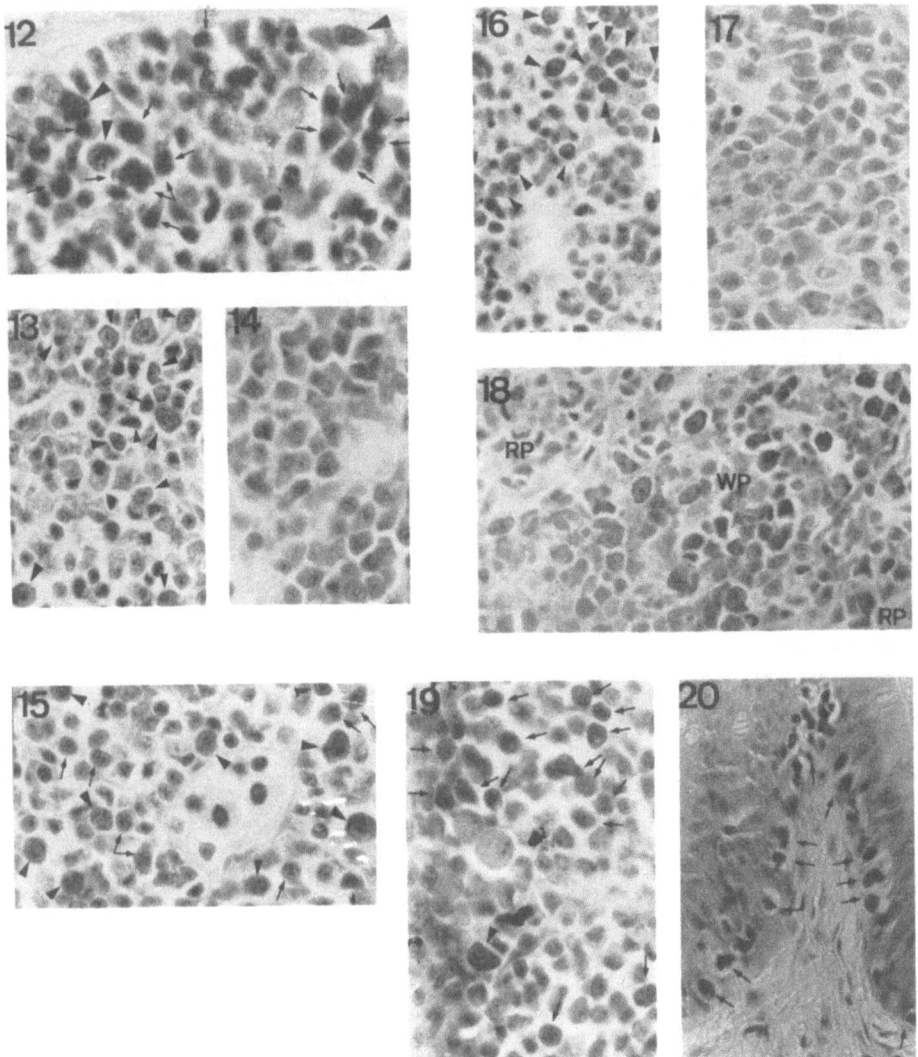

Plate II. Pyroninophilic cells in bullfrog lymphomyeloid organs(MP)

Arrow : plasma cell, Arrowhead : PLC. See text for details.
Abbrevations : (N) = unimmunized, (HI) = hyperimmunized.

Fig.12 Thymic peripheral cortex(HI)   Fig.13 JB;cortical region(N)
Fig.14 JB;cortical region,abundant plasma cells(HI)   Fig.15 JB;
medulla(HI)   Fig.16 PPCB;cortical region(N)   Fig.17 PCB;abundant
plasma cells(HI)   Fig.18 Splenic white pulp;abundant PLC(HI)
Fig.19 Bone marrow(HI)   Fig.20 Pyroninophilic cells in intestinal
lamina propria(HI)

of plasma cells could be demonstrated in the spleen, even if in hyperimmunized animals (Fig. 18). Plasma cells and PLC were also encountered in the bone marrow and lamina propria of the intestine, and plasma cells increased in these tissues by immunization (Figs. 18-19). Nodular accumulations of lymphoid cells were occasionally found in lamina propria, and abundant plasma cells were demonstrated in the nodular structure after repeated antigen injection. Consequently, plasma cells increased in various LM organs by immunization, while PLC did not.

DISCUSSION AND CONCLUSION

Marked increase in plasma cells after hyperimmunization was shown in the branchial lymphoid organs, thymus, and marrow, each of which was demonstrated to contain abundant PFC. The spleen was, however, unusually scarce of both plasma cells and PFC. Active lymphocytopoiesis in the peripheral cortex of thymus observed in the present work might be comparable with the similar observations in mammals (14-17), indicating that the anuran thymus also has a role of central lymphoid organ. The occurrence of PFC and plasma cells in the bullfrog thymus coincides with the observations on PFC and plasma cells in the thymus of the larval bullfrog (10), and on antibody-forming cells in the thymi of adult anurans (18, 5). The diffrences of the outer and inner regions of the JB, which has been indicated by Baculi and Cooper (6), was further studied, and the more complicated structure of this organ has become known. This organ was found to be composed of three different tissue areas: the cortical region, periarteriolar lymphoid accumulations, and 'medulla'. High mitotic activity and marked pyroninophilia in the CR were demonstrated, and the latter agreed with the result of Cowden et al. (19). The present data substantiated the active antibody production in anuran bone marrow which has been recently suggested in the genus Rana (3, 9). The question remains to be solved whether or not anuran bone marrow is a central lymphoid tissue, although active hemopoiesis was shown by a high mitotic activity. The spleen was rather inactive in antibody production in the adult bullfrog; however, it seems to be reasonable to recognize this fact as a specialized character in this species (3), because active antibody production in the spleens of other anurans (5, 8, 9) and larval bullfrogs has been reported (10). Stimulated mitotic activities in carbon-injected bullfrogs demonstrated in this work seem to be related to the enhanced antibody production after carbon injection in toads (20).

In conclusion, increase of PFC and/or plasma cells after hyperimmunization occurred in the thymus and bone marrow as well as in the JB, PPCB and PCB in the bullfrog. The thymus was found to have an architechture of central lymphoid organ from the aspects of lymphocytopoiesis. The JB consisted of the three histologically different areas; cortical region, periarteriolar lymphoid accumulations, and medulla. High mitotic activity and marked pyroninophilia were remarkable in the cortical region of the JB.

ACKNOWLEDGEMENTS

The authors wish to thank Dr. A. Hagiwara for valuable suggestions and kind encouragement during this work. They also acknowlege Dr. Y. Honma for reading the manuscript. They express their thanks to Mrs. J. Nagashima for preparing the manuscript. This work was partly supported by a Scientific Research Grant from Japan Ministry of Education.

LITERATURES

1. Gaup, E., A. Ecker's und R. Wiedersheim's Anatomie des Frosches, 3. Abt., 964 S., Braunschweig, F. Vieweg und Sohn (1904).
2. Braunmühl, A. von, Z. Mikr-Anat. Forsch. 4: 635 (1925).
3. Engle, R.L., Woods, K.R., Biol. Bull. 113: 363 (1957).
4. Kent, S.P., Evans, E.E. and Attleberger, M.H., Proc. Soc. Exp. Biol. Med. 116: 456 (1964).
5. Evans, E.E., Kent, S.P., Bryant, R.E. and Moyer, M., in : Smith, R.T. and Good, R.A. (eds.), Phylogeny of Immunity, p. 218, University of Florida Press, Gainsville, Florida (1966).
6. Baculi, B.S. and Cooper, E.L., J. Morph. 126: 463 (1968).
7. Ohnishi, K., Zool. Mag. 78: 53 (1969)(Abstr.)(in Jap.).
8. Ambrosius, H. and Hanstein, R., Acta Biol. Med. Germ. 27: 771 (1971).
9. Cowden, R.R. and Dyer, R.F., Amer. Zool. 11: 183 (1971).
10. Motiska, E.G., Brown, B.A. and Cooper, E.L., J. Immunol. 110: 855 (1973).
11. Jerne, N.K. and Nordin, A.A., Science, 140: 405 (1963).
12. Sever, J.L., J. Immunol. 88: 320 (1962).
13. Snedecor, G.W. and Cochran, W.G., Statistical Methods, 6th ed., Chapter 4, Iowa State University Press, Ames (1967).
14. Kindred, J.E., Amer. J. Anat. 67: 99 (1940).
15. Kindred, J.E., Amer. J. Anat. 71: 207 (1942).
16. Poste, M.E., and Olson, I.A., Immunology 24: 691 (1973).
17. Clark, S.L., Jr., in : Davies, A.J.S., and Carter, R.L. (eds.), Contemporary Topics in Immunobiology, Vol. 2, pp. 77-100, Plenum Press, New York, N.Y. (1973).
18. Kapa, E., Oláh, I. and Törő, I., Acta Morph. Acad. Sci. Hung. 19: 203 (1968).
19. Cowden, R.R., Gebhardt, B.M. and Volpe, E.P., Z. Zellforsch. 85: 196 (1968).
20. Turner, R.J., J. Reticuloendoth. Soc. 8: 434 (1970).

LYMPHOID ORGANS AND AMPHIBIAN IMMUNITY

Bruce A. Brown, Richard K. Wright, and Edwin L. Cooper

Department of Anatomy, School of Medicine, University of California, Los Angeles, California 90024

INTRODUCTION

Immunological responses are physiological mechanisms which endow an animal with the capacity to recognize foreign materials and to eliminate them. In order to execute the functions of immunity, a ubiquitous cell system has evolved within the verte-brates known as the lymphoreticular system. This collection of cellular elements is distributed strategically throughout the body and housed primarily in various lymphoid organs. Observations on the morphological development of the vertebrate lymphoid system (1) reveals that as one examines the phylogenetic scale from agnathans to birds and mammals, the number, location and diversity of lymphoid organs increases. By analyzing the lymphoid system of primitive vertebrates, one can thus gain answers as to how the immune system of advanced vertebrates evolved.

Amphibians occupy a critical point in the evolution of terrestrial vertebrates, and for this reason recent reviews have focused on the potentialities of their immune system (2, 3, 4). In addition to their phylogenetic position, their larval stages are not confined to an _in utero_ development, they have a prolonged development (relative to birds but not marsupial mammals) and are readily available in the free living state. Thus, they are con-venient models for explaining the ontogeny and phylogeny of the functional components of terrestrial vertebrate immune systems.

LYMPHO-MYELOID ORGANS OF LARVAL RANA CATESBEIANA

The amphibian used in our studies is the larval stage of the

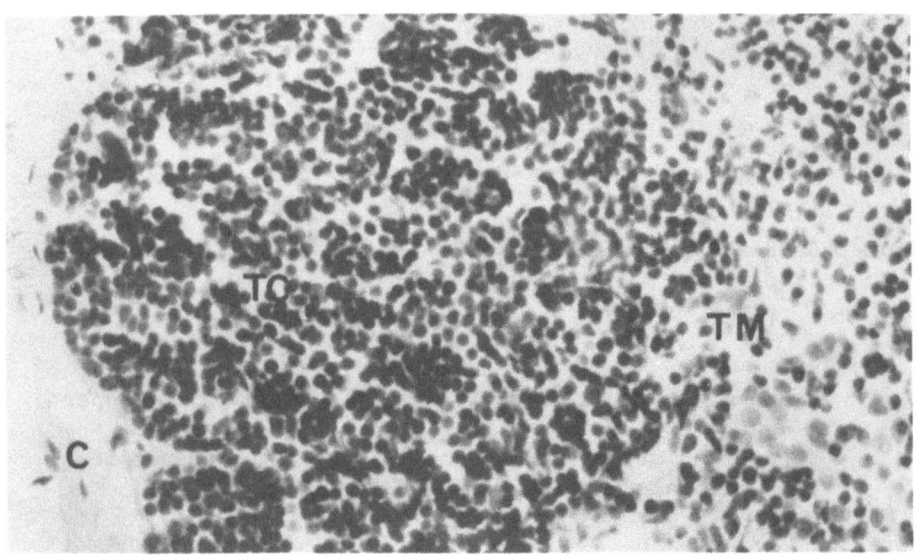

Figure 1.   Tadpole thymus, stage 26.   The loose connective
tissue capsule (C), dense cortical thymocytes (TC) and medullary
region (TM) are visible.

American bullfrog, Rana catesbeiana.   Its lympho-myeloid organs
consist of the thymus, spleen, lymph gland and accumulations of
lymphocytes in the liver, and kidney.   Bone marrow is absent until
after metamorphosis at which time the lymph gland disappears
(5, 6).   The thymus is the first organ to become lymphoid (7)
followed one month later by extra-thymic lymphopoiesis that gives
rise to the spleen and lymph gland (6).

The thymus is a bilateral organ located in the branchial
cavity adherent to the quadrate cartilage (Figure 1).   It is surrounded by a loose fibrous connective tissue capsule containing
blood sinuses and capillaries.   The parenchyma is divided into a
cortex and medulla.   The cortex is characteristically dense due to
its large compact homogeneous population of small lymphocytes.   In
contrast, the medulla appears diffuse, secondary to its sparce
lymphocyte population and numerous epithelial elements.   Swirls of
thymic myoid cells, reminiscent of mammalian Hassall's corpuscles,
are present within the medulla.

The lymph gland is a bilateral structure also located in the
branchial cavity in close association with the gill vasculature
(Figure 2).   It is surrounded by a fibromuscular capsule that contains melanin laden pigment cells and occasional myeloid elements.

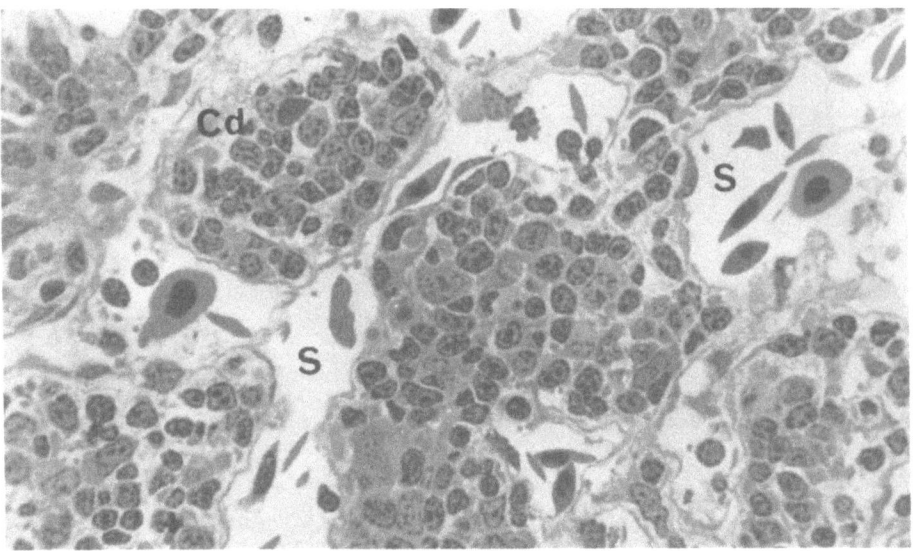

Figure 2. Tadpole lymph gland, stage 26. Multiple sinusoids
(S) surround lymphoid cords (Cd) containing blast cells. Reticuloendothelial cells line the sinusoids. Erythrocytes and lymphocytes
can be seen within the sinusoids, 670x.

The parenchyma is composed of a distinct lymphoid population arranged as cords of lymphocytes separated by sinusoids lined with
phagocytic reticuloendothelial cells. Support for the lymphocytes
within the cords is provided by abundant reticular fibers. Blast
cells are often located centrally in the cords, an arrangement suggesting a germinal center with the more mature cells splayed out
along a maturation gradient from the center to the periphery (8).
Myeloid and erythroid elements are not contained within the
parenchyma.

The spleen is surrounded by a thin capsule which overlies
numerous subcapsular vessels and sinusoids lined by phagocytic
reticuloendothelial cells (Figure 3). Its general appearance is
consistent with a typical lymphomyeloid organ. The parenchyma
contains lymphoid and myeloid elements supported by a stroma composed principally of reticuloendothelial elements (9). White and
red pulp have a characteristic morphologic relationship. The
white pulp, composed of blast cells and lymphocytes in various
stages of maturation, is organized around central arteries and is
supported by a reticulum net. This arrangement becomes more
prominent as larvae mature. The red pulp is composed of sinusoids
and a myriad of hematogenic cell types.

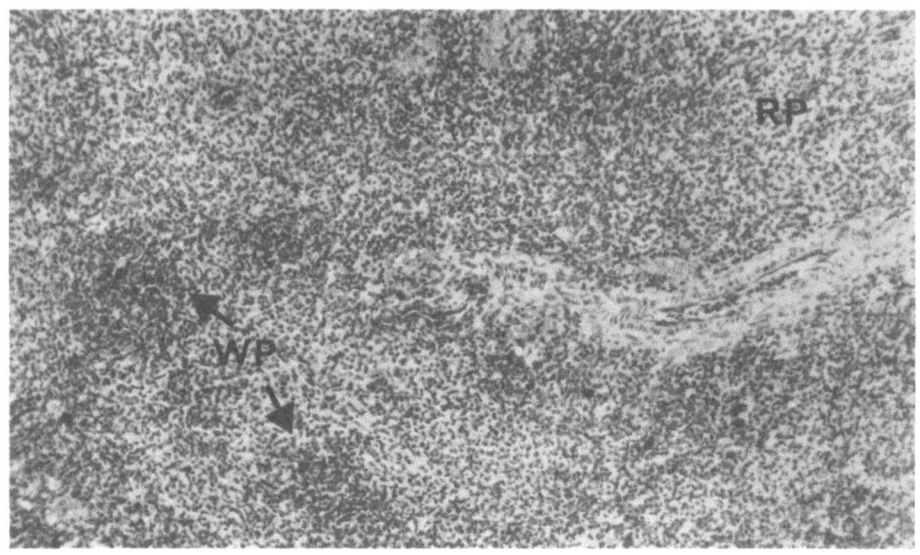

Figure 3. Tadpole spleen, stage 26. Accumulations of white pulp (WP) scattered amid the red pulp (RP) are visible, 165x.

PARAMETERS FOR DETERMINING THE FUNCTION(S)
OF LARVAL LYMPHO-MYELOID ORGANS

Rana catesbeiana larvae become immunologically mature at 30-45 days post hatching and reject orthotopic skin allografts. Later they can synthesize immunoglobulins to a variety of antigens. The thymus exerts its greatest influence on allograft rejection during the first month of larval life (7) and the lymph gland appears to control antibody synthesis (10). Studies aimed at defining the role of each lympho-myeloid organ in 6 month or older larvae have shown that removal of the spleen, lymph gland, or thymus does not affect allograft survival (11). Removal of the lymph gland or spleen however leads to slightly depressed antibody synthesis to sheep erythrocytes (9, 12).

To assess the function(s) of each lympho-myeloid organ more precisely, two experimental approaches have been used: autogeneic and allogeneic reconstitution. Owing to the lack of syngeneic bullfrog larvae, techniques have been developed for the surgical removal of each lympho-myeloid organ (5, 10) and their temporary maintenance in vitro (13). Previous studies from our laboratory have shown that larvae can be rendered immunoincompetent by 1000 R ^{60}Co total body irradiation (TBR) (14). Thus, removal of the lympho-myeloid organ under investigation followed by TBR and re-implantation of the organ (autogeneic reconstitution) allows one to determine the humoral and cellular immune potentials of the organ's cell population. Similarly, irradiation followed by implantation of an organ from an unrelated donor (allogeneic reconstitution) should also allow an evaluation of that organ's immune potential for evoking a graft-versus-host reaction. Using these two procedures, each organ's relative contribution to humoral or cellular immunity can be defined. Three immune parameters have been used in conjunction with autogeneic or allogeneic reconstitution in testing for the function(s) of each lympho-myeloid organ: 1) antibody synthesis to a single subcutaneous injection of sheep erythrocytes (SRBC), 2) orthotopic skin allograft rejection, and 3) graft-versus-host reactions.

AUTOGENEIC RECONSTITUTION STUDIES

The results obtained from our autogeneic reconstitution studies (9, 12, 14, 15) of spleen, lymph gland, or thymus are summarized in Table 1. Spleen and lymph gland reconstituted larvae can mount a humoral immune response to SRBC. Antibody synthesis, however, is delayed by 7-11 days. These results suggest that the spleen and lymph gland are sources of lymphocytes that can differentiate into antibody forming cells after antigenic challenge.

Table 1. Autogeneic Reconstitution, Antibody Synthesis to SRBC, and Skin Allograft Rejection, 25°C, in Bullfrog Larvae 6 months or older.

Reconstituting Organ	Antibody Synthesis to SRBC	Allograft Rejection, MST $\pm$ S.E. (days)[a]
None, controls	Peak titer[b] 5.8; day 10	11.5 $\pm$ 0.5
Spleen	Peak titer 5.0; day 21	>30[c]
Lymph gland	Peak titer 4.0; day 17	24.6 $\pm$ 1.5
Thymus	-ND[d]	>30[c]

[a]Mean survival time $\pm$ standard error; [b]log base 2 reciprocal of last serum dilution showing SRBC agglutination; [c]no signs of rejection during the experimental period; [d]not done.

Additional supporting evidence for this conclusion comes from the fact that readily demonstrable plaque forming cells to sheep erythrocytes occur in the spleen and lymph gland following anti-genic stimulation (16).

In contrast to the ability of the spleen and lymph gland to reconstitute humoral immunity, only the lymph gland can reconsti-tute a cell mediated component of immunity as evidenced by the rejection of skin allografts. Rejection however requires approx-imately twice the time typical of control graft destruction. The prolonged allograft rejection time in lymph gland reconstituted larvae and the delay in antibody synthesis in spleen and lymph gland reconstituted larvae probably reflects the time necessary for emigrating lymphocytes from these organs to repopulate, respond to antigen, and generate a population of immuno-competent cells in the lymphoid organs damaged by irradiation.

ALLOGENEIC RECONSTITUTION STUDIES

When a graft of foreign tissue contains immunologically competent cells, the graft effects an immunological attack against the host, especially if the host is immunologically deficient. This constitutes a graft-versus-host (GVH) reaction. The type of reaction may be localized (14, 17, 18) or it may be systemic, seriously injuring or killing the host (19). Thus, the GVH reaction can be used as another indicator of lymphocyte function.

To determine whether the three major lympho-myeloid organs can elicit a GVH reaction, irradiated larvae were reconstituted with lympho-myeloid organs from allogeneic donors, as summarized in Table 2. The responses to implants were characterized by a localized induration, erythema and edema at the area of reconsti-tution that appeared 5-6 days after implantation (Figure 4). This was followed by ulceration and pigment cell destruction within the skin overlying the organ and then death of the larvae. Of the three organs, only the spleen and lymph gland evoked a localized response. We have not determined if death results from systemic effects.

FUNCTIONS OF LARVAL LYMPHO-MYELOID ORGANS

By means of extripation and in combination with total body irradiation, we have assessed the functional significance of the lympho-myeloid organs of 6 month old pre-metamorphic Rana catesbeiana larvae (Table 3). At least three types of immune reactions can be restored by these organs in immunologically crip-pled larvae: 1) antibody synthesis, 2) allograft rejection, and

Table 2.   Allogeneic Reconstitution Resulting in Graft-Versus-Host Reaction in Bullfrog Larvae 6 months or older.

Allogeneic Organ	GVH Reaction	LD_{50} [a] (days)
None, $1000R^{60}Co$	–	16
Spleen	Yes	12
Lymph gland	Yes	10
Thymus	No	14

[a] Time at which 50% of the larvae were dead.

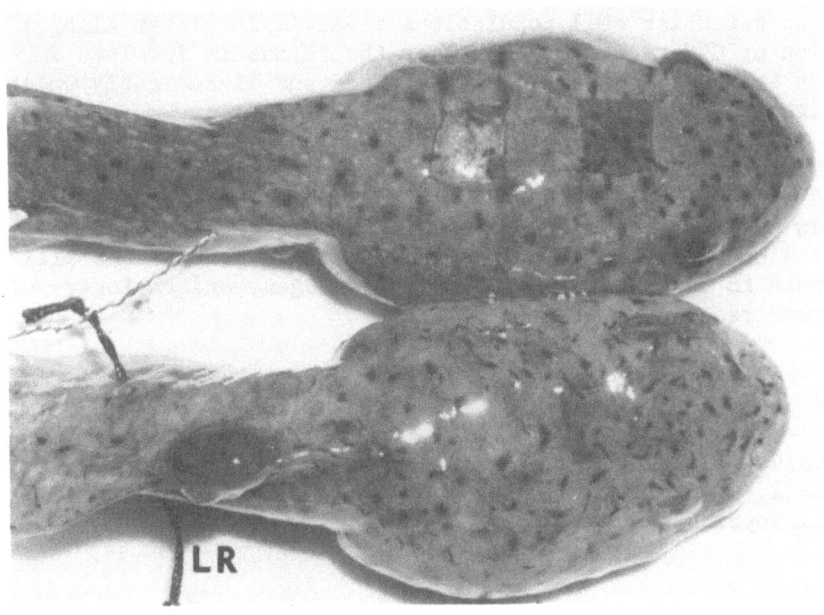

Figure 4.   Top, control larvae showing well healed skin autograft (right) and rejected skin allograft (left). Bottom, total body irradiated larva with a well healed allograft and localized reactions (LR) to an allogeneic spleen graft 6 days after splenic implantation.

Table 3. Function(s) of Lympho—myeloid Organs of Pre-
metamorphic Bullfrog Larvae (6 months or older) Assessed by
Extirpation, Irradiation, and Reimplantation.

Lympho—myeloid Organ	Antibody Synthesis	Allograft Rejection	GVH Reaction
Spleen	Yes	No	Yes
Thymus	?	No	No
Lymph gland	Yes	Yes	Yes

3) graft—versus—host reactivity. The lymph gland can restore all
three immunologic responses suggesting that it is a source of stem
cells which differentiate into cells effecting humoral and cellular
immune reactions (12). The spleen appears to contain a population
of cells capable of synthesizing antibodies and evoking a localized
GVH; it does not, however, appear to contain a cell population that
effects graft rejection. By contrast, the thymus is apparently
unable to refurbish cell populations involved in either allograft
rejection or GVH reactions. Whether the thymus is involved in
antibody synthesis has not been evaluated and is currently under
investigation.

The functional diversity observed in the different lympho-
myeloid organs suggests that the origins of immunologic diversity
found in the advanced vertebrates are present in amphibians.
Extension of these findings to other primitive vertebrates will
contribute to our understanding of the ontogeny and phylogeny of
the immune response.

ACKNOWLEDGEMENTS

Supported in part by NSF grant GB—17767, NIH grant 1R01
HD09333—01, and a grant from the Brown—Hazen Corporation.
Send all reprint requests to E. L. Cooper.

REFERENCES

1. Good, R. A., Finstad, J., Pollara, B., and Gabrielsen, A., in
    Phylogeny of Immunity, p. 149 (University of Florida Press,
    Gainesville, 1966).

2. Cooper, E. L., in Contemporary Topics In Immunobiology, 2:
    13 (1973).

3. Du Pasquier, L., in Current Topics In Microbiology and
    Immunology, 61: 37 (1973).

4. Cooper, E. L., in Physiology of Amphibia, 3 (1975, in press).

5. Cooper, E. L., J. Morphol., 122: 381 (1967).

6. Horton, J. D., J. Morphol., 134: 1 (1971).

7. Cooper, E. L., and Hildemann, W. H., Transplantation, 3:
    446 (1965).

8. Cooper, E. L., Brown, B. A., and Baculi, B. S., in Morphol-
    ogical and Fundamental Aspects of Immunity, p. 1 (Plenum
    Press, New York, 1971).

9. Brown, B. A., and Cooper, E. L., submitted for publication
    (1975).

10. Cooper, E. L., Anat. Rec., 162: 453 (1968).

11. Baculi, B. S., and Cooper, E. L., J. Exp. Zool., 183: 185
    (1973).

12. Cooper, E. L., Brown, B. A., and Wright, R. K., Am. Zool.,
    15: 85 (1975).

13. Riviere, H. B., and Cooper, E. L., Proc. Soc. Exp. Biol. Med.,
    143: 320 (1973).

14. Brown, B. A., Ph.D. Dissertation, University of California,
    Los Angeles (1974).

15. Wright, R. K., and Cooper, E. L., Fed. Proc., 33: 768 (1974).

16. Moticka, E. J., Brown, B. A., and Cooper, E. L., J. Immunol.,
    110: 855 (1973).

17. Warner, N. L., Aust. J. Exp. Biol. Med. Sci., 43: 417 (1964).

18. Ford, W. L., Brit. J. Exp. Pathol., 48: 335 (1967).

19. Elkins, W. L., Progr. Allergy, 15: 78 (1971).

CELLULAR ASPECTS OF HUMORAL IMMUNE RESPONSIVENESS IN <u>CHELYDRA</u>

Myrin Borysenko

Department of Anatomy
Tufts Medical School
Boston, Massachusetts

Some general evolutionary trends are now emerging from comparative studies on representative species of the vertebrate classes with respect to the occurrence and morphological features of lymphoid organs and cells, their reactivity to antigenic stimulation and the species' capacity for humoral immune responsiveness. From the wealth of information in this symposium, it is evident that all vertebrates can mount adaptive immune responses and show some form of immunological memory to a variety of antigens, under properly controlled laboratory conditions.

Agnathans, the first vertebrate class phylogenetically, presents us with an enigma, since their well-demonstrated repertoire of humoral immune responses and production of IgM-type immunoglobulin (1-4) is not paralleled by the presence of definitive lymphoid organs or organized lymphoid tissue, to which one could attribute the role of immunocompetent cell production (5-8). Furthermore, plasma cells are apparently absent, even in immunized animals of this class. Although small lymphocytes of peripheral blood of the hagfish have been demonstrated as effector cells, producing specific antibody (2), their source has not been elucidated beyond the simple observation of the presence of small foci of lymphoid cells along the lamina propria of the gut and in the pronephros (5-7). Peripheral lymphocytes from immunized lampreys have been shown to undergo blast transformation <u>in vitro</u> in response to stimulation with specific hapten-serum conjugates or the mitogen PHA (9). Although direct evidence is still lacking, these studies suggest that antigenic stimulation probably results in proliferation of immunocompetent lymphocytes in diffuse microenvironments and that effective immune response can be mounted in the absence of definitive lymphoid organs.

A well-organized thymus and spleen, as well as kidney-associated lymphoid aggregates appear at the level of Osteichthyes and Chondrichthyes, and the immunocompetence of cells derived from these organs has been clearly demonstrated. Plasma cells have also been found in advanced elasmobranches and in chondrostean and teleost fishes (6, 10-15). These lymphoid organs and cells reach a higher level of organization in the Amphibian class, in which the emergence of lymph nodes (jugular bodies) and a lymphopoietic bone marrow (16, 17) also occurs. A very rough evolutionary line from the fishes to the amphibians reflects phylogenetic parallels toward more efficient and reproducible immune responses and the diversification of immunoglobulins into distinct immunochemical classes. In anurans, for example, immunological tasks are generally shared by lymph nodes, spleen and anterior kidney. Immune responses are generally prompt, at high titers and involve two distinct immunoglobulin classes (18-21).

Two orders of reptiles, the Chelonia (turtles) and Squamata (lizards) have received serious immunological consideration. Species of both orders possess an extensive lymphoid complex including a well-organized thymus, spleen and lymph nodes as well as an array of lymphoid aggregates of lesser organization (22-26). The spleen, as a peripheral lymphoid organ, is the largest, most highly developed and most important immunologically (22, 27, 28).

Reptiles and amphibians are capable of good secondary immune responses, at least to some antigens, and IgM-type antibody production is generally followed by the IgG-type. The latter immunoglobulin type is usually associated with the secondary response (20, 24, 28-31). Although not extensively studied, cellular proliferation and differentiation in peripheral lymphoid organs has been observed following primary antigenic stimulation. Secondary challenges did not produce new or further histological changes (28, 32-35). It has, in fact, been widely observed that "germinal centers", so closely associated with secondary immune responsiveness and IgG antibody production in mammals (36), are conspicuously absent in the peripheral lymphoid organs of ectothermic vertebrates (37). These observations pose some interesting problems regarding the cellular kinetics associated with humoral antibody production, particularly with respect to immunological memory.

We utilized the snapping turtle, Chelydra serpentina, as a reptilian model for in situ morphological and immunological studies of cells and cell populations in the spleen, following primary and secondary antigenic stimulation. The turtle spleen is large, well-organized, easily accessible to antigen by way of intracardiac injection and probably contains the primary supply of immunocompetent cells.

METHODS AND RESULTS

Both routine paraffin sections of normal (unstimulated) spleen stained with methyl green-pyronin Y, and 1   plastic (epon) sections stained with methylene blue, show the splenic parenchyma to be composed of distinct white and red pulp regions. The white pulp is composed primarily of densely packed small lymphocytes, surrounding central arterioles as fairly uniform "cuffs", corresponding to the periarteriolar lymphocyte sheath in mammals (38). Blast cells are seen occasionally within the lymphocyte sheaths as lightly pyroninophilic or metachromatic cells, depending on the histological preparation. In addition to their staining properties, they are easily identified by their large size, large euchromatic nuclei, prominent nucleoli and "grainy" cytoplasm. These cells are found in small numbers and are apparently randomly distributed throughout the white pulp (Figs. 1 and 2).

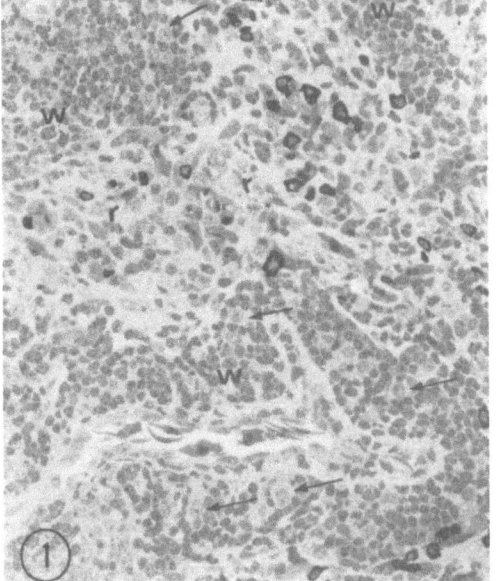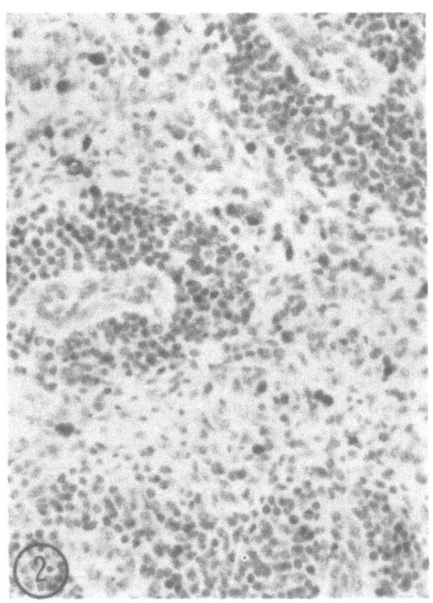

Fig. 1.   1µ epon section of normal spleen showing red (r) and white (w) pulp regions. A random distribution of large blast cells is seen in the white pulp (arrows). Methylene blue.   X 235

Fig. 2.   Section of normal spleen, showing appearance of white pulp, consisting of lymphocyte sheaths. The surrounding red pulp contains a number of darkly stained plasma cells. Methyl green-pyronin Y.   X 225

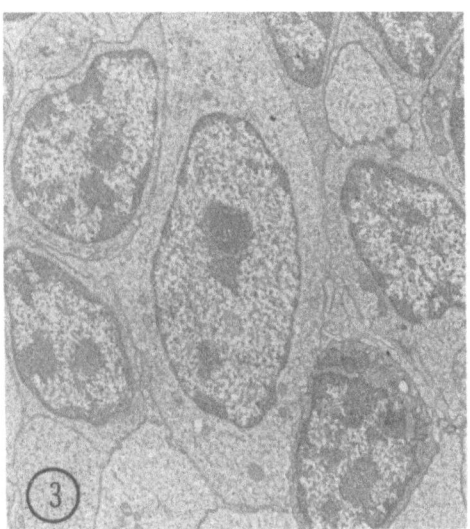 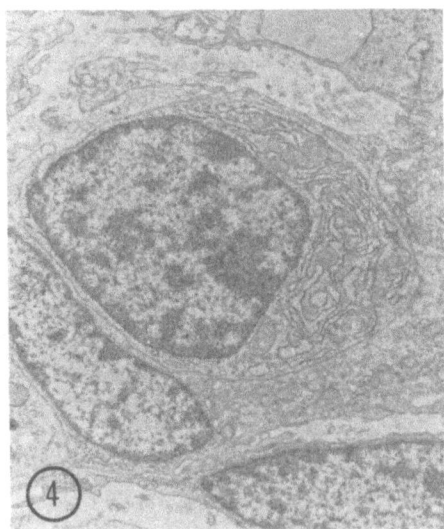

Fig. 3.   EM section of normal white pulp showing a large blast
           cell surrounded by numerous small lymphocytes. X 4000
Fig. 4.   EM section of normal red pulp showing a typical plasma
           cell. X 5000

On the electron microscopic level, small lymphocytes possess
intensely heterochromatic nuclei, abundant free ribosomes and a
cluster of mitochondria, usually at one pole of the cell. The
much larger blast cells are characterized by nuclei in which
small amounts of dense chromatin are adherent to the nuclear
envelope, and a cytoplasm filled primarily with polyribosomes.
In addition, sparse mitochondria and a few short segments of
rough endoplasmic reticulum are also seen in most blast cells
(Fig. 3).

The red pulp is seen as a system of cords and sinuses,
containing all the cellular elements of peripheral blood and a
random scattering of plasma cells which have heterochromatic
nuclei and intensely pyroninophilic, bright orange-red cytoplasm
(Fig. 2). Fine structural observations reveal the layered
pattern of rough endoplasmic reticulum (RER) typical of plasma
cells (Fig. 4). In addition, macrophages with numerous
pseudopodia and prominent lysosomal organelles are commonly seen
in the cords and sinuses of the red pulp.

Cells which adhere to glass, such as lymphocytes and
macrophages, can be studied topographically with the transmission
electron microscope by shadowing dried preparations with platinum-
palladium under vacuum (39). Surface replicas of spleen cell

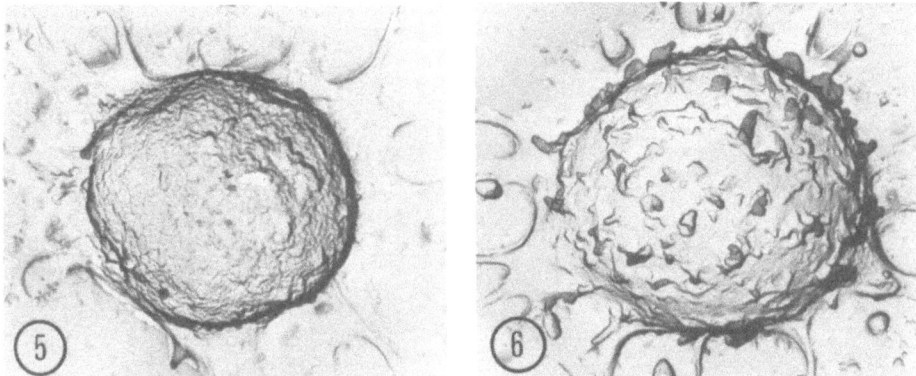

Fig. 5.   Surface replica of a smooth-surfaced splenic lymphocyte.
           X 6300
Fig. 6.   Surface replica of a rough-surfaced splenic lymphocyte.
           X 7200

suspensions prepared in this manner reveal the presence of two
morphologically distinct lymphocyte populations. The majority of
splenic lymphocytes are smooth surfaced (Fig. 5). A small
percentage (<10%) are rough surfaced, showing numerous microvillus
projections (Fig. 6). Whether such cells represent T and B cells,
respectively, as has been demonstrated in some mammals, using
scanning electron microscopy (40, 41) remains to be determined.
Macrophages are also easily identified by this method and are
often preserved in the act of crawling and phagocytizing particles
or bacteria (Fig. 7). We are presently doing a lymphoid organ
survey to determine the distribution of the two lymphocyte
populations and plan to study their mitogen and antigen-binding
capacities and other surface phenomena by direct visualization,
using this technique.

     The morphological pattern of reticular cells and fibers is of
particular interest as it relates to the antigen trapping
mechanism. Paraffin sections processed with a silver stain
reveal an intricate pattern of reticular fibers projecting from
the central arterioles outward through the white pulp. At the
marginal zone, they interlace with reticular fibers which are
arranged circumferentially around the white pulp. In the red
pulp itself, the fibers form a fine network throughout the cords
and along the sinuses. Reticular cells are found in close
association to the fibers. Intracardiac injection of colloidal
carbon results in the entrapment of carbon particles throughout
the red pulp and along the marginal zones. Little or no carbon is
found in the white pulp regions (Fig. 8). This trapping pattern
is similar to that of mammals, where macrophages, reticular cells
and fibers play a major role in particle and antigen trapping.

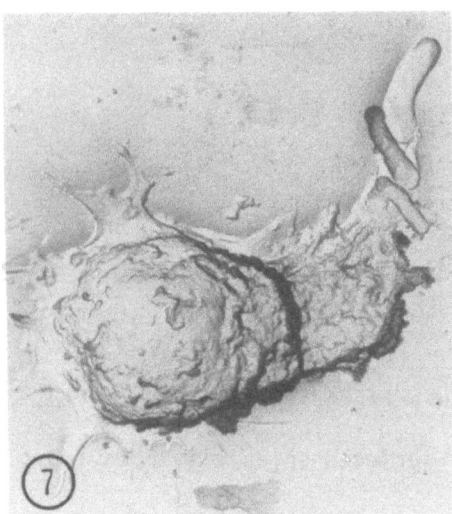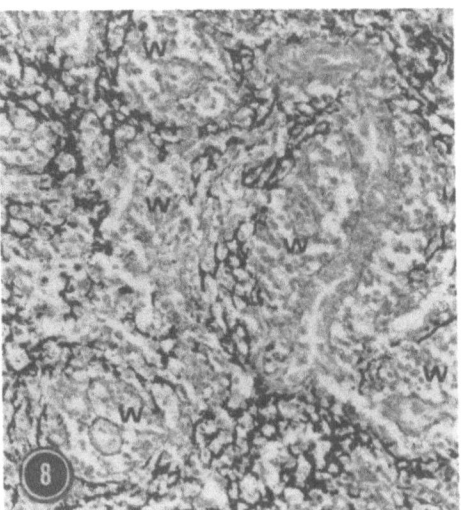

Fig. 7.   Surface replica of a splenic macrophage, caught intthe
           act of ingesting bacteria. X 3200
Fig. 8.   Section of spleen showing reticulum architecture and
           colloidal carbon trapping pattern in the red pulp and
           marginal zones. Note that the white pulp regions (w)
           are relatively free of carbon. Gridley's reticulum
           stain. X 220

Although carbon particles were not seen in the white pulp, soluble
antigens may very well be brought into the white pulp from the
marginal zone. Localization of antigen on reticular cells of
jugular bodies has been demonstrated in Bufo and may be related
to efficient sensitization of immunocompetent cells (18). A
proper assessment of the spleen's antigen-trapping mechanism
requires a time-course study, using labelled antigens.

   The differential staining characteristics of blasts and
plasma cells with methyl green pyronin, in addition to the
ultrastructural analysis of the lymphoid cell line, provide good
tools for a detailed in situ study of histological and cytological
changes in response to antigenic stimulation.

   At 30°C, a single intracardiac injection of .5-1mgKLH/10-15
gms body wt. results in significant splenic enlargement 8-12 days
post-immunization. Histological analysis shows many small foci
of blast cells developing in the white pulp (lymphocyte sheaths)
at about day 5. Progressive enlargement of these foci continues
and peaks at days 8-12, resulting in marked expansion of the
white pulp regions. These centers generally form in one side of
the lymphocyte sheath and expand into the adjacent red pulp,

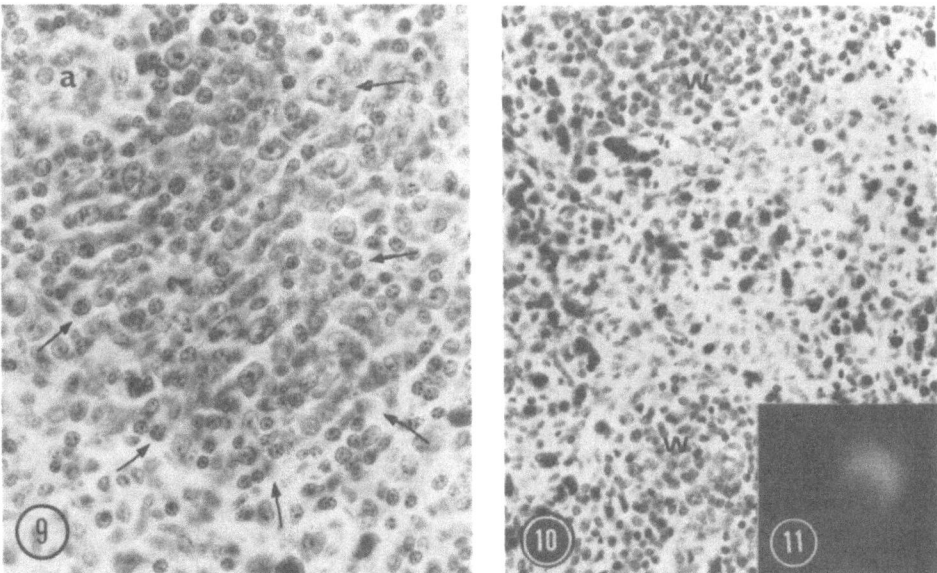

Fig. 9.   Section of immunized spleen at day 10, through a center
           of blast cell proliferation in the lymphocyte sheath
           (arrows) near the central arteriole (a). Methyl green-
           pyronin Y. X 420
Fig. 10.   Section of immunized spleen at day 18, showing the
           somewhat depleted appearance of white pulp (w) and a
           marked increase of plasma cells in red pulp. Methyl
           green-pyronin Y. X 320
Fig. 11.   Section of red pulp of immunized spleen at day 15,
           showing a fluorescein-labelled plasma cell containing
           anti-KLH antibody. X 1100

often joining other white pulp regions (Fig. 9). It is not
uncommon to see vast confluent proliferative areas which include
5-10 arterioles and their lymphocyte sheaths. Ultrastructural
analysis of proliferative foci shows that the blast cells are in
most respects similar to those seen in normal spleen, except for
a somewhat higher incidence of short segments of rough
endoplasmic reticulum, apparently reflecting the acquisition of
machinery for production of protein for export.

     At 15-20 days post-immunization, one sees a gradual
diminution of the white pulp until the periarteriolar sheaths
reach a normal or somewhat depleted appearance. At the same time,
there is a marked increase in the number of pyroninophilic cells
in the red pulp (Fig. 10). Most of these cells were determined
to be plasma cells by their morphological and staining features,
although larger, lighter staining blast-like cells were also of

common occurrence. These cells were not organized in groups in
the red pulp, but appeared to be randomly distributed.
Immunofluorescent studies, using a paraffin embedding technique,
confirmed the specificity of this population of cells. Sections
treated sequentially with KLH, rabbit anti-KLH and fluorescein
isothiocyanate-labelled goat anti-rabbit immunoglobulin, revealed
a scattering of fluorescent cells in the red pulp, producing
anti-KLH antibody (Fig. 11).

    Ultrastructural observation of the red pulp during this
period was particularly revealing. Plasma cells are seen in
various stages of maturation. Very immature plasma cells resemble
blast cells with respect to size and nuclear features. However,
their nuclei are somewhat more eccentrically placed and longer
segments of rough endoplasmic reticulum are present in the
cytoplasm. As in blast cells, polyribosomes are still the
predominant organelles (Fig. 12). An increase in the
RER/polyribosome ratio and the acquisition of more condensed
chromatin (heterochromatin) reflects progressive maturation of
the plasma cell, which finally contains an extensive rough
endoplasmic reticulum, a well-developed Golgi complex and very
few polyribosomes (Fig. 13). On this basis, the red pulp contains
many intermediate stages of maturing plasma cells as well as some
mature cells. Cells of the plasma cell line, including immature
cells, contain dilated cisternae of rough endoplasmic reticulum,
containing a slightly electron dense material, presumably

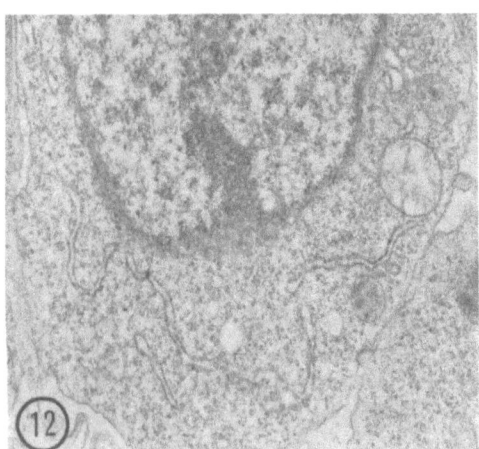 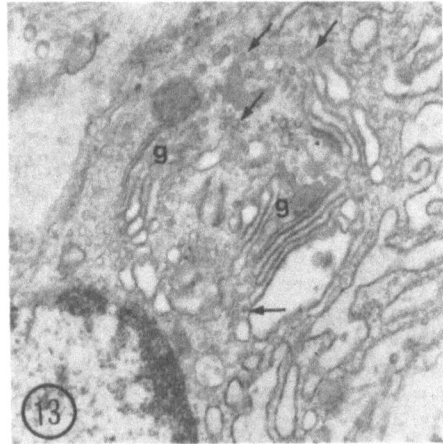

Fig. 12.   EM section of an immature plasma cell, containing some
           long segments of RER and many polyribosomes. X 9500
Fig. 13.   EM section of part of a mature plasma cell, showing
           extensive dilated cisternae of RER and a well-
           developed Golgi complex (g) with secretory vesicles
           (arrows). X 17000

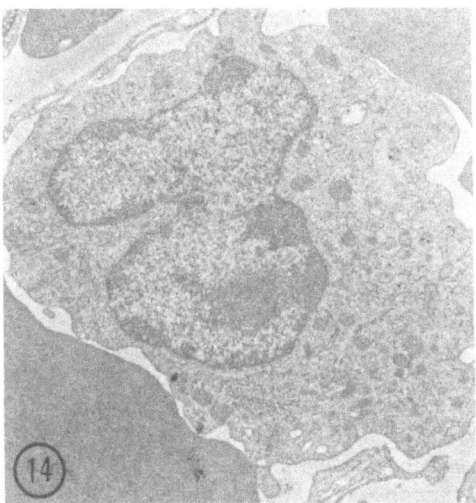 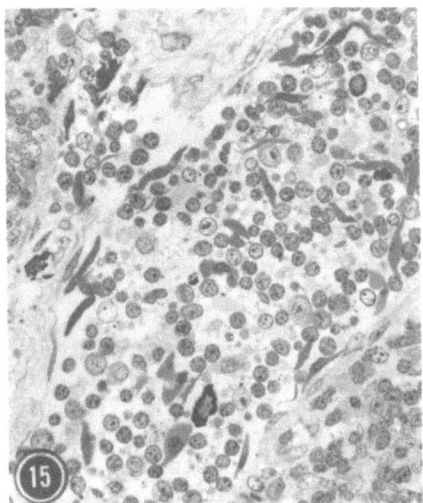

Fig. 14.   EM section of a monocyte or immature macrophage in
           immunized spleen. X 6300
Fig. 15.   1μ epon section of a major vein of an immunized spleen,
           containing a variety of lymphoid cells leaving the
           organ. Methylene blue. X 400

immunoglobulin.   Our immunofluorescent study, paralleled with
fine structural observations, seems to confirm the heterogeneity of
the plasma cell line where both immature and mature cells are
capable of synthesizing and storing significant amounts of specific
antibody. An increase in the number of immature macrophages and
monocytes in the red pulp is also observed, although their
presumptive role (if any) in the immune mechanism is uncertain
(Fig. 14).

The number of pyroninophilic cells in the red pulp is
reduced to normal (unimmunized) levels by day 25. Histological
sections through the major splenic veins show large numbers of
lymphoid cells in circulation, apparently migrating out of the
spleen (Fig. 15). These cells include large numbers of small
lymphocytes, plasma cells and some blast-like cells (probably
immature plasma cells). In addition, electron micrographs often
show plasma cells in the red pulp sinuses as free cells. No
further changes were observed during the remainder of the 60 day
observation period of the primary response.

Secondary antigenic challenge 20, 40 and 60 days after
primary immunization (separate groups) resulted in no further
proliferative activity in the spleen. White pulp regions
remained unaffected and plasma cell counts in the red pulp

remained relatively constant during the 40 day observation
period, although there was some variation between individual
animals.

DISCUSSION

The initial cellular events of the primary response in
Chelydra, namely blast cell proliferation in periarteriolar
lymphocyte sheaths, followed by migration and differentiation of
blast cells into plasma cells in the red pulp and production of
specific antibody, suggests an evolutionary advance toward the
immunological systems of endothermic vertebrates (42, 43). There
are, however, notable differences between Chelydra and most
endotherms. First of all, in Chelydra spleen, plasma cells do not
take up long term communal residence in the red pulp, but are a
rather transient population of cells which are randomly distributed
throughout the red pulp, while in the organ. Mature plasma cells
are seen in the spleen in small numbers. The presence of large
numbers of lymphocytes and pyroninophilic cells in the splenic
circulation and a concomitant depletion of these cells in the red
pulp suggests a cellular migration from the spleen to other sites.
Moreover, upon further antigenic stimulation, no new proliferative
response is observed in the spleen.

The kinetics of the primary blast cell response and lack of
responsiveness following secondary challenge correlates well
with observations in Xenopus (33, 43), Bufo (32), and Rana (35),
although in these amphibians the proliferation of blast cells is
more random, involves the red pulp to a greater extent, and
mature plasma cells are said to be of rare occurrence in both
immunized and unimmunized animals. Other studies have demonstrated
specific antibody forming cells by adherence and plaque assays
of spleen cells in the toad, Bufo (18, 44), and the tortoise,
Agrionemys (45), and have characterized these cells as a
heterogeneous population of immature plasma cells. Our
observations in Chelydra suggest that the rare occurrence of
mature plasma cells may be attributable to the efflux of most
plasma cells from the spleen prior to full maturation, although
cells which are maturing to some extent within the spleen are
already capable of synthesizing (and storing) specific antibody.

Since the blast cell foci observed in Chelydra are of short
duration and do not appear following secondary antigenic
stimulation, they do not fit the mammalian criteria for
"germinal centers". Furthermore, immunized spleens which are
silver stained for reticulum do not show any regions of white
pulp relatively free of reticular fibers, which could be
considered "nodules". Although detailed kinetic studies have not
been performed on other reptilian species, the absence of

germinal centers has been reported in immunized lizards (24, 28, 46) and toads (32, 34). In spite of this apparent deficiency, recent serological evidence shows that anurans (20), several species of lizards (24, 28, 30), the tortoise (31) and the alligator (29) produce good secondary responses that are quantitatively higher and/or qualitatively different from the primary response.

Although the evidence is still somewhat sketchy for definitive conclusions regarding the apparent lack of correspondence between humoral immunological memory and secondary cellular activity in peripheral lymphoid organs, there is at least circumstantial evidence leading to the hypothesis that there has been a progressive evolutionary trend toward the "centralization" of immunocompetent cell production into primary and peripheral lymphoid organs. The first vertebrate class, the agnathans, represents a completely decentralized system where cells develop and respond to antigenic stimulation in microenvironments in connective tissue regions of the body. Further up the phylogenetic tree, lymphoid organs appear, become larger and more complex. Immune induction at this level can now be attributed to the thymus (and other lymphoid organs?). Peripheral lymphoid organs maintain cells primarily responsive to primary antigenic stimulation. In reptiles at least, the primary response, involving the periarteriolar lymphocyte sheath, is in many respects similar to that of most endothermic animals. Secondary cellular responses, however, still occur in microenvironments outside of the lymphoid organs, up through the reptilian class. The endotherms represent a further evolutionary centralization of immune function, that of the secondary cellular response (immunological memory), into the peripheral lymphoid organs, corresponding to the appearance of nodules and germinal centers.

It is interesting in this respect that ontogenetic studies of immune development show that the fetal lamb is capable of an array of immune responses prior to the development of peripheral lymphoid organs. IgM is produced in the absence of peripheral lymphoid organs, while IgG is produced prior to the appearance of germinal centers (47). Other ontogenetic studies have suggested that such microenvironmental alternative pathways can function in establishment of immunocompetence in the absence of primary lymphoid organs in birds and mammals (48). If ontogeny recapitulates phylogeny in this instance, these developmental studies support the above hypothesis. The complex lymphoid structure of endotherms may, therefore, reflect a greater efficiency and diversity in immune responsiveness, rather than their simple capacity to elicit primary and secondary reactions.

We must, however, take into account other possible mechanisms which may function in the immune responses of ectothermic vertebrates. For example, ultrastructural analysis of reptilian and amphibian plasma cells (45, 49) suggests that they are capable of storing large quantities of immunoglobulin and that this may represent a physiological mechanism for antibody storage and release, possibly controlled by temperature, antigen levels and antibody levels. If this were so, it is conceivable that a secondary antigenic challenge could trigger such a release mechanism, which would result in rapid increase of antibody at high levels. However, unless there was also a mechanism of modulation, without new cellular proliferation, one would expect to find antibodies of the same immunoglobulin class in both primary and secondary responses. At any rate, special care must be taken to cover all parameters when testing the hypothesis.

These findings invite further research to bring together more precisely the relationship between cellular proliferative responses in lymphoid organs and microenvironments, the mechanism of antibody synthesis and release, and the kinetics of IgM-type and IgG-type immunoglobulin production in primary and secondary immune responses.

ACKNOWLEDGEMENTS

This investigation was supported by U.S. Public Health Service Grant AI 10679. The author is indebted to Marilyn Powers for her expert technical assistance.

REFERENCES

1. Thoenes, G.G. and Hildemann, W.H., In: Developmental Aspects of Antibody Formation and Structure, p. 711, (Czechoslovak Academy of Sciences, Prague, 1970).

2. Linthicum, D.S. and Hildemann, W.H., J. Immunol., 105: 912 (1970).

3. Boffa, G.A., Fine, J.M., Drilhon, A. and Amouch, P., Nature, 214: 700 (1967).

4. Marchalonis, J. and Edelman, G.M., J. Exp. Med., 127: 891 (1968).

5. Jordan, H.E. and Speidel, C.C., Amer. J. Anat., 46: 355 (1930).

6. Good, R.A., Finstad, J., Pollara, B. and Gabrielsen, A.E., In: Phylogeny of Immunity, p. 149, (Univ. of Florida Press, Gainesville, 1966).

7. Fange, R., In: Phylogeny of Immunity, p. 141 (Univ. of Florida Press, Gainesville, 1966).

8. Fichtelius, K.E., Finstad, J. and Good, R.A., Lab. Invest., 19: 339 (1968).

9. Cooper, A.J., In: Fourth Leukocyte Culture Conference, p. 137 (Appleton-Century-Crofts, New York, 1971).

10. Finstad, J. and Good, R.A., In: Phylogeny of Immunity, p. 173, (Univ. of Florida Press, Gainesville, 1966).

11. Clawson, C.C., Finstad, J. and Good, R.A., Lab. Invest., 15: 1830 (1966).

12. Smith, A.M., Potter, M. and Merchant, E.B., J. Immunol., 99: 876 (1967).

13. Chiller, J.M., Hodgins, H.O., Chambers, V.C. and Weiser, R.S., J. Immunol., 102: 1193 (1969).

14. Chiller, J.M., Hodgins, H.O. and Weiser, R.S., J. Immunol., 102: 1202 (1969).

15. Ortiz-Muniz, G. and Sigel, M.M., J. Retic. Soc., 9: 42 (1971).

16. Baculi, B.S., Cooper, E.L. and Brown, B.A., J. Morph., 131: 315 (1970).

17. Cooper, E.L., In: Morphological and Functional Aspects of Immunity, p. 13 (Plenum Press, New York, 1973).

18. Diener, E. and Marchalonis, J., Immunology, 18: 279 (1970).

19. Marchalonis, J.J., Allen, R.B. and Saarni, E., Comp. Biochem. Physiol., 35: 49 (1970).

20. Lin, H.H., Caywood, B.E. and Rowlands, D.T., Immunology, 20: 373 (1971).

21. Acton, R.T., Evans, E.E., Weinheimer, P.F., Niedermeier, W. and Bennett, J.C., Biochemistry, 11: 2751 (1972).

22. Borysenko, M. and Cooper, E.L., J. Morph., 138: 487 (1972).

23. Kanakambika, P. and Muthukkaruppan, V., Proc. Ind. Acad. Sci.,
     B78: 37 (1973).

24. Wetherall, J.D. and Turner, K.J., Aust. J. exp. Biol. med.
     Sci., 50: 79 (1972).

25. LeFebre, M.E., Reincke, U., Arbas, R. and Gennaro, J.F.,
     Anat. Rec., 176: 111 (1973).

26. Johnston, M.R.L., J. Morph., 139: 431 (1973).

27. Kanakambika, P. and Muthukkaruppan, V., Experientia, 28: 1225
     (1972).

28. Kanakambika, P. and Muthukkaruppan, V., J. Immunol., 109:
     415 (1972).

29. Lerch, E.G., Huggins, S.A. and Bartel, A.H., Proc. Soc.
     Exp. Biol. Med., 124: 448 (1967).

30. Wright, R.K. and Shapiro, H.C., Herpetologia, 29: 275 (1973).

31. Ambrosius, H., Hemmerling, J., Richter, R. and Schimke, R.,
     In: Developmental Aspects of Antibody Formation and
     Structure, p. 727 (Academic Press, New York, 1970).

32. Diener, E. and Nossal G.J.V., Immunology, 10: 535 (1966).

33. Manning, M.J. and Turner, R.J., Comp. Biochem. Physiol.,
     42A: 735 (1972).

34. Turner, R.J. and Manning, M.J., J. Exp. Zool., 183: 21 (1973).

35. Moticka, E.J., Brown, B.A. and Cooper, E.L., J. Immunol.,
     110: 855 (1973).

36. Thorbecke, G.J., Romano, T.J. and Lerman, S.P., Prog.
     Immunol. II, 3: 25 (1974).

37. Pollara, B., Finstad, J. and Good, R.A., In: Lymphatic
     Tissue and Germinal Centers in Relation to Phylogenesis,
     p. 1 (Plenum, New York, 1969).

38. Weiss, L., The Cells and Tissues of the Immune System -
     Structure, Functions and Interactions. (Prentice-Hall,
     New Jersey, 1972).

39. Smith, S.B. and Revel, J., Devel. Biol., 27: 434 (1972).

40. Lin, P.S., Tsai, S. and Wallach, D.F.H., In: Second
     International Symposium on Metabolism and Membrane
     Permeability of Erythrocytes, Thrombocytes and Leukocytes,
     p. 438 (Stuttgart, Verlag, 1973).

41. Lin, P.S, Cooper, A.G. and Wortis, H.H., New Eng. J. Med.,
     289: 548 (1973).

42. Neher, G.H. and Siegel, B.V., Int. Arch. Allergy, 39: 133
     (1970).

43. Nossal, G.J.V. and Ada, G.L., Antigens, Lymphoid Cells and
     the Immune Response (Academic Press, New York, 1971).

44. Kraft, N. and Shortman, K., J. Cell Biol., 52: 438 (1972).

45. Ambrosius, H. and Hoheisel, G., Acta biol. med. germ., 31:
     733 (1973).

46. Marchalonis, J.J., Ealey, E.H.M. and Diener, E., Aust. J.
     exp. Biol. med. Sci., 47: 367 (1969).

47. Fahey, K.J., Prog. Immunol. II, 3: 49 (1974).

48. Bryant, B.J., Prog. Immunol. II, 3: 5 (1974)

49. Cowden, R.R. and Dyer, R.F., Amer. Zool., 11: 183 (1971).

BURSAL AND THYMIC ALLOANTIGEN EXPRESSION IN LYMPHOID TISSUES OF THE CHICKEN

N. Donnelly[*], A. Brand[†] and D. G. Gilmour[†]

[*]University of Rochester School of Medicine & Dentistry, Rochester, New York 14642. [†]New York University School of Medicine, New York, New York 10016

Aves represent that point on the evolutionary tree where separation of lymphoid tissues into thymus-dependent (T cell) and thymus-independent (B cell) lymphoid systems has been compartmentalized to its fullest. Two primary lymphoid organs control differentiation of immunity in birds - the thymus governs development of lymphocytes primarily mediating cellular immune functions, while the bursa of Fabricius controls the maturation of antibody-forming cells (1,2). The division into T and B cell systems is not as anatomically distinct in other vertebrates, but studies in a number of species indicate that functionally such compartmentalization does exist (3-6). Thus, although Aves present a unique opportunity for studying the relative contribution of T and B cells to immune functions, knowledge gained in this model system has far wider applicability.

Antigenic differences between thymus- and bursa-dependent lymphocytes in chickens have been repeatedly demonstrated by antisera raised in other species (7-11); these heteroantisera are proving valuable tools in studies of the structural and functional composition of the immune system (additional ref. 12-18). However, the recent progress in dissection of the major histocompatibility complex in mice has demonstrated the superior discriminatory capacity of alloantisera prepared by immunization between inbred strains of the same species. If we are to take maximum advantage of the chicken as a model for studying ontogeny and phylogeny of immunity, it is imperative that we develop comparable alloantisera. In this report we describe the first production of alloantisera specific for bursal or thymic lymphocytes in an avian species. These sera were used to analyze the cellular composition of

central and peripheral lymphoid tissues, and to follow alloantigen
expression on cells from thymic and bursal suspensions during
maturation.

PREPARATION AND CHARACTERIZATION OF ALLOANTISERA

Antisera which specifically recognize bursa- and thymus-dependent alloantigens were prepared by reciprocal immunizations between chickens of East Lansing lines 6_3 (EL6) and 7_2 (EL7). Both
lines are 99% inbred, and they share several of the known chicken
cell surface antigens. They are syngeneic for the major blood
group-histocompatibility locus (B^2/B^2), and for three other blood
group loci, A, C and L. The antigenic products of A and C are expressed on lymphocytes. These two particular lines were paired on
the basis of several functional differences they exhibit (Table 1).
It was hypothesized (by D.G.G.) that these differences may reflect
the existence of distinct lymphocyte surface alloantigens.

Females ranging from 3-4 months of age received 4 weekly intra-
muscular and intraperitoneal injections of bursa or thymus cells
from 7- to 12-week donors of the other line. High titered, specific antisera were obtained after 2 courses of injections separated by a 3-month rest. (A manuscript detailing immunization procedures and genetic analysis of the inheritance of these alloantigens is in preparation, Gilmour et al.) Cytotoxic antibody activity was assayed by trypan blue dye exclusion in a system using the

TABLE 1. Characteristics of East Lansing Lines 6_3 and 7_2

1. Line 6_3 is homozygous susceptible to infection by subgroup A
   and B leukosis/sarcoma viruses (tva and tvb loci).
   Line 7_2 is homozygous resistant (19).

2. Line 6_3 is relatively resistant to induction of leukosis (i.e.,
   to transformation).
   Line 7_2 carries dominant gene(s) for susceptibility (20,21).

3. Line 6_3 is relatively resistant to induction of Marek's Disease.
   Line 7_2 is highly susceptible (22).

4. Line 6_3 is a high responder in delayed hypersensitivity reactions.
   Line 7_2 is a low responder (23).

5. Line 6_3 is a low responder in graft-vs-host reactions.
   Line 7_2 is a high responder (23,24).

Stolfi method of complementation (25). In this technique, anti-complementary factors are precipitated from the un-heat-inactivated antiserum, and a mixture of chicken C'1 and guinea pig C'2-9 is used as complement. Titers are expressed as a cytotoxic index (CI) which is calculated according to the following formula:

$$CI = \frac{\% \text{ dead cells (test)} - \% \text{ dead cells (controls)}}{\text{average } \% \text{ live cells in controls}} \times 100$$

Although antisera were successfully raised against both EL6 and EL7 cells, the work described here is confined to anti-line EL7 sera. Fig. 1 shows cytotoxic titrations of an anti-EL7 bursa and thymus serum. None of the EL6 anti-EL7 sera tested were cytotoxic for cells of EL6 bursa or thymus, indicating no formation of detectable autoantibodies in this system. Both anti-bursa and anti-thymus sera consistently showed reduced CI at dilutions of 1/10 or less, probably due to residual anticomplementary factors.

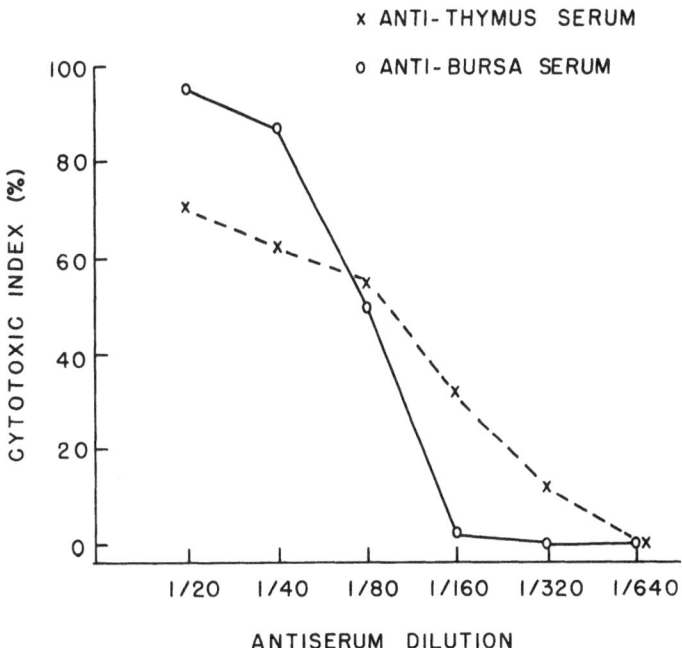

Fig. 1. Titration of anti-EL7-bursa and thymus serum. Equal volumes (0.05 ml) of antiserum, chicken C'1, and cell suspension (5 x 10^6/ml) were mixed and incubated 20 min at 30°. One volume guinea pig C'2-9 was added and the reaction transferred to 37° for 45 min. Cytotoxicity was determined after addition of 1 volume 0.32% trypan. Each point represents the mean of 3 determinations.

Several anti-bursa sera showed a maximum CI of 95% when tested against suspensions from 4-week EL7 bursa, with only 1-2% activity against 4-week EL7 thymus. That this specificity was obtained without the need for prior absorption sharply distinguished these alloantisera from heteroantisera. Absorption of the anti-bursa serum (whose titration profile appears in Fig. 1) with thymus cells from 3- to 4-week chickens did not alter its cytotoxic activity, an indication that there were no significant subthreshold cross-reactivities. Its absorption with bursa cells, however, removed all cytotoxicity.

The following data indicate that this anti-bursa serum is not directed against surface immunoglobulin. Repeated gel diffusion analysis with varying concentrations of NaCl and heavy metal ions (which facilitate precipitation of chicken antigen-antibody complexes) revealed no precipitin band formation between anti-bursa serum and normal EL7 serum. In addition, anti-bursa serum activity was unaffected by absorption with normal EL7 serum, even at ratios as high as 2 mg normal gamma globulin per ml antiserum diluted 1/20. Similar absorptions at ratios of 0.5 mg normal gamma globulin per ml antiserum remove all cytotoxic activity from known anti-chicken-immunoglobulin sera (8).

Our most potent anti-thymus serum (Fig. 1) had a CI of 69-70% when tested against thymus cells from 4-week chickens. Reactivity for bursa cells from chickens of this age was less than 1%; thus this serum was also highly specific with no need for absorption. In analyzing the cytotoxic profile of this anti-thymus serum, we can not yet discriminate between the possibilities that 1) it identifies a specific subpopulation of cells within thymic suspensions, or 2) it identifies an alloantigen(s) expressed on all thymus cells, but our assay is not sufficiently sensitive to detect that antigen(s) below a certain threshold concentration. We plan to use both anti-thymus and anti-bursa sera in fluorescent antibody studies for a more exact determination of the number of cells expressing alloantigen, and quantitation of antigen expression per cell.

ALLOANTIGEN EXPRESSION IN CENTRAL LYMPHOID TISSUES DURING MATURATION OF THE CHICKEN

There is a high rate of cellular proliferation and seeding to peripheral organs during the first weeks after hatching, but in EL7 chickens, both the bursa and thymus size peak at 10-12 weeks of age and begin to atrophy by 14 weeks. Alloantigen expression on bursa and thymus cells during the first 14 weeks of age was determined using the 2 antisera whose titration profiles are shown in Fig. 1. Despite the known maturational changes which occur during this period, cells from both the bursa and thymus exhibited relatively

constant expression of their respective alloantigens. The CI of
anti-bursa serum on bursa cells was 95% from hatching through 6
weeks of age. At 6 weeks it decreased to 90% and remained at this
slightly reduced level. Reactivity of anti-thymus serum against
thymus cells was 69-74% throughout the entire period of study.

    In contrast, there were very definite age-related changes in
subpopulations of lymphocytes within the thymus or bursa which expressed alloantigens of the opposite type (i.e., B cells in the
thymus and visa versa). Fig. 2 shows the development of lymphocyte
subpopulations in the thymus which expressed bursa-specific alloantigen. Between 2 and 4 days after hatching, the level of allo-
antigen-bearing B cells in thymic suspensions began to increase
from a background of 1-2% to a peak of 16.4% by 2 weeks of age. This
population was not present in hormonally bursectomized chicks, and
thus is truly bursa-dependent. In addition, it was not identified
by a rabbit anti-bursa serum (CI for bursa = 95%) which was tested
simultaneously with our alloantisera. In 3-week old chickens this
bursa-dependent subpopulation was no longer detectable. Indeed, 6
separate CI determinations at this age were 0 (Fig. 2). The

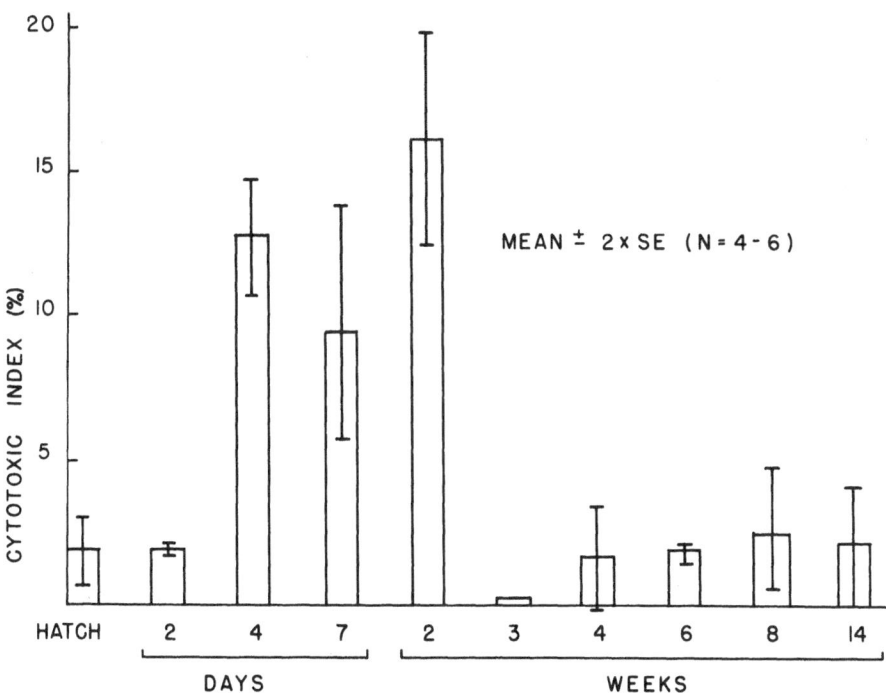

Fig. 2. Bursal antigen expression in thymus cell suspensions from
chickens of various ages.

appearance of this subpopulation suggests an interaction between B and T cells during the early development of the immune system. Droege has also demonstrated bursa-dependent cells within the thymus of young chicks. In his study, which used the parameters of size and electrophoretic mobility, he correlated this subpopulation with suppressor cell activity and postulated that it may be involved in establishment of tolerance during the neonatal period (26). A second phase of cells expressing bursa alloantigen began at 4 weeks of age, but never exceeded 5% of the total thymus population.

Figure 3 shows the results of a parallel search for thymus-dependent lymphocyte subpopulations in bursal suspensions. In contrast to the previous pattern in which we observed an early influx of B cells into the thymus, T cell subpopulations within the bursa were not observed until relatively late - 6 weeks of age. By 14 weeks the CI of anti-thymus serum on bursal suspensions was 9.8%. Previous studies have shown that evidence of cell traffic between the thymus and bursa can be seen in chickens older than 4 weeks (27,28). The late phases of contamination observed in both tissues probably reflect this cellular exchange.

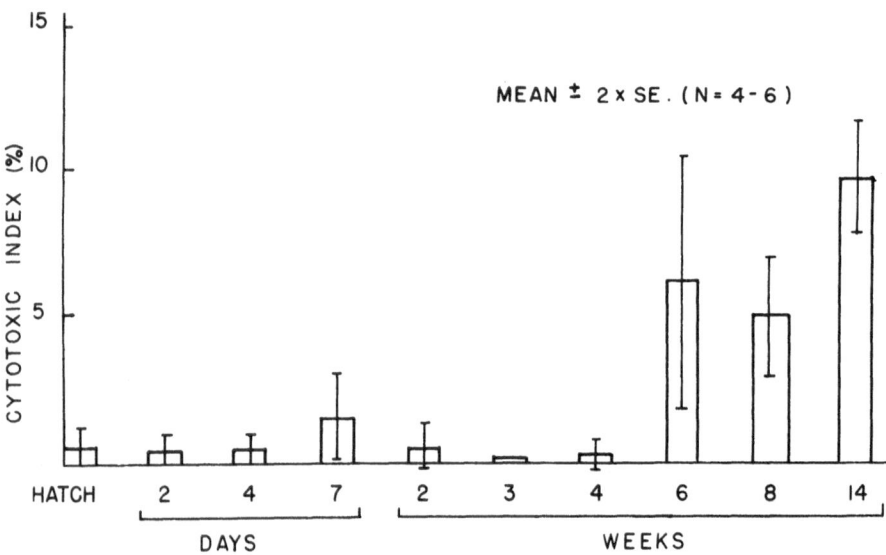

Fig. 3. Thymic antigen expression in bursa cell suspensions from chickens of various ages.

COMPARISON OF EL7 ALLOANTIGEN EXPRESSION IN
CENTRAL AND PERIPHERAL LYMPHOID TISSUES

Fig. 4 compares alloantigen expression in the bursa and thymus (central lymphoid tissues) with that seen on lymphocytes from the spleen, bone marrow and peripheral blood (peripheral lymphoid tissues). All experiments used 4-week birds, a developmental age when the bursa and thymus contain essentially "pure" populations of B and T cells, respectively. It is evident from Fig. 4 that both the anti-bursa and anti-thymus sera detect antigens found on cells in peripheral as well as central lymphoid tissues. Specifically, 73% of spleen cells were susceptible to the cytotoxic action of these alloantisera, and T cells predominated in a ratio of 2:1. In contrast, very low CI were observed in assays of bone marrow suspensions, where B cells predominated (1.6:1). In peripheral blood, 48% of mononuclear cells (excluding erythrocytes, granulocytes and thrombocytes) could be identified by the alloantisera. Of these, 75% expressed thymus alloantigens. Thus, in no instance did the number of B and T cells identified in peripheral tissues account for 100% of the cell population. Similar observations have been made in studies using heteroantisera (10,11,15,16). This often substantial population of null cells in the peripheral tissues may represent undifferentiated precursors, or lymphocytes which have lost their bursa or thymus-specific differentiation antigens as a consequence of further maturation.

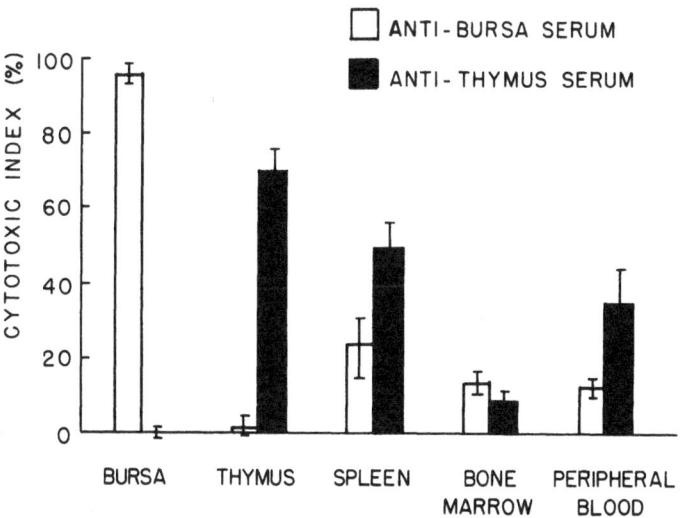

Fig. 4. Bursal and thymic antigen expression on cells from central and peripheral lymphoid tissues of 4-week chickens (Mean ± 2 x SE, N = 5-8).

The cell compositions of bursa, thymus and spleen were further
characterized by applying cytotoxic assays to purified cell populations separated by density gradient centrifugation (29). The
results of these studies on 4-week chickens are shown in Fig. 5.

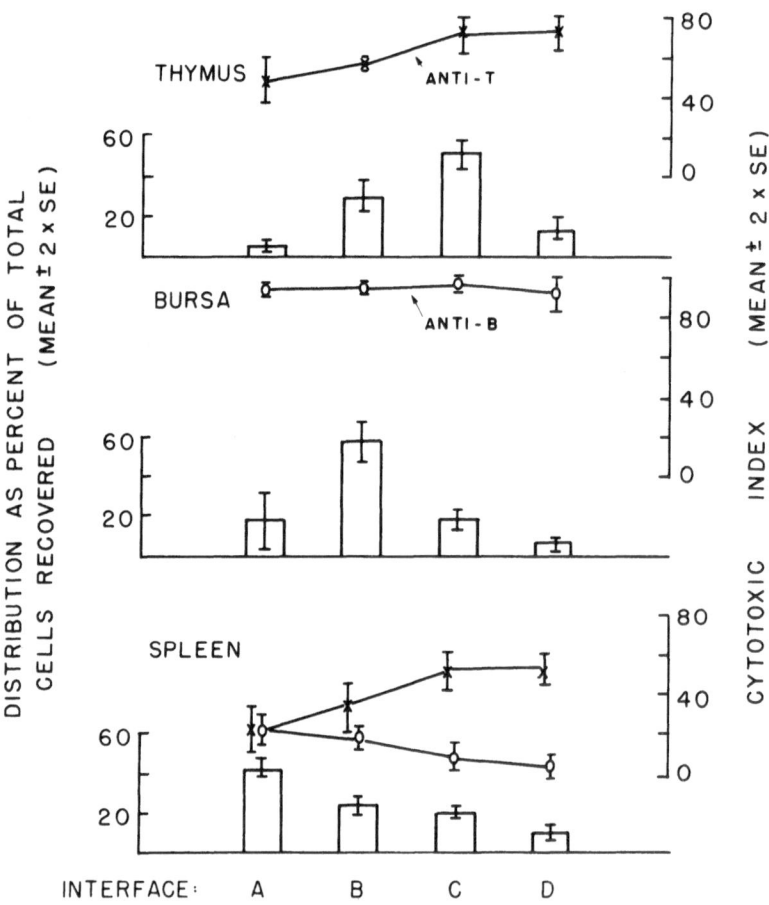

Fig. 5. Distribution of T and B cells in density gradients. Cells
were suspended in the top fraction of a 5-layer discontinuous BSA
gradient (BSA % = 13, 20, 23, 25, + 33; S.G. 33% BSA = 1.094).
After spinning 30 min at 20,000 g_{max}, cells were recovered from the
4 interfaces, washed twice, then assayed in cytotoxic tests with
anti-bursa and anti-thymus serum.   (N = 5-8).

The thymus was characterized by a predominantly dense population. Specifically, 51% of cells concentrated at the C interface (SG = 1.066-1.071), another 15% at D (SG = 1.071-1.094). Both fractions showed elevated CI when assayed with anti-thymus serum. This distribution profile did not change markedly with age until 14 weeks, when dense cells were more equally distributed between C and D. B cells found in thymic suspensions from chickens ≤ 2 weeks or >4 weeks of age were also dense; 65-75% of their total consistently banded at the C and D interfaces.

In contrast, B cells within the bursa itself were characteristically light. At all ages, 70-80% were recovered at the A and B interfaces (SG = 1.037-1.057 and 1.057-1.066, respectively). Cells banding at all 4 interfaces were equally susceptible to the cytotoxic action of anti-bursa serum. The T cells detected in bursal suspensions of older chickens were not concentrated at any particular interface.

The density distribution of spleen suspensions indicates that peripheralized cells in 4-week chickens tend to be light. The percentage recovery of spleen cells at the least dense A interface was greater than that observed even in bursal suspensions (43% vs 18%). Since we have yet to examine spleen suspensions from chickens at other ages, we do not know if this profile is related to maturational state of the lymphoid system. Cytotoxic tests with anti-bursa and anti-thymus sera revealed that B cells in the spleen exhibited the same density characteristics as B cells within the bursa. They were recovered primarily at the A and B interfaces and constituted less than 10% of cells collected at C or D. On the other hand, peripheralized T cells did show a density shift in that they were more evenly spread throughout the gradient than were T cells within the thymus itself.

ACKNOWLEDGEMENTS

We would like to thank Mr. Albert Richard Scafuri for excellent technical assistance, and Dr. Nicholas Cohen for critically reading this manuscript. This work was supported by U.S. Public Health Service Grant CA-14061 from the National Cancer Institute. N.D. is a Leukemia Society of America Fellow.

REFERENCES

1. Glick, B., Chang, T. S. and Jaap, R. G., Poultry Sci., 35:224 (1956).
2. Cooper, M. D., Peterson, R. D. A., South, M. A. and Good, R. A., J. Exp. Med., 123:75 (1966).

3. Waksman, B. H., Arnason, B. G. and Jankovic, B. D., J. Exp. Med., 116:187 (1962).
4. Cooper, M. D., Perey, D. Y., McKneally, M. F., Gabrielsen, A. E. Sutherland, D. E. R. and Good, R. A., Lancet 1:1388 (1966).
5. Parrot, D. M. V., deSousa, M. A. B. and East, J., J. Exp. Med., 123:191 (1966).
6. Cooper, M. D., Perey, D. Y., Peterson R. D. A., Gabrielsen, A.E. and Good, R. A., in Immunologic Deficiency Diseases in Man, Birth Defects Original Article Series, IV:7 (National Foundation Press, New York, 1968).
7. Forget, A., Potworowski, E. F., Richer, G. and Borduas, A. G., Immunol., 19:465 (1970).
8. McArthur, W. P., Chapman, J. and Thorbecke, G. J., J. Exp. Med., 134:1036 (1971).
9. Ivanyi, J. and Lydyard, P. M., Cell. Immunol., 5:180 (1972).
10. Wick, G., Albini, B. and Milgrom, F., Clin. exp. Immunol., 15: 237 (1973).
11. Hudson, L. and Roitt, I. M., Eur. J. Immunol., 3:63 (1973).
12. Lydyard, P. and Ivanyi, J., Transplantation, 12:493 (1971).
13. Potworowski, E. F., Richer, G., Borduas, A. G. and Forget, A., J. Immunol., 106:1416 (1971).
14. Wick, G., Kite, J. H. and Cole, R. C., Int. Arch. Allergy, 40: 603 (1971).
15. Potworowski, E. F., Immunol., 23:199 (1972).
16. Albini, B. and Wick, G., J. Immunol., 112:444 (1974).
17. Evans, G. H. and Ivanyi, J., Cell. Immunol., 14:402 (1974).
18. Wick, G., Albini, B. and Johnson, W., Immunol., 28:305 (1975).
19. Crittenden, L. B., Stone, H. A., Reamer, R. H. and Okazaki, W., J. Virol., 1:898 (1967).
20. Crittenden, L. B. and Briles, W. E., Transpl. Proc., 3:1259 (1971).
21. Crittenden, L. B., personal communication to D.G.G., 1974.
22. Crittenden, L. B., Poultry Sci., 51:261 (1972).
23. Gilmour, D. G., unpublished observations.
24. Longenecker, B. M., Pazderka, F., Law, G. R. J. and Ruth, R. F., Transplantation, 14:424 (1972).
25. Stolfi, R. L., Fugmann, R. A., Jensen, J. J. and Sigel, M. M., Immunol., 20:299 (1971).
26. Droege, W., Malchow, D. and Strominger, J. L., Eur. J. Immunol., 2:156 (1972).
27. Thorbecke, G. J., Gordon, H. A., Wostman, B., Wagner, M. and Reyniers, J. A., J. Infect. Dis., 101:237 (1957).
28. Woods, R. and Linna, T. J., Acta Pathol. Microbiol. Scand., 64: 470 (1965).
29. Raidt, D. J., Mishell, R. I. and Dutton, R. W., J. Exp. Med., 128:681 (1968).

VERTEBRATE IMMUNOLOGY

Mitogen Responsiveness, MLC Reactions, and Lymphocyte Heterogeneity

IN VITRO RESPONSES OF URODELE LYMPHOID CELLS: MITOGENIC AND MIXED LYMPHOCYTE CULTURE REACTIVITIES

Nancy H. Collins, V. Manickavel and Nicholas Cohen

Division of Immunology, Department of Microbiology,
University of Rochester School of Medicine & Dentistry
Rochester, New York 14642

In vitro studies of lymphocytes activated by mitogens and allogeneic cells have provided valuable information about the immunologic function of this cell type. In the Amphibia, such studies have been restricted to cells from anurans (1,2). There are substantive immunologic differences between the order, Urodela (salamanders), and the phylogenetically more advanced order, Anura (frogs and toads) which relate to increased complexity of the lymphoid system, increased number of immunoglobulin classes, and rapidity of graft rejection (3-6). Such differences have made us aware of the pitfalls of generalizing about the immunologic capability of a vertebrate class from data collected from one order. Thus, to understand the biology of the amphibian lymphocyte and the evolution of immunity within this pivotal class of vertebrates, it is necessary to characterize the lymphocytes from salamanders in terms of the kinetics and magnitude of their responses to mitogens. To better understand the phylogeny of histocompatibility systems, it is necessary to analyze the reactivity of urodele lymphocytes in MLC. This paper presents our initial attempts to so characterize splenocytes and peripheral blood leukocytes (PBL) from representatives of the families Ambystomatidae and Salamandridae.

MITOGEN STUDIES

Methods. Partially inbred Ambystoma mexicanum (axolotls), obtained from the DeLanney colony (7), were maintained at 22°C and were fed chopped beef heart. Notophthalmus v. viridescens (newts) were collected from one pond in Cattaragus County, N. Y. They were kept in continually filtered water at 25°C and were fed with Tubificid worms.

Animals were anesthetized with 1% MS-222 (ethyl m-aminoben-zoate methanesulfonate, Eastman) or with 0.3% chloretone. Blood was drawn from the ventricle of the axolotl into a heparinized syringe that contained 0.4-0.6 ml heparin (10 U/ml) diluted with phosphate buffered amphibian saline (PBS). The blood was separated into a fraction rich in leukocytes by a modified Ficoll-Hypaque procedure (8). Aseptically removed spleens were minced and then forced through nylon sieves to obtain suspensions of single cells. Cells were thrice washed in Hank's balanced salt solution (HBSS; diluted to amphibian tonicity) and kept at $4^{o}C$ until they were dispensed into cell culture. Cell number was determined in a hemo-cytometer and viability was assessed by trypan blue dye exclusion. Cells were dispensed in 96-well Linbro U bottom plates at a cell concentration of 0.5×10^5 in 0.2 ml of 200-220 mOsm L-15 medium (Leibovitz) that contained 100 U penicillin/ml, 100 μg streptomycin/ml, and 12.5 mM HEPES buffer (GIBCO). This standard medium was supplemented with one of the following: 1) 10% heat-inactivated fetal calf serum (FCS); 2) 10% FCS plus 0.01 M $NaHCO_3$; 3) 5×10^{-5} M 2-mercaptoethanol (2-ME); 4) 2-ME plus 0.01 M $NaHCO_3$. Mitogens were diluted in PBS and were added to triplicate cultures; control cultures received only the PBS diluent. Cultures containing $NaHCO_3$ were incubated in an atmosphere of 5% CO_2 + 95% air; other cultures were incubated in air. All cultures were incubated at $26^{o}C$.

At various times of culture, DNA synthesis was measured by pulsing the cultures for 6-7 hours with either 10 or 8.33 μci tritiated thymidine (New England Nuclear; S.A. = 2 Ci/mMole). The cultures were harvested onto glass fiber filters with a multiple sample precipitator. The radioactivity incorporated into TCA pre-cipitable material was solubilized and evaluated by liquid scintil-lation spectrometry. Stimulation indices (SI) were determined by dividing the cpm in mitogen stimulated cultures by the cpm of PBS containing cultures.

Reactivity to Mitogens. In mice, phytohemagglutinin-P (PHA) and soluble concanavalin A (Con A) preferentially stimulate T-cells while lipopolysaccharide (LPS) stimulates B-cells (9). Spleen cells from the axolotl responded to T-cell mitogens in a dose de-pendent fashion but there were striking quantitative differences between the urodele, the mammalian, and even the anuran responses. Spleen cells from both the axolotl and the newt responded to the B-cell mitogen in a manner similar to that of the higher species in magnitude and kinetics.

Fig. 1 depicts a typical dose response profile of splenocytes from a strain B axolotl cultured with varying amounts of PHA in L-15 supplemented with 10% FCS plus $NaHCO_3$. By 3 days of culture, the peak SI was only 1.4 at 25 λPHA/ml. By 7 days, the response had increased to a SI of 2.3 which occurred at 6.25 λPHA/ml. Con-trol cultures in this and in other experiments showed remarkably

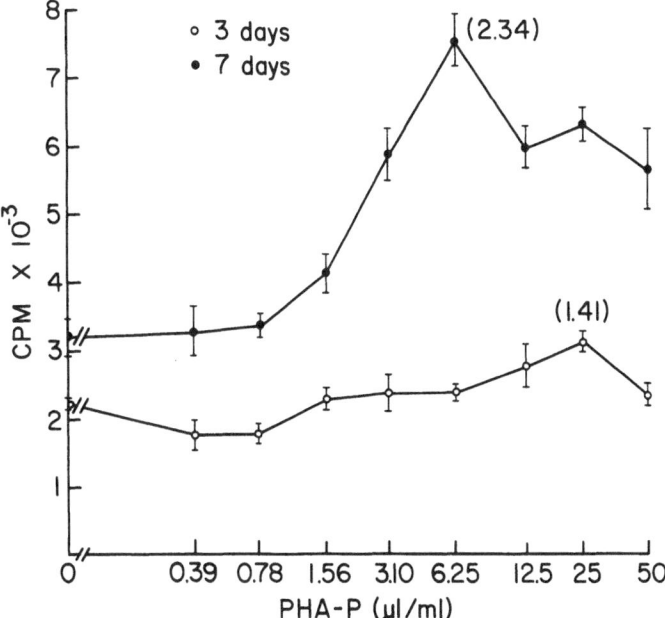

Fig. 1. Uptake of tritiated thymidine by splenocytes from a strain B axolotl incubated with various concentrations of PHA. Cultures were pulsed with 8.33 μci of tritiated thymidine for 7 hours before harvest on days 3 and 7 of culture.

consistent thymidine incorporation until 11 days when the cpm decreased. The cpm of PHA-treated cells from this animal had increased even more by 11 days, which, when coupled with the lower control value, resulted in a SI of 7 at 25 λPHA/ml. The 11 day results are not shown in Fig. 1 since there is considerable variation in the dose response profile and magnitude of the peak response at this time for cells from other animals.

PHA stimulation was also detected in cells from the C^{wis} and N strains of axolotls. Their response was also low by mammalian or anuran standards. Only for cells from 2 of 16 animals studied were SI of greater than 5 seen (SI = 15,20). We have as yet been unable to significantly increase the typically low SI by adding media supplements such as 2-ME with or without $NaHCO_3$. In fact, when FCS was removed from the cultures, the cpm in the control and PHA-treated cultures were reduced and the SI was decreased.

In one series of experiments, splenocytes from the anuran Rana pipiens were cultured in parallel with axolotl cells. The anuran cells displayed a higher peak SI than the urodele (11.5 versus 2.3). Additionally, the peak response for the anuran cells occurred at day 4, which is earlier than seen for urodele cells.

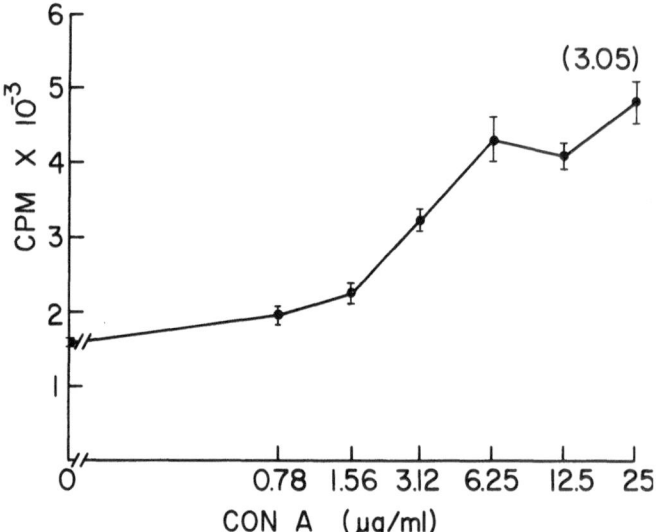

Fig. 2. Stimulation of tritiated thymidine uptake by splenocytes from a strain B axolotl exposed to various concentrations of Con A. Cultures were pulsed with 8.33 μci of tritiated thymidine for 7 hours prior to harvest on day 4 of culture. SI ranged from 1.25 to 3.05.

Con A is also mitogenic for salamander lymphoid cells. Although the Con A response is less well characterized than the PHA response, it is evident that the stimulation indices seen are also less than those described for endothermic vertebrates (10) and for other amphibia (2). Fig. 2 describes the reactivity of splenocytes from a strain B axolotl cultured with Con A for 4 days in L-15 supplemented with 2-ME plus NaHCO₃. Stimulation was seen with all six doubling dilutions of Con A tested and the SI increased as the concentration of the mitogen increased. Significant stimulation was noted earlier with Con A than with PHA (day 4 versus day 7). Indeed, by day 7 when PHA responses had increased relative to day 4, incorporation of thymidine in Con A stimulated cultures fell off both in terms of absolute cpm and the SI. Also, axolotl lymphocytes were reactive over a wider dose range of Con A than is normally seen for cells from higher species (10). When FCS was added to the medium, either with or without NaHCO₃, the Con A response was clearly diminished.

In striking contrast to the low stimulation achieved with PHA and Con A, urodele cells were highly reactive to the presumptive B cell mitogen, LPS. Axolotl cells, cultured for 4 days in L-15 supplemented with 2-ME plus NaHCO₃, responded vigorously to LPS extracted

from E. coli 0111:B4 by a Westphal extraction (Table 1). A clear-
cut but diminished response was seen on day 7. Similar results
over a more restricted dose range were seen for newt splenocytes
with this and other Westphal-extracted LPS preparations. Newt
cells harvested on day 4 responded less dramatically to a Boivin-
extracted LPS from the same bacterial strain (Table 1). The Boivin
preparation contains less of the mitogenic component, Lipid A, on
per weight basis than does the Westphal-extracted material (11).
As was seen in the Con A cultures, FCS added to the medium effectively decreased the response to Con A over the dose range tested.
There are similar findings for anuran cells in the same culture
system (2).

Lymphoid cells from anurans and mammals respond to mitogens
in an analogous fashion (2). While definitive proof of the existence of T and B cells in the Amphibia is lacking, the range
and magnitude of the anuran response to selective mitogens imply
parallel heterogeneity at the level of cell activation in vitro.
Thus, it is not surprising that salamanders also react to mitogens.
Indeed, PHA has been used previously to induce mitosis for karyo-
type analysis of urodele cells (12). What is surprising, however,
is that the response to T-cell mitogens is not more striking.
This delayed and quantitatively smaller response of urodele cells
compared with similarly cultured cells from the frog might reflect
basic differences between the reactive cell populations (T-cell?)
of these two amphibian orders. It is not known whether these
differences result from biochemical or temperature requirements for
stimulation, relative numbers of cells necessary for reactivity, or
the responding cell type itself.

TABLE 1. Stimulation of axolotl and newt splenocytes with LPS[*]

Species	LPS	Concentration (μg/ml)	cpm ± S.E.[**]	Stimulation index
Axolotl (B strain)	E. coli 0111:B4 (Westphal)	0	1,591 ± 55	1.0
		200	22,642 ± 1,537	14.2
		666	29,893 ± 349	18.8
Newt	E. coli 011:B4 (Boivin)	0	571 ± 38	1.0
		2	2,489 ± 105	4.4
		20	2,154 ± 90	3.8
		200	1,330 ± 112	2.3

[*] Cells were cultured in L-15 supplemented with 2-ME plus $NaHCO_3$ for 4 days.

[**] Axolotl cells were pulsed for 7 hours with 8.33 ci 3HTdR; newt cells, for 6 hours with 10 μci 3HTdR.

Recent studies of Ruben et al. (13), which show a hapten-carrier effect in the newt, imply that lymphocyte heterogeneity exists at the level of the Salamandridae. Indeed, in our hands, the LPS response is more easily demonstrable than the PHA response in this species. Similarly, the response of axolotl lymphoid cells to the B-cell mitogen was earlier and greater than the response to the T-cell mitogens. In the absence of sufficient hard data, it is tempting to speculate that the LPS reactive cells (B-cells?) of urodeles exist in greater numbers in the spleen and/or that preferential activation by a bacterial polyclonal B-cell activator offers the salamander a great survival value.

MIXED LYMPHOCYTE CULTURE STUDIES

Methods. Splenocytes and PBL from axolotls, and splenocytes from newts were prepared as described for mitogen studies. Control cultures, containing only cells from each partner, were plated in triplicate; mixed cultures containing equal numbers of cells from each partner were plated in quadruplicate. Both control and mixed cell cultures contained 0.5×10^5 leukocytes in 0.2 ml. In 1-way cultures, DNA synthesis in mitomycin C-treated stimulator cells (14) was inhibited more than 90%. Viabilities were unaffected by mitomycin C. Stimulation indices (SI) for 2-way MLC's were calculated by dividing the cpm of the mixed culture by one-half the sum of the cpm of the corresponding control cultures. SI for 1-way MLC's were calculated by dividing the cpm of the MLC by the cpm of the responder control culture which was incubated with autologous mitomycin-treated cells. SI of ≥ 1.6 were considered positive; from 0.6-<1.6, nonstimulatory; and <0.6, possibly suppressive.

Reactivity in Mixed Lymphocyte Cultures. The axolotl study was undertaken to further define the histocompatibility characteristics of several strains of partially inbred axolotls (C^{wis}, B, M, N) in the DeLanney colony (7). Results, detailed elsewhere in this volume (7), are summarized as follows:

1. Axolotl lymphoid cells were capable of responding and stimulating in 2-way MLC. Positive SI's could be obtained in interstrain combinations, but not every interstrain combination resulted in stimulation. No stimulation was recorded in the four C^{wis} (F_{11} generation) intrastrain combinations examined.

2. The kinetics of the MLC reaction were delayed when compared with Con A or LPS responses. The magnitude of the MLC response increased with increased culture time.

3. SI's were generally lower than stimulation that is seen in murine MLC's where the allogeneic cells differ at the major histocompatibility complex (MHC). They were, however, comparable to SI's

TABLE 2.   Effects of Cell Source and Medium Supplementation on MLC Reactivity in Axolotls

Pair[*]	Strain Combination[+]	Cell Source	Medium Supplement	cpm ± S.E.[‡]		SI
1	$C_1^{wis}+M_1$	PBL	FCS	c^{wis}:	21,058 ± 603	
				M:	19,367 ± 1,269	
				$c^{wis}+M$:	44,733 ± 1,256	2.21
		Spleen	FCS	c^{wis}:	607 ± 57	
Effect of cell source				M:	2,150 ± 161	
				$c^{wis}+M$:	1,590 ± 39	1.15
2	$C_2^{wis}+C_3^{wis}$	Spleen	FCS	c^{wis}:	2,005 ± 53	
				c^{wis}:	4,159 ± 369	
				$c^{wis}+c^{wis}$:	3,274 ± 104	1.06
			FCS + NaHCO₃	c^{wis}:	1,731 ± 162	
Media effects in intrastrain combination				c^{wis}:	4,920 ± 426	
				$c^{wis}+c^{wis}$:	2,974 ± 146	.89
			2-ME	c^{wis}:	226 ± 28	
				c^{wis}:	797 ± 48	
				$c^{wis}+c^{wis}$:	402 ± 7	.78
			2-ME + NaHCO₃	c^{wis}:	1,199 ± 82	
				c^{wis}:	1,919 ± 109	
				$c^{wis}+c^{wis}$:	1,260 ± 110	.80
3	$C_4^{wis}+M_2$	PBL	FCS	c^{wis}:	858 ± 576	
				M:	10,244 ± 708	
				$c^{wis}+M$:	16,408 ± 736	1.80
			FCS + NaHCO₃	c^{wis}:	6,520 ± 115	
Media effects in interstrain combination				M:	10,401 ± 29	
				$c^{wis}+M$:	14,529 ± 288	1.70
			2-ME	c^{wis}:	4,227 ± 252	
				M:	2,084 ± 123	
				$c^{wis}+M$:	3,696 ± 192	1.17
			2-ME + NaHCO₃	c^{wis}:	4,497 ± 269	
				M:	3,212 ± 102	
				$c^{wis}+M$:	5,060 ± 359	1.31

[*]Pair = allogeneic combination
[+]Subscript number after strain designation refers to individual animals.
[‡]Cells were cultured for 7 days and harvested after a 7 hour pulse with 8.33 µCi tritiated thymidine.

obtained in MLC's when the cocultured murine cells differ only at minor H-loci.

4. Positive reactivity was dependent on the tissue source of the cultured cells. PBL usually gave a higher stimulation than splenocytes from the same animals (e.g., Table 2).

5. Detection of an MLC reaction is dependent on culture conditions. Table 2 demonstrates that in the nonstimulatory $C^{wis}+C^{wis}$ splenocyte combination, the SI varied from 0.78 in medium supplemented with 2-ME to 1.06 in medium that contained FCS. In the marginally stimulatory combination, $C^{wis}+M$, SI for PBL varied from 1.17 to 1.80 in medium supplemented with 2-ME or FCS, respectively. Thus, as in mammalian systems (15), MLC reactivity depends on both the stimulating alloantigens and the conditions of culture.

Like the axolotl, MLC's of newt splenocytes stimulated in some combinations but not in others. In kinetic studies that spanned 3-9 days, maximal responses (SI = 1.6-3) occurred on days 6-8 (Fig. 3) as they did for axolotls. One-way MLC's allowed us to visualize the differential responses of newts to alloantigens. For example, in Fig. 3, cells from animal #4 responded more vigorously to cells from animal #3 than did #3 to #4 (SI of 3.1 versus 1.7). If the genetic and cellular bases of MLC reactivity in urodeles and endotherms are analogous, then differential stimulatory responses

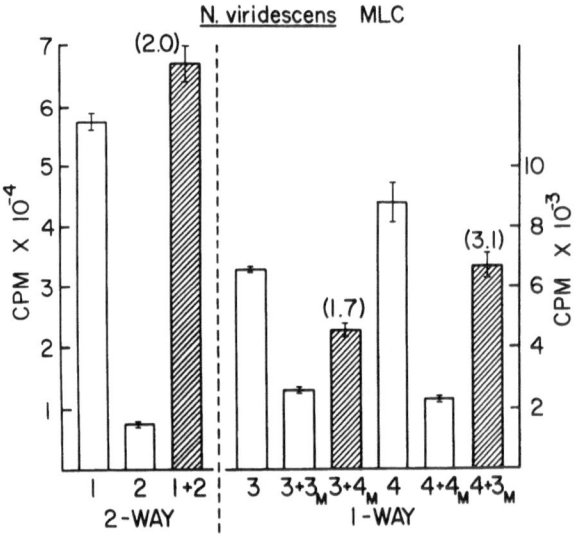

Fig. 3. The activity of newt splenocytes in 2-way and 1-way MLC's. Newts were collected from one location. Their cells were cultured for 7 days in L-15 supplemented with FCS. The cultures were pulsed with 10 μCi tritiated thymidine for 6 hours.

may be indicative of variability of shared antigens, cumulative stimulatory effects of multiple loci, or differential stimulatory capacities of the alloantigens.

MLC reactivities of cells from several anuran species are well-established (1,17). Indeed, based on his correlative analyses of graft rejection, erythrocyte alloantigens, and MLC reactivities within families, du Pasquier (17) recently proposed that the primitive anuran, Xenopus laevis, has a major histocompatibility complex. However, based primarily on analysis of the typically chronic rejection reactions of urodeles, it has been hypothesized that representatives of this order lack the functional and/or structural equivalent of the mammalian MHC. Since MLC reactions in mice can result from differences at minor H-loci and since such reactions are usually marked by relatively low stimulation indices, demonstration and definition of salamanders' MLC reactivities may help to identify the nature of the urodeles' histocompatibility systems. In our culture system MLC responses in two urodele species are quantitatively lower but not qualitatively different from those obtained with cocultured cells from advanced anurans or mice which differ at the MHC. This provides another argument that the "classic" MHC in salamanders does not exist.

ACKNOWLEDGEMENTS

The research cited has been supported by grants HD-07901 (to N.C.) from the USPHS and grant IN-18 (to N.H.C.) from the American Cancer Society to the University of Rochester. N.H.C. is a predoctoral trainee supported by Training Grant 5T01-GM-00591. V.M. is a postdoctoral fellow supported by USPHS grant HD-07901. N.C. is a recipient of USPHS Research Career Development Award AI-70736. The authors gratefully acknowledge Dr. L. E. DeLanney for providing us with axolotls and S. N. Goldstine for excellent advice. The expert technical assistance of Mary Horan is gratefully appreciated. We thank F. R. Ogg, Jr. and Sally Mander for continuing inspiration.

REFERENCES

1. Goldshein, S. J. and Cohen, N., J. Immunol. 108:1025 (1972).
2. Goldstine, S. N., Collins, N. H. and Cohen, N., Adv. Exp. Med. & Biol. (this volume) (1975).
3. Cooper, E. L., Contemp. Topics. Immunobiol. 2, 366 pp. (Plenum Press, New York, 1973).
4. Goldstine, S. N., Manickavel, V. and Cohen, N., Amer. Zool. 15: 107 (1975).
5. Hildemann, W. H., Transplant. Rev. 3:5 (1970).
6. Cohen, N., in Comparative Immunology, J. J. Marchalonis (ed.) (Blackwell, Oxford, 1975).

7. DeLanney, L. E., Collins, N. H., Cohen, N. and Reid, R., Adv.
    Exp. Med. & Biol. (this volume) (1975).
8. Weiss, N. and du Pasquier, L., J. Immunol. Methods 3:273
    (1973).
9. Andersson, J., Sjöberg, O. and Möller, G., Transplant. Rev. 11:
    131 (1972).
10. Stobo, J. D., Transplant. Rev. 11:60 (1972).
11. Milner, K. C., Rudbach, J. A. and Ribi, E., in Microbial
    Toxins, vol. IV, G. Weinbaum, S. Kadis and S. J. Ajl, (eds.),
    473 pp. (Academic Press, New York, 1971).
12. Seto, T. and Rounds, D. E., in Methods in Cell Physiology,
    Vol. III, D. M. Prescott (ed), 387 pp. (Academic Press,
    New York, 1968).
13. Ruben, L. N., van der Hoven, A. and Dutton, R. W., Cell. Im-
    munol. 6:300 (1973).
14. Bach, F. H. and Voynow, N. C., Science 166:545 (1966).
15. Peck, A. B. and Click, R. E., Transplantation 16:331 (1973).
16. Festenstein, H., Transplant. Rev. 15:62 (1973).
17. du Pasquier, L., Chardonnens, X., Miggiano, V. C., Immuno-
    genetics 1:482 (1975).

TRANSPLANTATION IMMUNOGENETICS AND MLC REACTIVITIES OF PARTIALLY INBRED STRAINS OF SALAMANDERS (*A. Mexicanum*): PRELIMINARY STUDIES

Louis E. DeLanney[1], Nancy H. Collins[2], Nicholas Cohen[2], and Robert Reid[1]
[1]Department of Biology, Ithaca College, Ithaca, N.Y.;
[2]Division of Immunology, Department of Microbiology, University of Rochester School of Medicine and Dentistry, Rochester, N. Y. 14642

Allograft rejection in field collected representatives from at least 11 different genera of urodele amphibians is typically chronic in that median survival times (MSTs) range from approximately 30-50 days (1). Although such chronicity may be experimentally varied by temperature or by the criterion selected as a survival end point (2), it is more important that it reflects donor - host antigenic disparities at what appear to be the urodelean equivalents of murine "minor" histocompatibility or H-loci (3). In the absence of appropriate breeding studies we have only been able to speculate as to the number of H-loci in a given population or species, the number of alleles at each locus, and the frequency of alleles within any population under analysis. Similarly, in the absence of testable criteria other than graft survival times we have only been able to speculate as to whether urodeles really lack a major histocompatibility complex (MHC) comparable in its complexity, polymorphism, and immunologic relevance to the H-2 system of mice (4) or the HL-A complex of man (5). Currently we are aware of two potential sources of urodeles typed for histocompatibility factors. These are the Pleurodeles waltlii developed by Gallien and now being used in immunologic studies by Charlemagne and Tournefier (6) and the DeLanney colony of Ambystoma mexicanum (axolotls; 7). The purpose of this paper is to provide preliminary data derived from these partially inbred strains of axolotls that concern the number of H-loci in this species and the immunogenicity of their products.

BRIEF HISTORY OF THE DELANNEY AXOLOTL COLONY

The first animals in this colony were received in 1957 from R. R. Humphrey but their geneologies were unrecorded. Since at that early point in the recent history of comparative immunology, it was of interest to simply establish whether these neotenic urodeles were immunocompetent, they were reciprocally skin grafted. Although immune rejection was noted, the genetic uniqueness of each animal was not apparent in all instances since the animals could be grouped into acceptor and rejector categories. This observation was in marked contrast to results from subsequent studies with wild-caught axolotls in which all animals rejected all transplants. The latter observation is consistent with the presence of multiple histocompatibility alleles or loci segregating in wild populations; the former is not, and suggested that some genetic selection had occurred in the Humphrey lines. Matrix-analysis grafting with Humphrey's animals allowed them to be distributed into three major groups and breeding studies were begun (7-9). At this time the effort and space required to establish and define a number of different strains was sacrificed in favor of developing the C strain for analyzing lymphosarcoma-associated transplantation antigens (7). A protozoan (Oodinium) infestation further helped to reduce the number of representative animals in several strains. However, with the recognition of the potential usefulness of the axolotl for immunogenetic analyses of transplantation immunity of a phylogenetically pivotal order of primitive vertebrates (10) has come an expansion of the inbreeding program. The strains currently available in the DeLanney colony that are now being sibling or back-cross inbred are from Humphrey as well as from other sources. They are[*]: 1) B strain dark (Humphrey-Holtfreter derived) @ F_6; 2) B strain white (DeLanney) @ F_4; 3) Mexican melanoids (m/m) @ F_6; 4) $C^{nonWistar}$ @ F_6; 5) C^{Wistar} @ F_{11-12}; 6) Netherlands @ F_{3-4} and 7) London whites (DeLanney imports) @ F_3.

SOME IMMUNOGENETIC ANALYSES OF TRANSPLANT REJECTION

In the following studies full thickness skin grafts were transplanted to the epaxial trunk or head according to established procedures. Since in many instances grafts were exchanged between white animals, melanophore breakdown could not be used as the criterion of total graft destruction (2,3). Instead, survival end points were based on criteria associated with the definitive onset of rejection, namely epidermal sloughing, vasodilation, and hemostasis. All animals were maintained at 20°C.

The following data speak to the Mendelian segregation and codominance of histocompatibility genes, to the minimum number of H-loci currently detectable by transplantation rejection, and to differential chronic rejection times associated with these genetic

---

[*]Strains numbered 1)-7) will be referred to in the subsequent text as: 1) B^{DD}: 2) B^{dd}; 3) M; 4) C; 5) C^{wis}; 6) N and 7) LW.

differences. Tables 1 and 2 present the results of two replicate experiments in which grafts from F_2 progeny of a mating of (C^{wis} x B^{DD})F_1s were transplanted to typing hosts thought to have the C and B^{DD} parental and (C x B)F_1 genetic backgrounds. The typing hosts in each experiment were derived from different matings as were the parents of the F_2 donors. Grafts exchanged between parental strains C $\rightleftharpoons$ B and C^{wis} $\rightleftharpoons$ B^{DD} were always rejected; grafts between C^{wis} $\rightleftharpoons$ C were always accepted. Results of a chi square comparison between the predicted (1:2:1) and observed segregation ratio of genotypes in the F_2 (Table 1) and the predicted and observed per cent of F_2 grafts accepted:rejected by each typing host in each experiment (Table 2), are consistent with the hypothesis

TABLE 1. F_2 Progeny Analysis of a (B^{DD} x C^{wis}) F_1 Cross

Four possible survival patterns of F_2 grafts on typing hosts			Number of F_2 graft showing each survival pattern on typing hosts in				Proposed F_2 genotype
			Exp. 1 (n=20)		Exp. 2 (n=30)		
B^{DD}	C	(B^{DD}xC)F_1	Pre-dicted	Ob-served	Pre-dicted	Ob-served	
#1 A*	R**	A	5	4	7½	5	B/B
#2 R	R	A	10	10	15	13	B/C
#3 R	A	A	5	6	7½	11	C/C
#4 A	A	A	0	0	0	1	?

* A = accepted
**R = rejected

TABLE 2. Ratio of the % of F_2s rejected: % accepted by typing hosts in:

	Exp. 1 (n=30 F_2s)			Exp. 2 (n=20 F_2s)		
	B^{DD}	C	(B^{dd}xC)F_1	B^{DD}	C^{wis}	(B^{dd}xC)F_1
Expected	75:25	75:25	0:100	75:25	75:25	0:100
Observed	80:20	60:40	0:100	80:20	70:30	0:100

that B^{DD} and C^{wis} axolotls are two homozygous strains which differ
from each other by alleles at one H-locus or at several closely
linked H-loci. The single exception was that grafts from one F_2
donor were accepted by all typing hosts (Table 1).

The possibility cannot be dismissed, however, that B^{DD} and
C^{wis} differ from each other by more than one H-locus but that the
alloantigens coded for by genes at the other loci either failed to
elicit a detectable rejection reaction (as in the case of certain
H-Y antigens in mice; 11) or would have been rejected had the
grafts been observed longer than 12 weeks. In this regard, perhaps
temperatures higher than 20°C (2) might have increased the per cent
rejected. Similarly, since chronic rejection seems to be in part
a function of active enhancement, we are currently determining
whether preferential elimination of this immunoprotective response
to H-alloantigens with cytosine arabinoside (12) might also reveal
destructive immunity as it does across the H-Y barrier in C_3H mice
(Manickavel and Cohen, unpublished).

Fig. 1 depicts another approach to testing the isogenicity of
several spawnings. If we assume that because the C^{wis} line (derived from one pair of animals and kept separate since 1935) was

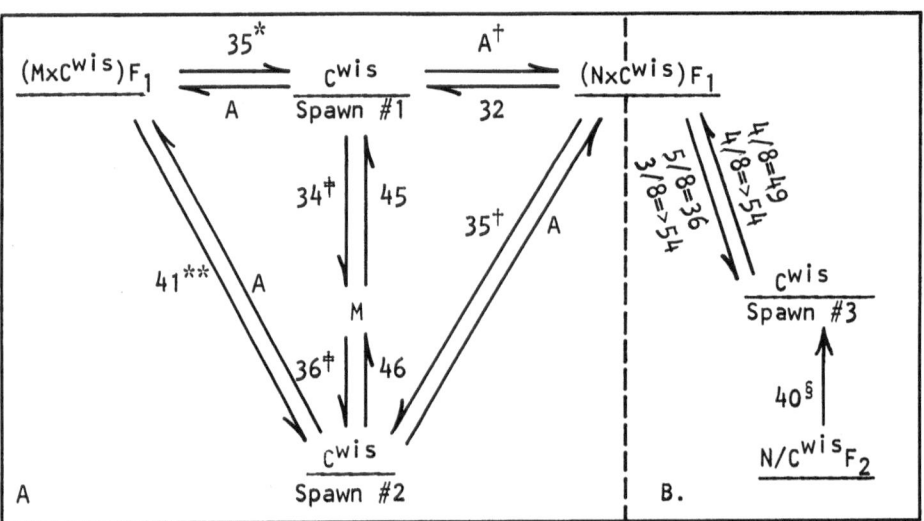

Fig. 1. Allografting to test the isogenicity of the progeny of
several of the C^{wis} strains. Numbers next to arrows = median
survival times; A = accepted for >54 days. Number of grafts transplanted in each direction in a combination:

*= 13; **= 15; †= 5; ‡ = 10; §= 12

inbred for 11 generations it should be homozygous or else be approaching homozygosity for its H-loci, then the grafting procedure depicted in Fig. 1 should reveal such homozygosity. As seen in Fig. 1A, all reciprocal grafts between the three parental strains (N, M, C^{wis}) were rejected as were grafts from the F_1 hybrids to the C^{wis} parentals. All C^{wis} parental grafts were accepted by the $(C^{wis}xM)F_1$ hybrid. This is consistent with the homozygosity of C^{wis}. However, the following data presented in Fig. 1B reveal that C^{wis} has a minimum of two H-loci and is homozygous at only one of them. At least 50% of the grafts from C^{wis} (spawn #3) were chronically rejected by one of the three spawns of the $(C^{wis}xN)F_1$ hybrid. The remaining four grafts were still viable at >54 days. These data suggest that C^{wis} is not yet homozygous and has a minimum of two H-loci. This conclusion is supported by the rejection of all F_2 grafts (N/C^{wis}) by the C^{wis} of spawn #3. Why none of the other F_1 hybrids involving a C^{wis} parent failed to detect the heterozygosity at an additional locus (loci) is speculative at this time. Suffice it to say that additional inbreeding and P → F_2 grafting studies are in progress so that the number of H-loci in the axolotl can be more accurately estimated.

MIXED LYMPHOCYTE CULTURE (MLC) REACTIONS

In mammals, proliferation of allogeneic lymphoid cells in MLC is stimulated by differences in defined regions of the genome of the cell donors (13). In the mouse, these regions have been located in the MHC (4), the minor or non-H-2 loci (14) and in other non-H-2-linked regions (15). Distinctions between major and minor H-loci, originally based on the rapidity of graft rejection (16), may also relate to the magnitude of the stimulation observed in MLC. Differences in the MHC generally result in higher stimulation indices than those obtained when differences prevail only at the minor loci (17).

With this background information in mind, it was of interest to ascertain whether strains of partially inbred axolotls which differ by at least one H-locus and reject grafts chronically, might also differ at MLC determining loci. While it is too premature to ask if the MLC genes are linked to H-loci in the urodele, it is possible to compare the kinetics and magnitude of axolotl MLC reactivities with those of other genetically defined species which are known to result from differences at either major or minor loci.

Two-way MLCs were set up in microculture in three interstrain and in one intrastrain combination according to protocols detailed elsewhere in this volume (18). Briefly, spleen cells or peripheral blood leukocytes (PBL) were cultured with allogeneic cells from the same tissue source at a concentration of 0.5×10^5 in 0.2 ml in

220 mOsm L-15 supplemented with either: 10% fetal calf serum
(FCS); 10% FCS with 0.01 M $NaHCO_3$; 5 x 10^{-5} M 2-mercaptoethanol
(2-ME); or 2-ME with 0.01 M $NaHCO_3$. Cultures were incubated at
$26^{o}C$ in air or in 5% CO_2, and were harvested after 3, 7, and 11
days of culture with a semi-automatic multiple sample precipitator.
Thus, multiple observations were made for any combination (pair) of
allogeneic cells. DNA synthesis was measured prior to harvest by
a seven hour pulse with tritiated thymidine. Stimulation indices
(SI) were calculated by dividing the counts per minute incorporated in the MLC by one-half the sum of the counts per minute obtained in the corresponding control cultures. The cell number and
volume were equal in both mixed and control cultures. Stimulation
indices $\geq$ 1.6 were considered to be positive; from 0.6-<1.6 were
considered nonstimulatory; and from 0-<0.6 were judged as possibly
suppressive.

Table 3 summarizes the results of positive MLCs between cells
from 17 pairs of axolotls. Regardless of variables of culture
conditions, time of harvest, and cell source, leukocytes from four
of six pairs of animals studied in the $C^{wis}+$ M strains showed
positive SI from 1.7 to 2.8 in either spleen or blood. Positive
SI occurred after 7 or 11 days of culture in medium supplemented
with FCS (with or without $NaHCO_3$), or with 2-ME plus $NaHCO_3$.

In the C+N combination, leukocytes from only 1 of the 3 pairs
tested stimulated in MLC. This positive reaction was seen in a
seven day PBL culture in medium supplemented with 2-ME and $NaHCO_3$.
The spleen culture of that combination was negative in the same
medium and in medium supplemented with FCS with $NaHCO_3$. The other
two pairs of spleen cultures were also negative even after 11 days
in culture. In the C+B combination, cells from two of four pairs
were stimulated in MLC. Both were PBL cultures harvested at day
11 and cultured in 2-ME with $NaHCO_3$. All of the 15 spleen cultures
in other media harvested at 3, 7, or 11 days were nonstimulatory.

Finally, in the four $C^{wis}+C^{wis}$ combinations studied no positive SI were recorded. However, three of these were spleen cultures and all cultures were terminated on day seven. Therefore,
further experiments with longer culture times and more observations of PBL cultures are necessary before it can be stated
definitively that cells from the C^{wis} do not stimulate each other
in MLC.

The data presented in Table 3 demonstrate that SI greater than
1.6 can be obtained in axolotls and that these indices can be as
high as 3.0. Nevertheless, it is important that the strain differences were not always predictive of stimulation. That no
positive indices were noted with cells from two of the six C+M
pairs, two of three C+N pairs, and two of four $C^{wis}+$B pairs, even
though they were cultured under conditions comparable to those

TABLE 3. MLC Reactions in Axolotls

Positive MLC reactions with cells from:

Blood		Spleen			
CPM ± SE	SI	CPM ± SE	SI	Strain	Pair No.[*]
21,058 ± 603		78 ± 2		C^{wis}	
19,367 ± 1,269		1,434 ± 186		M	#1
44,733 ± 1,256	2.2	2,119 ± 55	2.8	C^{wis}+M	
		538 ± 23		C^{wis}	
Not done		2,642 ± 242		M	#2
		3,025 ± 79	1.9	C^{wis}+M	
3,204 ± 104		787 ± 48		C^{wis}	
957 ± 108		488 ± 10		M	#3
5,848 ± 860	2.8	1,382 ± 118	2.1	C^{wis}+M	
6,520 ± 115				C^{wis}	
10,401 ± 295		Not done		M	#4
14,529 ± 228	1.7			C^{wis}+M	
1,908 ± 106				C^{wis}	
990 ± 54		Not done		B	#1
3,989 ± 356	2.7			C^{wis}+B	
3,204 ± 104				C^{wis}	
990 ± 54		Not done		B	#2
5,379 ± 542	2.6			C^{wis}+B	
217 ± 21				C^{wis}	
488 ± 20		Not done		N	#1
905 ± 19	2.6			C^{wis}+N	

[*]Pair = allogeneic mix.
Number pairs stimulatory/number pairs studied in C^{wis}+M = 4/6; C^{wis}+B = 2/4; C^{wis}+N = 1/3; C^{wis}+C^{wis} = 0/4. Although only a few pairs were studied, multiple observations (upwards of eight) were made for each pair since each was studied with respect to culture medium, harvest time, and tissue origin of cells.

where positive reactions were seen in the same strain combinations, means that it is not possible simply to equate MLC reactivity with differences between partially inbred salamanders. While the data in Table 3 suggest that there may be a ranking of strain combinations with respect to the per cent that reveal positive reactions, they were collected from a limited number of animals.

The positive MLC response of the axolotl exhibits many of the same characteristics of MLC reactions in endotherms and anuran amphibians (18,19). For example, the maximum response is delayed relative to mitogen-induced proliferation (18-21). Variation in the response is dependent on the tissue source of the cells and on the medium employed. Fig. 2 depicts a typical response in the $C^{wis}+$ M combination harvested on day seven in each of two media. The response of PBL is greater than that of splenocytes from the same combination in both media and is itself affected by the medium used. Two conclusions may, therefore, be warranted. 1) The cell population(s) in blood and spleen are different. The PBL cultures are either richer in stimulator and/or responder cells or they lack an immunoregulatory cell or factor that is present in the splenic MLC (22). 2) The medium employed can either favor or mask the expression of potential MLC reactive cell populations. Therefore, considerable caution must be exercised in interpreting situations where the potential MLC reaction is not great. Thus, lack of or low stimulation may be the result of medium, serum source, other supplements (17) or source of the cells used. It may also reflect cell-to-cell inhibition, antigenic similarity of MLC products, lack or limited number of cells carrying appropriate receptors and limited distribution of appropriate receptors on lymphoid cells.

It has yet to be established whether MLC reactivity in the axolotl is associated with a single H-locus. If such linkage

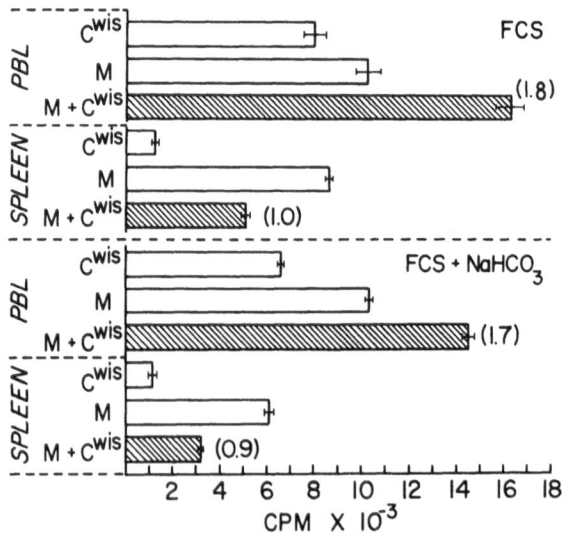

Fig. 2. Marginal MLC reacting between splenocytes and PBL from one pair of animals ($C^{wis}+M$) in two different media. Note that SI is highest with PBL.

becomes demonstrable then these data would suggest that a rather high degree of MLC determinants is shared between histoincompatible strains. If MLC reactivity results from the summation effects of differences at a number of H-loci (23), then the observation that not all interstrain combinations are stimulatory suggests a significant degree of H-locus polymorphism in the axolotl.

The magnitude of the axolotl MLC is in the range of mammalian responses that are marginally stimulatory and are associated with minor H-locus differences in mice (14,17). However, it is not yet possible to ascertain the "major" or "minor" character of the histocompatibility differences operative in axolotls simply by the magnitude of the stimulation index since under certain culture conditions multiple minor locus differences in mice may in fact lead to stimulation indices as large as or larger than those seen when the donors of the allogeneic cells differ at the MHC (24).

We plan further characterization of the capabilities of the urodele lymphocytes in MLC. The DeLanney colony of axolotls offers a unique opportunity to explore the responses of lymphoid cells in a variety of genetic situations and to combine such studies with transplantation analyses. Such efforts should move urodele immunogenetics from the realm of theory and speculation along the pathway towards fact and subsequent understanding of the phylogeny of histocompatibility systems.

ACKNOWLEDGEMENTS

Research cited has been supported by grants GM-05619, GM-15363 (to L.D.) and HD-07901 (to N.C.) from the USPHS and grant IN-18 (to N.H.C.) from the American Cancer Society to the University of Rochester. N.C. is a recipient of USPHS Research Career Development Award AI-70736; N.H.C. is a predoctoral trainee supported by Training Grant 5T01-GM-00591. The technical assistance of Ms. Mary Horan and Dr. Bryan Hamilton is gratefully appreciated.

REFERENCES

1. Cohen, N., Amer. Zool. 11:193 (1971).
2. Cohen, N., J. Exp. Zool. 163:231 (1966).
3. Cohen, N. and Hildemann, W. H., Transplantation 6:208 (1968).
4. Klein, J., Biology of the Mouse Histocompatibility-2 Complex (1975) 624 pp. Springer-Verlag, New York, N.Y.
5. Thorsby, E., Transplant. Rev. 18:51 (1974).
6. Charlemagne, J. and Tournefier, A., J. Immunogen. 1:125 (1974).
7. DeLanney, L. E. and Blackler, K., in Biology of Amphibian Tumors, M. Mizell, ed., Springer-Verlag, New York, N.Y. (1969) p. 399.

8. DeLanney, L. E., Amer. Zool. 1:349 (1961).
9. Meier, A. H. and DeLanney, L. E., Amer. Zool. 2:431 (1962).
10. Cohen, N., in Comparative Immunology, J. J. Marchalonis, ed., Blackwell, England (in press).
11. Goldberg, E., Boyse, E. A., Scheid, M. and Bennett, D. Nature (New Biol.) 238:55 (1972).
12. Manickavel, V. and Cohen, N., Transplant. Proc. 7:451 (1975).
13. Dutton, R. W., J. Exp. Med. 123:665 (1966).
14. Mangi, R. J. and Mardiney, M. R., Jr., Transplantation 11:369 (1971).
15. Festenstein, H., Transplant. Rev. 15:62 (1973).
16. Hildemann, W. H., Transplant. Rev. 3:5 (1970).
17. Peck, A. B. and Click, R. E., Transplantation 16:331 (1973).
18. Collins, N. H., Manickavel, V. and Cohen, N., Adv. Exp. Med. Biol. (this volume) (1975).
19. Du Pasquier, L., Chardonnens, X., Miggiano, V. C., Immunogenetics 1:482 (1975).
20. Goldshein, S. J. and Cohen, N., J. Immunol. 108:1025 (1972).
21. Goldstine, S. N., Collins, N. H. and Cohen, N., Adv. Exp. Med. Biol. (this volume) (1975).
22. Folch, H. and Waksman, B. H., J. Immunol. 113:140 (1974).
23. Graff, R. J., Hildemann, W. H. and Snell, G. D., Transplantation 4:425 (1966).
24. Katz-Heber, E., Peck, A.B. and Click, R. E., Eur. J. Immunol. 3:379 (1973).

MITOGENS AS PROBES FOR STUDYING TEMPERATURE EFFECTS ON THE

DEVELOPMENT OF IMMUNOCOMPETENT CELLS IN POIKILOTHERMIC VERTEBRATES

Richard K. Wright, A. Lakshma Reddy, and Edwin L. Cooper

Departments of Anatomy and Microbiology and Immunology,
School of Medicine and Dental Research Institute,
University of California, Los Angeles, California 90024

INTRODUCTION

Vertebrate physiological processes take place over a limited temperature range. With the poikilothermic vertebrates (fishes, amphibians and reptiles), their internal body temperature is closely linked to the environmental temperature with little regulation possible. In general, within the thermal tolerance limits of the organism, low temperatures depress, delay or inhibit antibody synthesis and increase allograft survival times whereas high temperatures increase or accelerate antibody synthesis and decrease allograft survival times (1-4).

The introduction of antigen into an animal is followed by complex events culminating in the development of immunocompetent cells and clearance or neutralization of the antigen. These stages can be delineated into three broad categories: 1) antigen recognition, binding, and processing; 2) lymphocyte activation; and 3) mitosis with the concomitant development of immunocompetent cell populations. Any one or all of these stages could be susceptible to low temperatures in a poikilothermic vertebrate.

During antigenic stimulation, only a small number of the total lymphocyte population initially responds. These cells are difficult to detect and quantitate in vivo. The use of various plant lectins to stimulate lymphocytes from various animals (5-10) to undergo morphological transformation and mitosis is however a promising approach. Although the response is non-specific, i.e., most if not all lymphocytes are stimulated to mature and divide, in many ways it is reminiscent of the specific response to antigen (11-14).

Assuming that mitogenic responses are equivalent to antigenic responses, then the three categories previously listed remain unchanged except for substituting antigen for mitogen in category 1. Since the in vitro response to mitogen occurs over a relatively short time span and can be quantitated by measuring protein or DNA synthesis (15), one can use mitogens as probes in determining the mechanism by which temperature influences the development of immunocompetent cells. Furthermore, the temperature sensitive stage or stages in the immune response continuum can be located chronologically.

IN VITRO RESPONSE OF RANA PIPIENS SPLEEN CELLS TO MITOGENS

Spleen cell suspensions from the leopard frog Rana pipiens are prepared by gently dissociating the spleen in a Kinitis homogenizer. The cells are washed, viability determined and cultures containing 1×10^5 cells in L-15 medium supplemented with 10% heat inactivated fetal cell serum and antibiotics are prepared in Microtest II culture plates. Mitogens are added at time zero. At selected time intervals, 2 μCi of tritiated thymidine (^{3}HTdR) are added; 18-24 hours later the cultures are harvested and processed for liquid scintillation. Radioactivity measurements in counts/ minute are obtained and the change in ^{3}HTdR incorporation caused by the mitogen is expressed for each culture as the stimulation index (S.I.) or ratio between counts per minute in cultures with and without mitogen.

Frog spleen cells give significant mitogenic responses to concanavalin A (Con A). At 22°C, maximum incorporation of ^{3}HTdR and stimulation occurs on day 4 of culture with 10 μg Con A. The magnitude and kinetics of these responses are similar to those reported for other vertebrates. Spleen cell responses to Con A are sensitive to temperature (Figure 1). At 4° and 15°C, no significant stimulation occurs over a six day culture period. Spleen cells cultured at 15 to 22°C for 3 to 5 days show that as the temperature is increased to 22-25°C, maximum incorporation of ^{3}HTdR and stimulation occurs. Thermal tolerance limits are reached at 28°C where no significant stimulation is observed. Thus, over a 10°C temperature range (15°-25°C) and four day culture period, the kinetics and magnitude of the response to Con A varies from no to maximum stimulation.

EFFECTS OF TEMPERATURE ON MITOGEN BINDING

Mitogenic stimulation of lymphocytes is dependent upon the binding of the lectin to glycoprotein receptors (16) on the cell surface. Kinetic studies on the effects of temperature (0-37°C) on the binding of [63]Ni-concanavalin A to SV40 transformed hamster cells have shown that the amount of lectin bound to the cell surface increases with temperature (17). Rat lymph node lymphocytes and mouse lymphoma cells however can bind sufficient amounts of some lectins to induce lymphocyte activation over temperatures ranging from 4-37°C (18). Preliminary studies from our laboratory using direct labeling techniques with fluorescein isothiocyanate conjugated concanavalin A (FITC-Con A) suggest that frog spleen

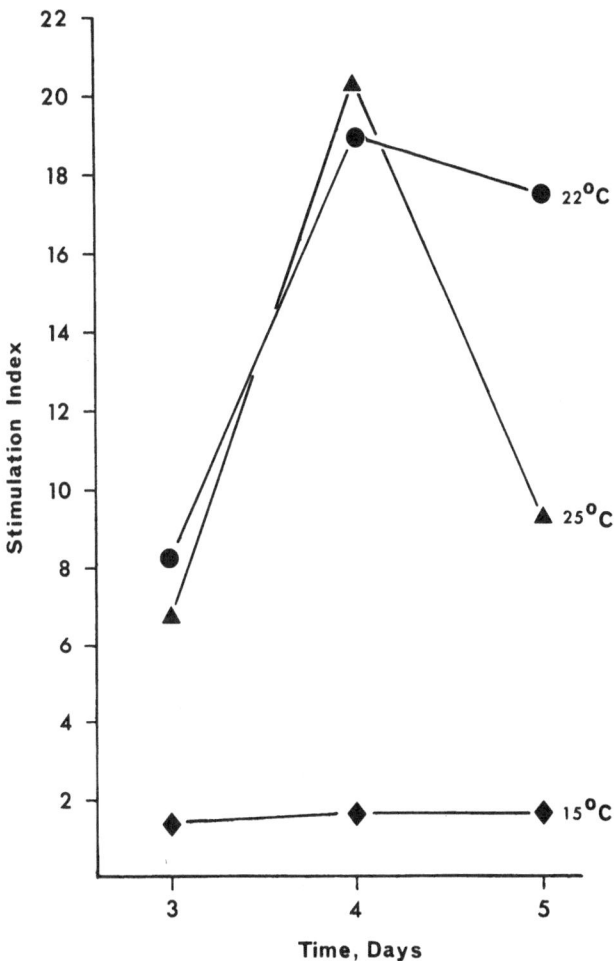

Figure 1. Effects of temperature on the response of frog spleen cells to 10 µg concanavalin A. Each point represents the mean of triplicate cultures from four different experiments.

lymphocytes can bind FITC-Con A over a 4-25°C temperature range.
While the above findings infer that low temperatures may influence
the kinetics of mitogen binding to the cell surface, temperature
does not appear to prevent the binding of sufficient amounts of
lectin to induce mitogenesis.

Mitogen binding to the cell surface is followed by cell
agglutination. Low temperatures (4°C) prevent the agglutination
of malignant transformed fibroblasts and rat lymphocytes by Con A
(19). In a poikilotherm system, frog spleen lymphocytes were
tested for agglutination by 10 μg Con A at 4, 15, 22 and 25°C.
They were agglutinated to the same extent at 15-25°C but did not
agglutinate at 4°C over a 24 hour culture period. If they were
incubated with Con A at 4°C for 24 hours and then transferred to
15-25°C, they became agglutinable.

These observations suggest that while a low temperature (4°C)
may affect Con A binding and cell agglutination, they do not
explain why spleen lymphocytes maintained at 15°C do not give a
mitogenic response (Figure 1). Since Con A binding and cell
agglutination occurs at 15°C, the temperature sensitive stage
affecting mitogen stimulation must be associated with later
events, i.e., lymphocyte activation and mitosis.

EFFECT OF TEMPERATURE ON LYMPHOCYTE ACTIVATION

Mitogen binding and cell agglutination are followed by complex
biochemical and morphological alterations that activate the cell
inducing it to undergo blast transformation and mitosis (20-26).
Lymphocyte activation and stimulation by Con A can be inhibited by
the addition of the saccharide α-methylmannoside. Detailed studies
on the kinetics of inhibition with mouse spleen cells have shown
that when the saccharide is added at various times up to 20 hours
after the addition of Con A, the incorporation of ^{3}HTdR and
stimulation is inhibited (27, 28). After 20 hours, no inhibition
is observed suggesting that those cells responding to the lectin
are committed within 20 hours after mitogen binding. Although
these studies have not been extended to the poikilothermic vertebrates, the kinetics and magnitude of their responses (5-10) imply
that the same time interval will apply.

The response of frog spleen lymphocytes to Con A varies from
no stimulation at 15°C to maximum stimulation at 25°C. Thus, one
can determine whether temperature interferes with lymphocyte
activation by manipulating the culture temperature over various
time intervals. If activation is affected by 15°C, then changes
in the kinetics and magnitude of the response should be observed
when the cells are transferred to 25°C. Conversely, if 15°C does

not affect activation, there should be no change in the kinetics
and magnitude of the response.

To test for the effects of temperature alterations, spleen
cells were maintained at 15°C for 24 hours and then transferred to
25°C. The response observed was similar to the kinetic response
of spleen cells kept at 25°C continuously (Figure 2). Stimulation
indices on days 2 and 3 were not significantly different and
maximum ^{3}HTdR incorporation occurred on day 4. The magnitude of
the response on day 4 however was lower. Increasing the exposure
time at 15°C to 48 hours and then transferring to 25°C however did
produce a change in the response kinetics by shifting the peak
response to day 5. Stimulation indices for these cells on days 3

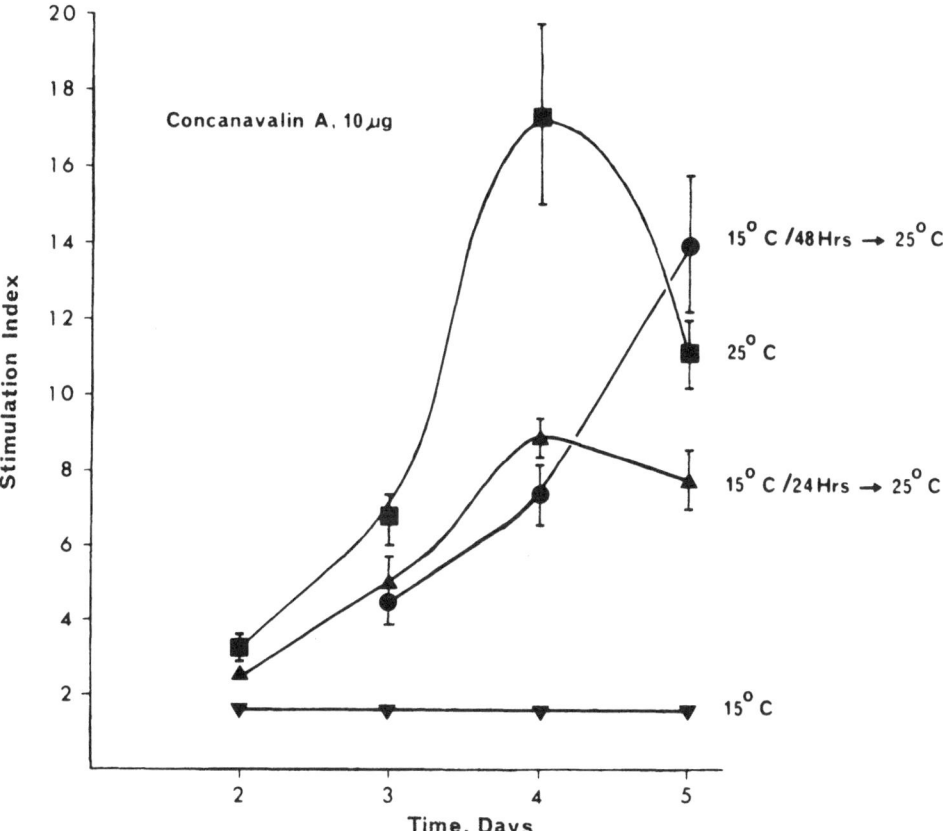

Figure 2. Effects of temperature changes (15° to 25°C) on
the response of frog spleen cells to 10 µg concanavalin A. Each
point represents the mean ± standard error of triplicate cultures
from six different experiments.

and 4 however were not significantly different and were of a
similar magnitude to those of spleen cells maintained at 15°C for
24 hours. Apparently lymphocyte activation is not affected by
incubation at 15°C. The inability of spleen cells maintained
continuously at 15°C to give a mitogenic response to Con A is
thus probably associated with mitosis.

EFFECT OF TEMPERATURE ON MITOSIS

In analyzing the effects of temperature on mitosis, we have
applied the same approach used for examining temperature effects
on lymphocyte activation. At 25°C, mitosis by mitogen stimulated
frog spleen cells as measured by ^{3}HTdR incorporation is apparent
by day 2 of culture. If mitosis is affected by temperature, then

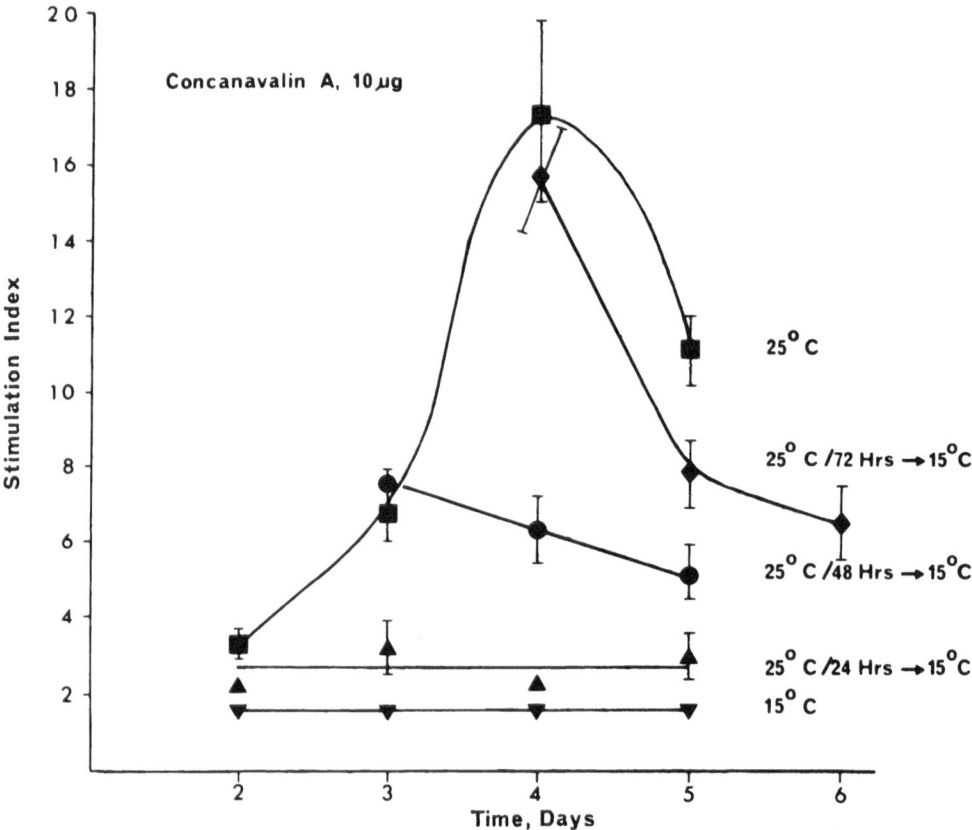

Figure 3. Effects of temperature changes (25°C to 15°C) on
the response of frog spleen cells to 10 μg concanavalin A. Each
point represents the mean ± standard error of triplicate cultures
from six different experiments.

changes in the kinetics and magnitude of the response should be observed when cells are transferred from 25°C to 15°C. The results of these experiments are shown in Figure 3.

Spleen cells maintained at 25°C with 10 µg Con A for 24 hours (when lymphocyte activation but not mitosis occurs) and then transferred to 15°C produce a kinetic response similar to spleen cells kept at 15°C continuously. Increasing the culture time at 25°C to 48 or 72 hours (mitosis is occurring) and following it by a transfer to 15°C also affects the kinetics and magnitude of the response as evidenced by decreased ^{3}HTdR incorporation and stimulation. These results suggest that by lowering the temperature from 25°C to 15°C, the mitotic process of frog spleen cells stimulated with Con A is retarded. Thus, the temperature sensitive event in the mitogenic response of frog spleen cells appears to be at the mitotic stage.

CHRONOLOGICAL DETERMINATION OF THE TEMPERATURE-SENSITIVE STAGE

The response of frog spleen cells to mitogens can be divided into three stages: 1) mitogen binding and cell agglutination, 2) lymphocyte activation, and 3) mitosis. The kinetics and magnitude of the response under optimal temperature conditions (22-25°C) suggest that mitogen binding and cell agglutination occur shortly after the exposure of spleen cells to the mitogen (day 0). Lymphocyte activation follows over the next 24-48 hours (days 1 and 2) resulting in blast transformation and mitosis (days 2-4) with maximum blastogenesis occuring on day 4 (Figure 4).

Mitogenic stimulation of frog spleen cells can be inhibited by low temperatures. At 15°C, no significant stimulation as measured by ^{3}HTdR incorporation occurs over a six day culture period. Preliminary studies with FITC-Con A show that at 15°C, the cells can bind the conjugated mitogen. Cell agglutination, a consequence of mitogen binding also occurs at 15°C. Manipulations of culture temperature (15°C to 25°C or 25°C to 15°C) over varying time intervals suggest that at 15°C lymphocyte activation occurs but cell division does not. This implies that the mechanism by which temperature interferes with mitogenic stimulation is by preventing mitosis. Thus, the temperature sensitive stage would be at day 2 when the cells first start dividing and undergoing blast transformation (Figure 4).

Do the results obtained from the effects of Con A on frog spleen cells in·vitro reflect what we know about the effects of temperature on the immune response of poikilothermic vertebrates in vivo? The detailed studies of Avtalion and his colleagues (4) on carp (Cyprinus carpio) and frogs (Rana ridibunda) immunized with non-microbial and microbial antigens provide us with some insight

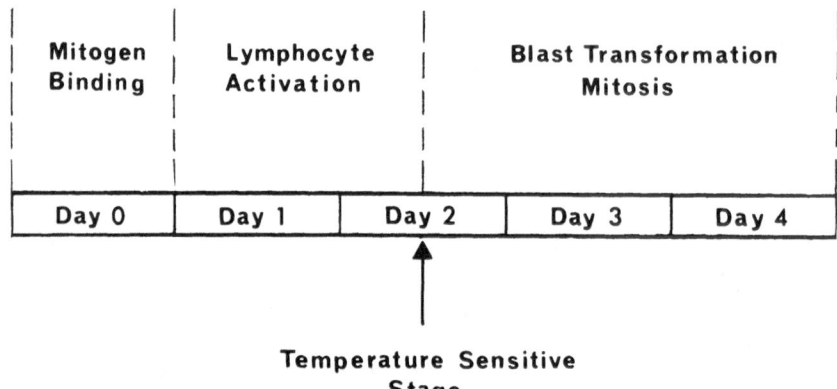

Figure 4. Schematic representation of the chronological stages and temperature sensitive stage in the response of frog spleen cells to concanavalin A.

into the effects of temperature on antigen processing and antibody synthesis. The experimental approach used was similar to that described in our mitogen studies, i.e., animals were immunized at 10–12°C or 25°C followed by manipulations of the temperature over varying time intervals. The results showed that phagocytosis and antigen clearance could take place at 12°C and suggested that the temperature sensitive stage occurs just before cellular multiplication, i.e., between the third and fourth day after antigen stimulation. Thus, there is close agreement between the effects of temperature on mitogen stimulation and the effects of temperature on antigen stimulation and antibody synthesis. The inhibition of mitosis in mitogen stimulated cultures by low temperatures suggests that the inhibition of antibody synthesis in vivo in animals maintained at low temperatures reflects their inability or retarded ability to generate a population of immunocompetent cells in response to an antigenic challenge. Extension of our studies using mitogens as probes should contribute to an understanding of temperature effects on the generation of immunocompetent cells, the phylogenetic development of the immune response, and how the immune response functions in poikilothermic vertebrates that inhabit wide temperature ranges.

ACKNOWLEDGEMENTS

Supported in part by NSF grant GB-17767 and NIH grant 1R01 HD09333-01. Send all correspondence to R. K. Wright, Department of Anatomy, School of Medicine, University of California, Los Angeles, California 90024.

REFERENCES

1. Hildemann, W. H. and Cooper, E. L., Fed. Proc., 22:1145 (1963).

2. Evans, E. E., Fed. Proc., 22:1132 (1963).

3. Evans, E. E., Kent, S. P. and Marie, H., Ann. N. Y. Acad. Sci., 126:629 (1965).

4. Avtalion, R. R., Wojdani, A., Malik, Z., Shahrabani, R. and Duczyminer, M., Current Topics Microbiol. Immunol., 61: 1 (1973).

5. Olsen, G. B., Fed. Proc., 26:357 (1967).

6. Goldshein, S. J. and Cohen, N., J. Immunol. 108:1025 (1972).

7. Lopez, D. M., Sigel, M. M. and Lee, J. C., Cell. Immunol., 10:287 (1974).

8. Wright, R. K. and Cooper, E. L., Amer. Zool., 14:1303 (1974).

9. Goldstine, S. N. and Collins, N. H., Fed. Proc., 34:966 (1975).

10. Etlinger, H. M., Hodgins, H. O. and Chiller, J. M., Fed. Proc., 34:966 (1975).

11. Bach, F. and Hirschhorn, K., Exp. Cell Res., 32:592 (1963).

12. Robbins, J. H., Science, 146:1648 (1964).

13. Ling, N. R., Lymphocyte Stimulation (North-Holland Publ. Co., Amsterdam, 1968).

14. Andersson, J. and Melchers, F., Proc. Natl. Acad. Sci., 70: 416 (1973).

15. Naspitz, C. K. and Richter, M., Progr. Allergy, 12:1 (1968).

16. Clarke, A. E. and Denbarough, M. A., Biochem. J., 121:811 (1971).

17. Huet, Ch., Lonchampt, M., Huet, M. and Bernadac, A., Biochem. Biophys. Acta, 365:28 (1974).

18. Inbar, M., Ben-Bassat, H. and Sachs, L., Exptl. Cell. Res., 76:143 (1973).

19. Inbar, M., Ben-Bassat, H. and Sachs, L., Proc. Natl. Acad. Sci., 68:2748 (1971).

20. van den Berg, K. J. and Betel, I., Exptl. Cell Res., 66: 257 (1971).

21. Hadden, J. W., Hadden, E. M., Haddox, M. K. and Goldberg, N. D., Proc. Natl. Acad. Sci., 69:3024 (1972).

22. Resch, K. and Ferber, E., Eur. J. Biochem., 27:153 (1972).

23. Yahara, I. and Edelman, G. M., Proc. Natl. Acad. Sci., 69: 608 (1972).

24. Yahara, I. and Edelman, G. M., Exptl. Cell Res., 81:143 (1973).

25. Edelman, G. M., Yahara, I. and Wang, J. L., Proc. Natl. Acad. Sci., 70:1442 (1973).

26. Ronco, D., Zabucchi, G., Jug, M., Miani, N. and Soranzo, M. R., Adv. Exp. Med. Biol., 55:273 (1975).

27. Novogrodsky, A. and Katchalski, E., Biochem. Biophys. Acta, 228:579 (1971).

28. Cunningham, B. A., Wang, J. L., Gunther, G. R., Reeke, G. N. and Becker, J. W., in Cellular Selection and Regulation in the Immune Response (Raven Press, New York, 1974).

SYNERGISTIC AND ANTAGONISTIC EFFECTS OF MITOGENS ON PROLIFERATION

OF LYMPHOCYTES FROM SPLEENS OF Rana pipiens

A. Lakshma Reddy and Richard K. Wright

Department of Microbiology and Immunology and Department of Anatomy, School of Medicine and Dental Research Institute, University of California, Los Angeles, 90024

INTRODUCTION

Phytomitogens such as phytohemagglutinin (PHA) and concanavalin A (Con A) bind to cell surface receptors of thymus-derived (T) and bone marrow-derived (B) lymphocytes but stimulate only T-cells to divide and transform into blast cells (1, 2, 3). These mitogens can also stimulate lymphocytes from fish (4, 5, 6, 7) and amphibians (8, 9, 10). In the absence of biological markers at this level of phylogeny, however, evidence is lacking as to whether the responding cells belong to specific lymphocyte subpopulations.

Conflicting reports appear in the literature regarding the selectivity of mitogenic stimulation by bacterial lipopolysaccharide (LPS). In some strains of mice, LPS induces mitogenesis in bone marrow-derived cells without T cell cooperation (11, 12, 13). Studies on lymphocytes from nude mice (14) and human peripheral blood lymphocytes (15), however, suggest that LPS activation of cell division involves the cooperation of thymus-derived cells. Activation of these cells required the addition of sub-mitogenic concentrations of Con A or PHA along with LPS to produce a mitogenic response.

Repeated investigations in our laboratory on LPS induced stimulation of Rana pipiens spleen cells consistently gave either no or minimal mitogenic responses. To see if a possible cell interaction is required in the induction of DNA synthesis to LPS, we have investigated the effects of various combinations of mitogens on producing synergistic or antagonistic effects on cell division of Rana pipiens spleen cells.

RESPONSE TO CON A, PHA, AND LPS

Details of the materials and methods used are described in the previous paper (10). Briefly, maximum proliferation as measured by ^{3}H-thymidine ([3]HTdR) incorporation occurs when 10^5 spleen cells are cultured in the presence of 10 μg Con A or 1 μg PHA for four days. In contrast, the response to varying concentrations (0.5-100 μg) of S. enteritidis LPS (Difco) was negligible suggesting that little blastogenesis had occurred.

RESPONSE TO MIXTURES OF CON A AND PHA

Concanavalin A and PHA are potent non-specific mitogens select-ively stimulating thymus-derived lymphocytes from humans, mice and rats in vitro. Results from our laboratory indicate that they also stimulate amphibian spleen lymphocytes. Evidence. however, is lack-ing at present that the responding cells are thymus-derived lympho-cytes. Experiments were initiated to determine whether PHA and Con A responding cells belong to the same or different cell populations by adding both mitogens to the same culture. If Con A and PHA res-ponding lymphocytes belong to two different populations then one would expect an additive effect on proliferation, i.e., more [3]HTdR incorporation in cultures containing both mitogens than those con-taining only one mitogen. Conversely, if the responding lymphocytes belong to the same population, then no synergistic effect should be observed.

To test for synergistic effects, spleen cells were maintained at 25°C in the presence of 1 μg PHA with varying concentrations (0.25-10 μg) of Con A (Fig. 1) or in the presence of 10 μg Con A with varying concentrations (0.12-1 μg) of PHA (Fig. 2). Cultures were pulsed with 2 μCi [3]HTdR 18-24 hours before harvesting on day 4. Control cultures of PHA or Con A alone gave characteristic dose res-ponse curves. In contrast, mixtures of Con A and PHA consistently showed marked inhibition of DNA synthesis as measured by [3]HTdR in-corporation. This suggests that Rana pipiens spleen lymphocytes responding to Con A or to PHA belong to the same population.

EFFECTS OF LPS ON CON A AND PHA

Mitogenic responses of frog spleen cells to various concentrations (0.5-100 μg) of LPS are consistently negative or minimal. To deter-mine whether LPS has an effect on the response to optimal concen-trations of PHA or Con A, experiments were performed similar to those described in the previous section. Low concentrations of LPS (0.5-1.0 μg) neither augmented nor inhibited the response to Con A and PHA (Fig. 3). Higher concentrations of LPS, however, inhibited the characteristic response usually obtained from PHA or Con A alone.

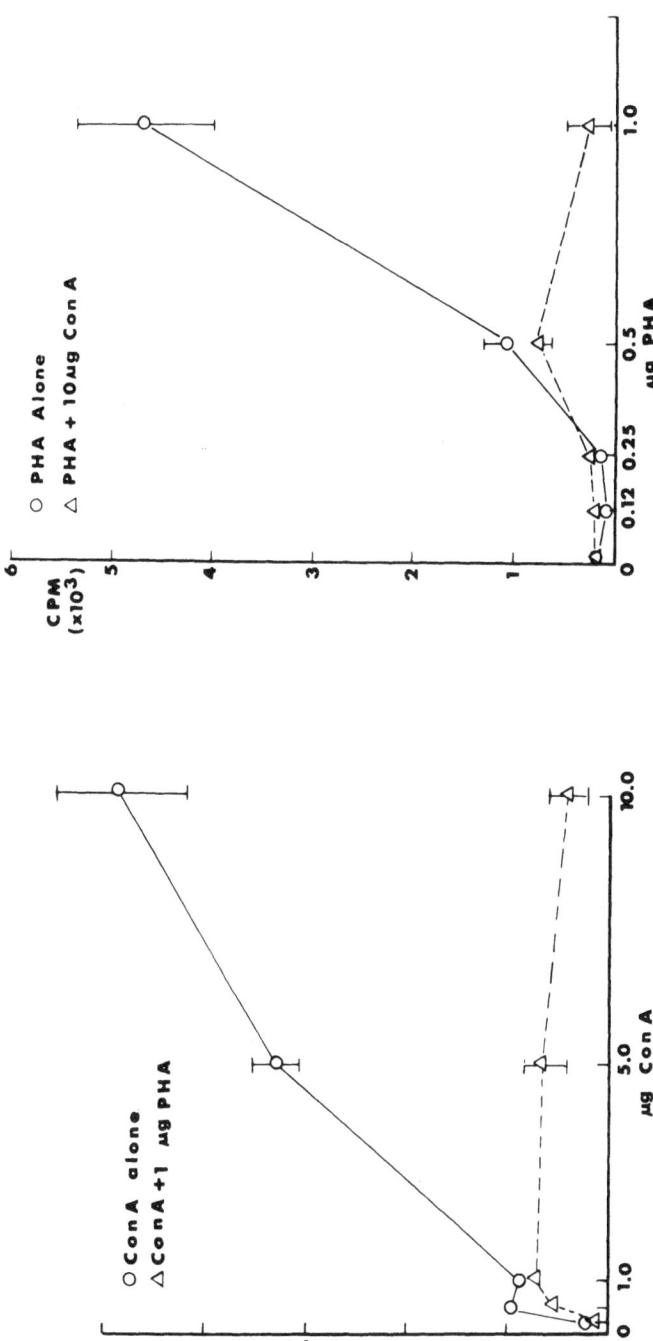

Figure 1. The effect of PHA with variable concentrations of Con A on *Rana pipiens* spleen lymphocytes (10^5) cultured for 4 days at 25°C in L-15 + 10% FCS and antibiotics. The incorporation of ^{3}HTdR present during the last 18 hours of culture is expressed as counts per minute (CPM) per culture. Each point is the mean ± standard deviation of triplicate cultures.

Figure 2. The effect of Con A with variable concentrations of PHA on spleen cell mitogenesis. For details see Fig. 1.

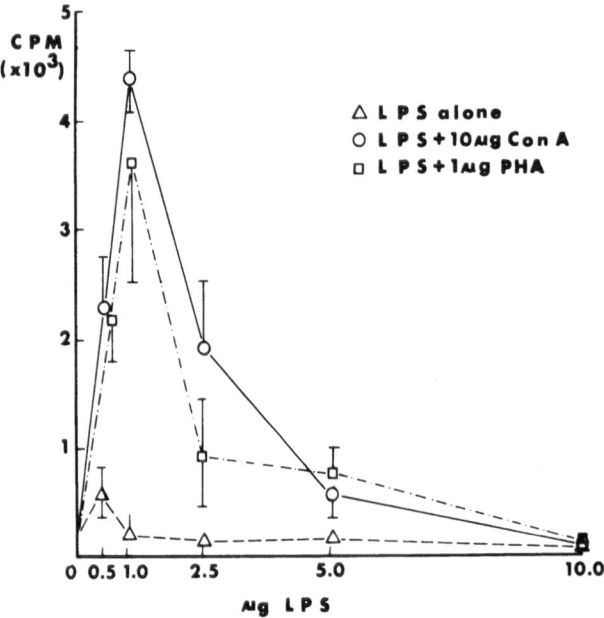

Figure 3. The effect of LPS with various concentrations of Con A or PHA on spleen cell mitogenesis. For details see Fig. 1.

EFFECTS OF CON A AND PHA ON THE RESPONSE TO LPS

Lipopolysaccharide activation has been shown to involve cell cooperation (15). Thus, it was of interest to examine the effects of variable suboptimal concentrations of PHA or Con A on a constant concentration of LPS (10 µg). If suboptimal concentrations of Con A or PHA influence the mitogenic response to LPS, then one would expect an increase in ^{3}HTdR incorporation in cultures containing both Con A (or PHA) and LPS. Conversely, if they have no effect, no increase should be observed. The LPS dose response curves to variable concentrations of PHA or Con A from two separate experiments are shown in Figs. 4 and 5.

The addition of suboptimal concentrations of Con A (Fig. 4) or PHA (Fig. 5) to cultures containing LPS produced a pronounced synergistic response. The incorporation of ^{3}HTdR observed with 0.25 µg Con A or PHA in combination with 10 µg LPS was significantly higher than the ^{3}HTdR incorporation obtained from 0.25 µg Con A, 0.25 µg PHS or 10 µg LPS alone. This synergistic effect decreased as the concentration of Con A or PHA increased. The addition of optimal concentrations (10 µg) of Con A to LPS cultures produced an antagonistic response and suppressed completely the proliferative

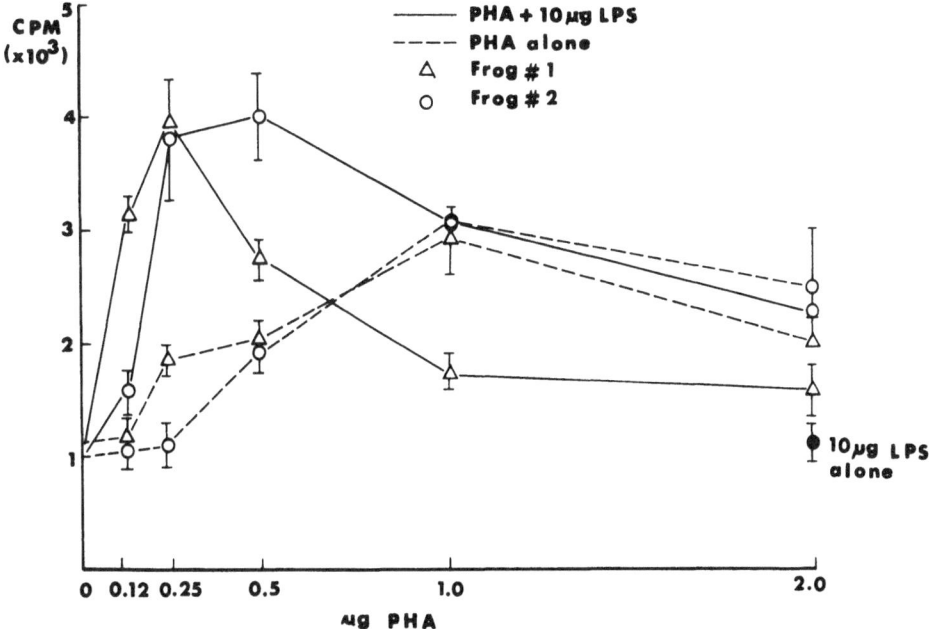

Figure 4. The effect of LPS on various concentrations of Con A. For details see Fig. 1. Each point represents mean of quadruplicate cultures ± standard deviation.

response observed in cultures containing Con A alone. Similar results were obtained with 1 µg PHA, but suppression was not as marked as with Con A.

DISCUSSION

Rana pipiens spleen lymphocytes are capable of responding in vitro to phytomitogens. In the present investigation, we have examined the capacity of two non-specific T cell mitogens, Con A and PHA, either alone or in combination to stimulate the proliferation of frog lymphocytes. Maximum stimulation of DNA synthesis was obtained at concentrations of 10 µg Con A or 1 µg PHA alone. Combinations of Con A and PHA either at optimal or suboptimal concentrations in the same culture produced an antagonistic response, i.e., depression of DNA synthesis. Analogous findings have been obtained with human peripheral blood lymphocytes (15) and rat thymocytes (16). Although our results do not exclude the presence of separate Con A and PHA responding spleen lymphocyte populations, the kinetics of the dose response curves suggest that the same population is stimulated by both mitogens.

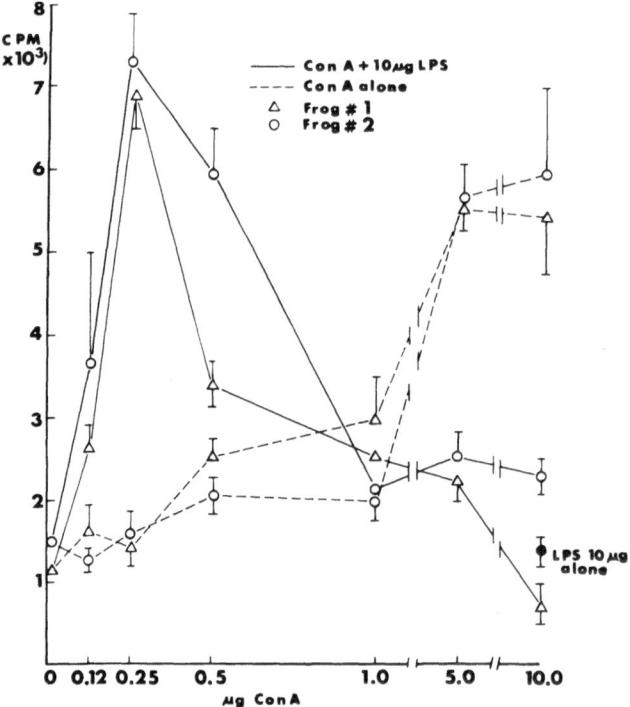

Figure 5. The effect of LPS on spleen cell mitogenesis to variable concentrations of PHA. For details see Fig. 1. Each point represents the mean ± standard deviation of quadruplicate cultures.

Findings of Goldstein and Collins (1975) that LPS can induce a positive blastogenic response in spleen lymphocytes from Rana pipiens and Bufo marinus. We have not been able to demonstrate with Rana pipiens spleen cells a mitogenic response to Salmonella enteriditis LPS at concentrations of 0.1-100 µg. This apparent discrepancy between their results and ours may be due to the use of different bacterial LPS extracts and tissue culture conditions. When submitogenic concentrations of Con A or PHA are added to spleen cultures containing 10 µg LPS, marked enhancement or a synergistic response occurs. This proliferation of cell division is significantly more than the sum of responses obtained from Con A, PHA or LPS alone. Similar results showing synergistic effects between Con A or PHA and LPS have been reported for human peripheral blood lymphocytes (15) and mouse thymocytes (17). The present results also show that lipopolysaccharide at low concentrations in combination with mitogenic doses of Con A or PHA induce neither suppression nor augment normal proliferative responses. Mitogenic concentrations of Con A or PHA with 10 µg LPS, however, exhibit marked suppression of DNA synthesis. Similar enhancement and suppressive effects have been observed in the primary antibody response of murine spleen cultures to sheep red cells in vitro when high or low concentrations of Con A are added (18, 19, 20).

The mechanism of synergistic and antagonistic responses induced by Con A or PHA in combination with LPS in Rana pipiens spleen cells in vitro cannot be explained from the present investigation. The failure of cells to respond to LPS alone in our studies suggests that cell cooperation is required for lymphocyte activation by LPS. Experimental evidence from mammals indicates that B cell activation and clonal expansion in response to some antigens requires T cell cooperation or helper activity (21). Different models have been suggested to explain the synergistic and antagonistic reactions induced by Con A or PHA and LPS in mammals. Studies with some strains of mice suggest that LPS activates B cells making them competent to be stimulated by T cell mitogens (22) or specific antigens (23, 24, 25). Alternatively, other studies indicate that low concentrations of Con A or PHA activate a subpopulation of T cells, most probably helper lymphocytes (17, 18, 26, 27) or macrophages (28, 29, 30, 31), which directly or indirectly through soluble factors influence B cells to respond to LPS or other antigens.

The biological surface markers on the surface of lymphocytes used to identify distinct T and B cell populations in birds and mammals have not been demonstrated in the lower vertebrates. Interactions or cooperation between cells, however, are implicated in the synthesis of antibody to sheep red blood cells in amphibians (32) and fish (33). Although the present study strongly implicates cell interactions in synergistic and antagonistic effects, other possibilities cannot be excluded to explain this phenomenon. The results reported in this paper, however, suggest the following points: (1) combinations of T cell mitogens (i.e., Con A and PHA) at optimal or suboptimal concentrations suppress DNA synthesis; (2) LPS alone is not mitogenic; (3) addition of submitogenic concentrations of Con A or PHA with LPS induces a synergistic response; (4) mitogenic concentrations of Con A or PHA with LPS suppresses the response to Con A or PHA alone. These findings plus those from other laboratories using plant mitogens strongly indicate the existence of functionally different subpopulations of lymphocytes in fish (5, 6, 7) and amphibians (8, 9, 10).

ACKNOWLEDGEMENT

This work was supported by National Institutes of Health grant AI-07070 to Professor W. H. Hildemann, Department of Microbiology and Immunology, University of California, Los Angeles, California 90024. A.L.R. was supported by a National Cancer Institute Postdoctoral Fellowship.

REFERENCES

1. Janossy, G. and Greaves, M.F., Clin. Exp. Immunol., 9: 483 (1971).
2. Greaves, M.F., Bauminger, S. and Janossy, G., Clin. Exp. Immunol.,
    10: 537 (1972).
3. Stobo, J.D., Rosenthal, A.S. and Paul, W.E., J. Immunol., 108:
    1 (1972).
4. Olsen, G.B., Fed. Proc., 26: 357 (1967)
5. Cooper, A.J., In Proced. Fourth Annual Leukocyte Culture
    Conference, Ed. O. R. McIntyre, p. 137 (1971).
6. Lopez, D.M., Sigel, M.M. and Lee, J.C., Cell. Immunol., 10: 287
    (1974)
7. Etlinger, H.M., Hodgins, H.O. and Chiller, J.M., Fed. Proc., 34:
    966 (1975).
8. Goldshein, S.J. and Cohen, N., 108: 1025 (1972).
9. Goldstine, S.N. and Collins, N.H., Fed. Proc., 34: 966 (1975).
10. Wright, R.K., Reddy, A.L. and Cooper, E.L., Adv. Exp. Med. Biol.,
    (these proceedings).
11. Andersson, B. and Blomgren, H., Cell. Immunol., 2: 411 (1971).
12. Smith, R.T., Transplant. Rev., 11: 178 (1972).
13. Aden, D.P. and Reed, N.D., Immunol. Communications, 2: 335 (1973).
14. Boyum, S., Scand. J. Clin. Lab. Inv., 21: Supp. 97 (1968).
15. Schmidtke, J.R. and Najarian, J.S., J. Immunol., 114: 742 (1975).
16. Karsenti, E.M., Bornens, M. and Avrameas, S., Eur. J. Immunol.,
    5: 73 (1975).
17. Forbes, J.T., Nakao, Y. and Smith, R.T., J. Immunol. 114: 1004
    (1975).
18. Dutton, R.W., J. Exp. Med., 136: 1445 (1972).
19. Rich, R.R. and Pierce, C.W., J. Exp. Med., 137: 649 (1973).
20. Sjoberg, O., Moller, G and Andersson, J., Clin. Exp. Immunol.,
    13: 213 (1973).
21. Miller, J.F.A.P. and Mitchell, G.F., Transplant. Rev. 1: 3 (1969).
22. Andersson, J., Moller, G. and Sjoberg, O., Eur. J. Immunol., 2:
    99 (1972).
23. Moller, G., Andersson, J. and Sjoberg, O., Cell. Immunol., 4:
    416 (1972).
24. Jones, J.M. and Kind, P.D., J. Immunol., 108: 1453 (1972).
25. Louis, J.A., Chiller, J.M. and Weigle, W.O., J. Exp. Med., 138:
    1481 (1973).
26. Watson, J., Epstein, R., Nakoinz, I. and Ralph, P., J. Immunol.,
    10: 43 (1973).
27. Rich, R.R. and Rich, S.S., J. Immunol., 114: 1112 (1975).
28. Hersh, E.M. and Harris, J.E., J. Immunol., 100: 1184 (1968).
29. Gery, I., Gershon, R.K. and Waksman, B.H., J. Exp. Med. 136: 128
    (1972).
30. Gery, I. and Waksman, B.H., J. Exp. Med., 136: 143 (1972).
31. Sjoberg, O., Andersson, J. and Moller, G., J.Immunol., 109: 1379
    (1972).
32. Ruben, L.N., Amer. Zool., 15: 93 (1975).
33. Stolen, J.S. and Makela, O., Nature, 254: 718 (1975).

MITOGENS AS PROBES OF LYMPHOCYTE HETEROGENEITY IN ANURAN AMPHIBIANS

S.N.GOLDSTINE, N.H.COLLINS, AND N.COHEN

Departments of Dental Research and Microbiology,
Division of Immunology, The University of Rochester,
School of Medicine and Dentistry, Rochester, New York 14642

Based on functional and structural properties, lymphocytes
from birds and mammals have been classified into thymus-derived T
cell and bursa- or bone marrow-derived B cell populations. Indeed,
we now recognize even further heterogeneity of each major population. For several years we have been interested in the phylogeny
of such immuno-competent cells. Since ontogenetically all lymphocytes of the anuran amphibian are derived from a single organ
source - the thymus (1) - we have focused our research efforts on
determining whether comparable heterogeneity exists at this level
of vertebrate evolution.

In this paper we will present results from some of our recent
in vitro studies on the biology of lymphocytes of the leopard frog,
Rana pipiens. Our basic tools have been mitogens which are selective for subpopulations of mammalian and avian cells in vitro (2).
The plants lectins, PHA (phytohemagglutinin) and Con A (concanavalin A), in their soluble form, are mitogenic for T cells; LPS
(bacterial lipopolysaccharide) and PPD (purified protein derivative)
are B cell mitogens (3,4).

MATERIALS AND METHODS

Field-collected Rana pipiens were housed for at least two weeks
before sacrifice, in our special facility (air temperature 28C,
water temperature 22 ± 2C) patterned after the Amphibian Facility
developed at Ann Arbor, Michigan by Dr. George Nace (5). Frogs were
fed on mealworms and crickets and appeared in good health at the
time of sacrifice. Animals were anesthetized with MS 222 or sacrificed by pithing.

Blood was collected in heparin (10 U/ml) from the ventricle
of the heart and the mononuclear cells were separated on Ficoll-
Hypaque gradients (6). Spleens were removed aseptically, minced,
and the fragments were forced through a nylon mesh to obtain suspensions of single cells. All cells were kept at 4C and washed at
least three times in a modified Hank's Balanced Salt Solution
(HBSS). Viable cell counts were done by trypan blue dye exclusion
in a hemocytometer under phase contrast microscopy.

Cells were resuspended in modified Leibovitz (L15) culture
medium (7) to the appropriate cell concentration. The L15 contained
12.5mM HEPES buffer, 100 U/ml penicillin and 100 μg/ml streptomycin.
Wash solution (HBSS), phosphate buffered salt solution (PBS) and
culture media (L15) were mammalian formulations (GIBCO) which were
diluted with glass-distilled water to the osmolarity of frog serum
(200-220mOsm) (7). Where cited, this stock L15 medium was further
supplemented so that it contained: 10% heat-inactivated fetal calf
serum (FCS - lot #A730702-GIBCO), 2-mercaptoethanol (2-ME, $5x10^{-5}$M),
hypoxanthine ($1x10^{-4}$M), or sodium bicarbonate ($1x10^{-2}$M). The cultures were incubated at 25C in air for 2-3 days. The bicarbonate
containing cultures were gassed with 5% CO_2 in 95% air, every 24
hours.

The cultures were assayed for mitogen-induced DNA synthesis
by a method modified from that described by Weiss and DuPasquier
(8). Briefly, cells were plated in 96-well microtiter plates
(Linbro) in a volume of 0.2 ml (usually $1-2x10^{-5}$ cells/well) and
freshly diluted mitogens or PBS (diluent) were added in a 10 μl
volume. Before harvesting, the cells were exposed to tritiated
thymidine (S.A. 2 Ci/mmole-New England Nuclear) for 7-18 hours.
The harvested cells were precipitated with cold 5% TCA on glass-
fiber filter paper with a multiple automatic precipitator. The
amount of tritiated thymidine incorporated into this precipitate
was counted at 50% efficiency in a liquid scintillation counter.
The standard error of the mean in triplicate cultures was approximately 10%. As a relative measure of mitogen-induced DNA synthesis,
the Stimulation Index (SI) was calculated by dividing the cpm in
mitogen-stimulated cultures by the cpm in control cultures to which
only the diluent (PBS) was added.

                    MITOGEN REACTIVITY

Splenocytes and peripheral blood lymphoid cells cultured in
L15 plus FCS respond to PHA in a similar dose-dependent fashion.
Optimal doses in the anuran system are similar to those in mammalian models (FIG 1). Under these culture conditions (and with a
single lot of FCS), the typical dose response profile seen in
figure 1 and the kinetics (peak responses at 3-4 days) of this

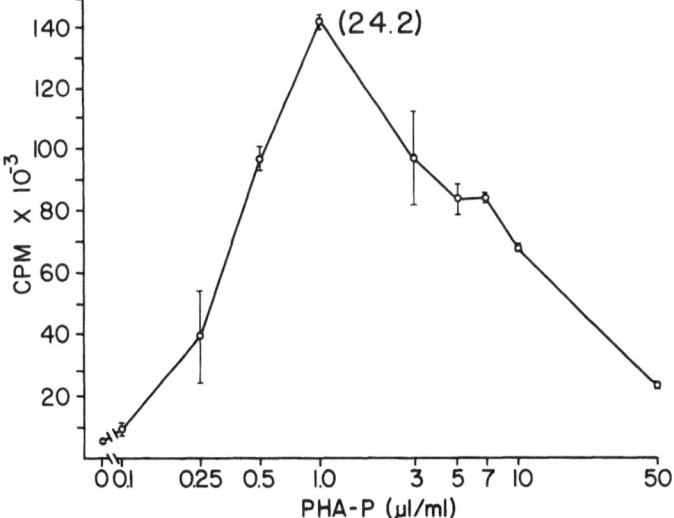

FIGURE 1. A typical PHA dose response of Rana splenocytes (splenocytes from one animal; 2×10^5 cells/culture; L15-10% FCS; 3 day culture; 18 hour pulse; SI in parentheses).

response was relatively invariable. However, substantial variation
in the absolute magnitude (SI) of the response was noted for cells
from individual animals.

Rana cells also respond vigorously to Con A in media supplemented with either FCS or 2-ME. Peak responses occurred on days
3-4 (as with PHA). The SI for a given dose of this mitogen, however, was dependent on the culture medium employed (FIG 2). For
example, at lower doses of Con A (2.5 or 5 µg/ml) the stimulation
indices were higher in the 2-ME medium than they were in media containing FCS. Only at higher doses of 50 µg/ml did cells in FCS respond to the same extent as they did without serum (SI = 11).
These effects of FCS on cultures with Con A have also been noted
for murine cells in culture by Coutinho and co-workers (9). They
have been attributed to the apparent binding of Con A to serum glycoproteins which would decrease the effective amount of mitogenic
Con A available for binding to appropriate cell surface receptor
sites.

Additional effects of media supplementation should also be
noted (FIG 2). When cells cultured in FCS were reactive to high
doses of Con A, the magnitude of the response could be increased by
at least 3 fold (SI = 36) by the addition of 2-ME. Identical
effects were noted with PHA but not with "B cell mitogens". The
mechanism by which 2-ME affects cells cultured with serum is unknown.
That it may directly affect the cells is suggested by observations

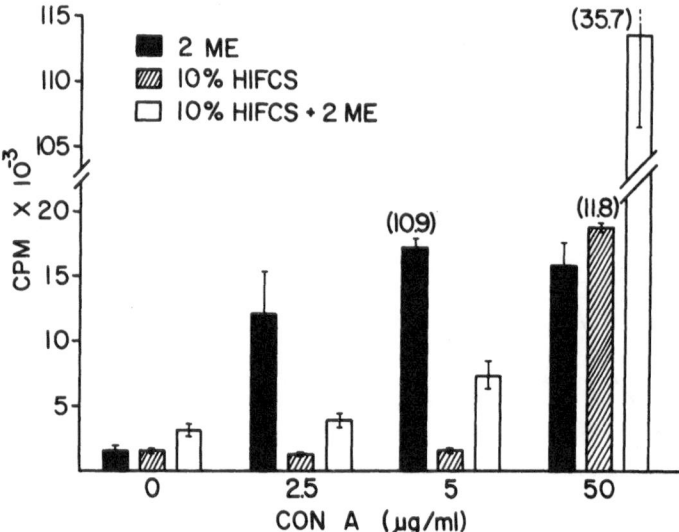

FIGURE 2. Effects of different media on the response to Con A. (splenocytes from one <u>Rana</u>; 2×10^5 cells culture; heat-inactivated (HI) FCS; 3 day culture; 18 hour pulse; SI in parentheses).

that 2-ME enhances growth and accelerates differentiation of lymphocytes (10,11). In this regard, our data indicate that by itself, 2-ME is not mitogenic and does not increase cell viabilities. However, the addition of 2-ME enhances Con A- and PHA-induced DNA synthesis in all media tested.

Effects of FCS on mitogen-induced DNA synthesis have also been noted with "B cell mitogens". Specifically, whenever LPS- or PPD-treated cells were cultured with FCS, stimulation indices were always low (SI = 2). Cells cultured with LPS or PPD in serum-free media supplemented with 2-ME, however, were associated with lower background counts, higher cpm at all doses tested, and significantly greater peak responses. A log plot of the cpm incorporated by LPS-stimulated cultures (FIG 3) makes it possible to see a small response (SI = 1.7-2.0) in serum-supplemented media at approximately the same LPS concentrations which effected maximal stimulation under serum-free conditions. Since the dose response profiles were similar in all three media tested, and since the FCS + 2-ME combined supplement failed to enhance LPS reactivity as it did with Con A, it may be that in some way FCS masks the potential DNA synthetic response to LPS.

PPD was also mitogenic for <u>Rana</u> cells. Concentrations that resulted in optimal stimulation were from 125 to 250 µg/ml. Kinetic

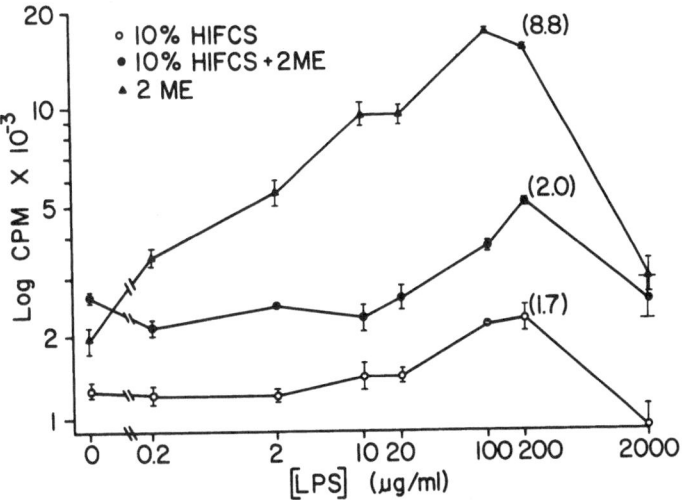

Figure 3. Effect of different media on the response to LPS.
(splenocytes from one Rana; 2×10^5 cells/culture; heat-inactivated
(HI) FCS; 2 day culture; 17 hour pulse; LPS derived from E. coli
055:B5 (Westphal preparation); SI in parentheses).

TABLE 1. Comparisons Between Mitogen Reactivities of
Rana Cells

Criterion	Mitogen Tested			
	PHA	CON A	LPS[c]	PPD
Reactivity in FCS [a]	yes	yes	no	no
Effects of FCS+2-ME [a]	increased reactivity		no effect	
Day of peak response [a]	3-4	3-4	2	2
Peak SI [a]	6-30	8-16	6-17	4-6
Peak SI [b]	16-36	12-31	5-13	3-6

a. Data from early experiments with L15-2-ME or L15-FCS media.
b. Data from experiments with L15-2-ME media supplemented with
   either hypoxanthine or sodium bicarbonate (see text).
c. Data include experiments with a variety of different
   preparations of LPS.

studies revealed that the peak response for PPD and LPS, at day 2, is earlier than that seen for Con A- or PHA-treated cultures.

HETEROGENEITY

Table 1 summarizes the reactivities of frog lymphoid cells to four mitogens. Results from these preliminary experiments suggest that mitogen reactivity may be grouped into two categories. One is associated with mammalian T cell mitogens (PHA and Con A); the other is associated with mammalian B cell mitogens (LPS and PPD). The following data describe other parameters that point out more dramatically that the mitogen-reactive cell populations of Rana are probably heterogeneous.

Our earlier observations that serum-free media consistently supported mitogenic reactivity to "B cell mitogens" but failed to do so with "T cell mitogens", suggested that there may be more than one mitogen-reactive cell population in Rana and that cells within these populations may differ with respect to the nutritive require- ments for mitogen-induced DNA synthesis.

These possibilities further suggested that there may be other selective media which would more clearly allow us to discriminate between lymphocyte populations in Rana. Purine supplementation of

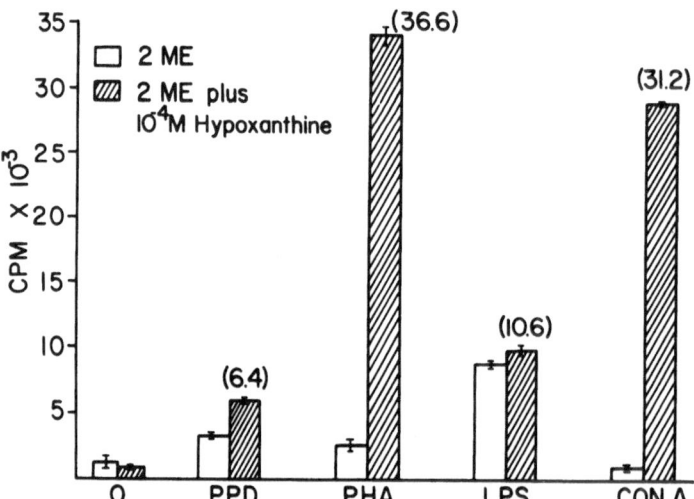

FIGURE 4. Purine enhancement of mitogen stimulation. (peripheral blood leukocytes from one Rana; 1×10^5 cells/culture; 2 day culture; 7 hour pulse; PBS diluent; PPD 250 µg/ml; PHA 0.8 µl/ml; LPS (E.coli 0111:B4) 667 µg/ml; Con A 3.1 µg/ml; SI in parentheses).

L15 media has been shown to enhance cell growth of <u>Rana</u> and mammalian cell lines (12,13). When we supplemented our basic L15-2-ME
culture medium with the purine, hypoxanthine, we found the following striking selective effect. Hypoxanthine markedly enhanced DNA
synthesis by cells stimulated with Con A or PHA up to 10 times that
seen in hypoxanthine-free media. No such enhancement was seen when
LPS or PPD were used (FIG 4). Hypoxanthine by itself was not mitogenic; nor did it affect the viabilities of control unstimulated
cells. It was possible to mimic the hypoxanthine effect by using
sodium bicarbonate in place of hypoxanthine. In these experiments,
CO_2/HCO_3^- probably serves as a required single carbon source for
purine synthesis, rather than as a buffer (13,14). With either
supplement, a differential effect was seen only with PHA- and Con A-
stimulated cells. Regardless of the synthetic steps or biochemical
pathways involved in this phenomenon, it is clear that there is a
marked purine requirement for the reactivity to only <u>one</u> class of
mitogens. The simplest interpretation of these data is that there
are at least two biochemically distinguishable cell populations,
and that selective "T and B cell mitogens" can be used to detect
each population. The validity of this interpretation must be
further tested with pure cell populations.

SUMMARY AND CONCLUSIONS

Cells from <u>Rana</u> react <u>in vitro</u> to classic "T and B cell mitogens" by enhanced DNA synthesis. Dose response and kinetic data
(TABLE 1) suggest lymphocyte heterogeneity at this phylogenetic
level. The biochemical requirements for DNA synthesis following
mitogen activation more strongly argue for the existence of at
least two populations of lymphoid cells which display differential
mitogen reactivity. Indeed, in terms of <u>in vitro</u> reactivities of
their cells, the frog does not differ radically from the mouse
(FIG 5). Our data, however, do not yet directly speak to the

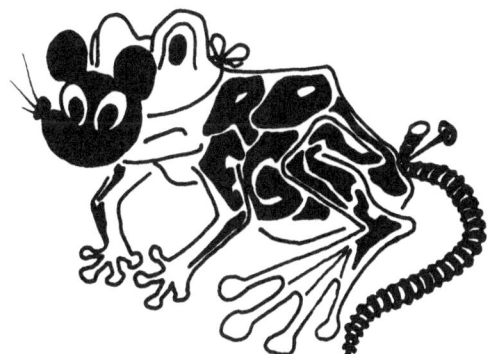

FIGURE 5. Sometimes frogs may appear to be mice, but at all times
frogs are still frogs. (Art work by Dr. W.M. Baldwin III)

existence of T and B cells in the frog. To demonstrate whether these cell types exist in Rana we are in the process of examining mitogen reactivities of lymphocytes treated with antithymocyte serum or harvested from larvally thymectomized animals (15).

T and B cells have been distinguished by multiple criteria which include: 1) their ontogeny from different sources; 2) differential reactivities to mitogens; 3) different functions; 4) different cell surface antigens. It is questionable whether all these criteria apply to Amphibia. Our in vitro experiments and the elegant in vivo larval thymectomy studies of Manning and colleagues (15) point out that by at least two of the above criteria (#2 and #3), comparable T and B cell heterogeneity probably exists in anuran amphibians. The recent developmental studies of Turpen, Volpe and Cohen (16) argue convincingly that during early ontogeny most, if not all of Rana's peripheral lymphocytes are thymus derived. Thus, not only must we recognize that as research tools frogs may, in certain instances, surpass mice (FIG 5), but we must also readjust our thinking to fit the concept that at least in this species, heterogeneity may not reflect organs of origin (15-17). Once the functional and structural heterogeneity of Rana lymphocytes is conclusively established, the important issue to resolve is when during ontogeny and where in the animal do these cells differentiate into functionally different populations.

ACKNOWLEDGEMENT

We thank Dr. G. Nace for his expert consul on the health, disease and maintenance of adult Rana. We are indebted to M. Horan and E. Schotman for technical assistance and advice. For their helpful discussions, we would like to acknowledge Drs. B. Ohlsson-Wilhelm, J. Kappler and P. Marrack.

S.N.G. is supported by 5-T01-DE00003, N.H.C. by 5-T01-GM00592 from the USPHS, and N.C. is a recipient of USPHS Research Career Development Award AI-70736. Research was supported by a grant HD 07901 from the USPHS.

REFERENCES

1. Turpen, J.B., Volpe, E.P. and Cohen, N., Science, 182:931 (1973).

2. Andersson, J., Sjöberg, O., and Möller, G., Transplant. Rev., 11:131 (1972).

3. Sultzer, B.M., and Nilsson, B.S., Nat. New Biol., 240:198 (1972).

4. Strong, D.M., Ahmed, A.A., Scher, I., Knudsen, R.C. and Sell, K.W., J. Immunol., 113:1429 (1974).

5. Amphibians: Guideline for the Breeding, Care and Management of Laboratory Animals, Nat. Acad. Sci., Washington, D.C., p. 64 (1974).

6. DuPasquier, L., Chardonnens, X., and Miggiano, V.C., Immunogenetics, 1:482 (1975).

7. Freed, J.J., and Mezger-Freed, L., Meth. Cell Physiol., 4:19 (1970).

8. Weiss, N., and DuPasquier, L., J. Immunol. Meth., 3:273 (1973).

9. Coutinho, A., Möller, G., Andersson, J., and Bullock, W.W., Eur. J. Immunol., 3:299 (1973).

10. Engers, H.D., MacDonald, H.R., Cerottini, J.-C., and Brunner, K.T., Eur. J. Immunol., 5:223 (1975).

11. Broome, J.D., and Jeng, M.W., J. Exp. Med., 138:574 (1973).

12. Sooy, L.E., and Mezger-Freed, L., Exp. Cell Res., 60:482 (1970).

13. Scheffler, I.E., J. Cell Physiol., 83:219 (1974).

14. McLimans, W.F., In: Growth, Nutrition, and Metabolism of Cells in Culture,Rothblat, G.H. and Cristofalo, V.J. (eds.) Academic Press, New York, N.Y. (1972) p. 137.

15. Manning, M.J., and Collie, M.H., Adv. Exp. Med. Biol. (this vol.) (1975).

16. Turpen, J.B., Volpe, E.P., and Cohen, N., Amer. Zool., 15:51 (1975).

17. Cohen, N., Amer. Zool., 15:119 (1975).

THYMIC FUNCTION IN AMPHIBIANS

Margaret J. Manning and Madeleine H. Collie

Department of Zoology
University of Hull, Hull, HU6 7RX, England

INTRODUCTION

The advantages of using anamniote vertebrates with free-living embryonic stages in studies on the ontogeny of the immune system are well known. Very young larval stages can readily withstand surgical intervention such as that of thymectomy and, unlike mammals, they are exempt from any possible maternal influence. Although experiments on the effect of early thymectomy have recently been reported in fish (1), most results of larval thymus extirpation come from amphibians. This class has many advantages: amphibians adapt well to conditions of laboratory aquaria and vivaria, in many species the early developmental stages are readily obtained and easy to manipulate, good cell markers can be produced by the creation of polyploid forms, inbred strains are available for some species (2) and convenient culture methods have been developed for the study of immune responses _in vitro_. Two groups which at present are being intensively studied, newts and anuran amphibians, have the additional advantage that the thymus originates in association with a single pair of pharyngeal pouches; in the newts the 5th pouch and in anuran amphibians, pouch 2. This contrasts with apodans, other urodeles and the remaining poikilotherm groups and it obviously facilitates experimental destruction of the thymic buds.

There is a present need to re-evaluate the role of the thymus in poikilotherms in its relationship to the peripheral lymphoid tissues (3). Recent work on experimentally produced triploid embryos of _Rana pipiens_ using orthotopic transplants of ploidy-labelled thymic anlagen indicates that most, if not all, of the amphibian lymphocytes originate from the thymic region, at least when traced sufficiently far back in their developmental history (4),

353

i.e., the thymus produces stem cells both for the establishment of its own lymphocytic population and for export. This may explain why there appears to be rather less distinction between the cellular populations of the thymus and of the peripheral lymphoid organs in anamniotes than in the more advanced phylogenetic groups. Thus production of antibody-forming cells in the thymus can be readily demonstrated following immunization of fishes (5) and of larval anurans (bullfrogs) (6). Moreover, the detection of immunoglobulin on the surface of a large percentage of the thymus lymphocytes in young adult fish (carp) (7) and in larval amphibians (Xenopus laevis) (8), strongly contrasts with the situation in homoiotherms where only a very small proportion of the thymus cells are labelled by the immunofluorescence techniques employed in these experiments.

Despite these differences, there is strong support for the fundamental homology of the amphibian immune system with that of higher vertebrates. Direct evidence for a division into "thymus-dependent" and "thymus-independent" components comes from the studies on antibody responses in thymectomized Xenopus discussed below (9). A dichotomy within the immune system is also revealed by the heterogeneity of lymphocytic populations in their in vitro responses to mitogenic stimulation (10) and by the existence of two cooperating cell populations in antibody production (11). This dichotomy probably extends to all jawed vertebrates (12). Functionally these populations behave like the T-cells and B-cells of mammalian systems but their origins in amphibia ("thymic-dependence" versus "thymic-independence") has yet to be established experimentally. We shall review the current data on the results of thymectomy with these considerations in mind.

RESULTS OF EARLY THYMECTOMY

Larval thymectomy has been performed in amphibians in a number of laboratories (reviewed by Cohen (12), Cooper (13), Du Pasquier (14)). This operation has the expected effect on alloimmune responses, i.e. it severely cripples the animal's ability to reject allografts. In thymectomized anurans, first-set skin grafts are usually eventually rejected although at a much slower rate than in normal animals while second-set alloimmunity is essentially unimpaired (15). On the other hand, in the possibly less advanced urodeles, larval thymectomy can result in specific and long-lasting survival of allogeneic skin grafts both in first-set (16,17) and in second-set (18) experiments.

Studies on antibody formation show that the response to foreign erythrocytes is impaired in thymectomized urodeles (19) and anurans (14,20,21). Suppression of antibody production to a soluble protein antigen (human gamma globulin) has also been demonstrated (21, 22). In sharp contrast, the response of thymectomized Xenopus to

TABLE 1. EFFECT OF THYMECTOMY ON ANTIBODY RESPONSES IN <u>XENOPUS LAEVIS</u>

Antigen	Operation	Antibody class	
		IgM	IgG
HGG	sham-oper.	+	+
	thymectomy	−	−
		(total suppression)	(total suppression)
SRBC	sham-oper.	+	−
	thymectomy	−	−
		(total suppression)	
LPS	sham-oper.	+	−
	thymectomy	+	−
		(normal)	

<u>Escherichia</u> <u>coli</u> lipopolysaccharide remains normal (9), while in partially thymectomized bullfrog larvae antibody production to haemocyanin may be enhanced (23).

THYMUS-DEPENDENT AND THYMUS-INDEPENDENT ANTIBODY RESPONSES

Table 1 summarizes recent results from our laboratory (9,21) on the humoral responses of Xenopus which were thymectomized early in larval life and immunized as toadlets some 5-9 months later. At the time of thymectomy, 7-8 days post-fertilization, the lymphoid organs are still rudimentary; the thymus contains fewer than 2,000 cells and is about 100 µm in diameter. The antigens used were: 1) human gamma globulin (HGG), a soluble protein antigen to which Xenopus forms both IgM and IgG antibody but which requires the use of an adjuvant for effective immunization (it was administered in Freund's complete adjuvant (FCA) in these experiments); ii) sheep erythrocytes (SRBC), a particulate antigen which in our toadlets elicits only IgM production and iii) E. coli lipopolysaccharide (LPS) extracted by the Westphal method from E. coli 055 B5 (Difco, Detroit), this also elicits only IgM. In mammals the first two antigens (HGG and SRBC) require thymic influence for full expression of the antibody response, while LPS is a thymus-independent antigen. Table 1 shows that this is also true for Xenopus. Thus in the amphibian, as in mammals, thymic depletion suppresses the IgG response. In Xenopus it also entirely abolishes IgM production to the thymus-dependent antigens while leaving thymus-independent (anti-LPS) antibody formation completely intact. The dichotomy is thus more clear-cut in Xenopus than in "nude" (thymus-less) mice, since in "nude" mice production of IgM antibody to thymus-dependent antigens has been detected at various levels (24-26). This difference may be technical rather than phylogenetic - a consequence of the early and effective

TABLE 2. SERUM ANTIBODY TITRES IN <u>XENOPUS</u> TOADLETS THYMECTOMIZED EARLY IN LARVAL LIFE, AND IN CONTROL ANIMALS, AFTER IMMUNIZATION WITH LPS

Operation	Anti-LPS antibody (reciprocal log-2 passive haemagglutination titre)						
	6	7	8	9	10	11	12
Intact		III	II	IIIIIII	II	I	
Sham-oper.		II	IIIIIII	IIIIII	IIII	II	II
Thymectomy	I	II	III	IIIIII	IIII	II	IIIII

I = score for one animal

removal of the thymic influence in our model.

Further information on antibody responses to <u>E. coli</u> LPS in <u>Xenopus</u> thymectomized at one week post-fertilization is incorporated in Table 2. Anti-LPS antibody was titrated by a passive haemagglutination technique and the specificity of the agglutination was checked using sera from all three groups (thymectomized, sham-operated and intact) against both uncoated SRBC and SRBC coated with the non-cross-reacting <u>Salmonella typhosa</u> LPS (9). These controls, and also titrations of sera from non-immunized animals, were uniformly negative. From Table 2, it can be seen that the antibody titres in the thymectomized group fall within a normal range. The animals are certainly capable of positive responses to LPS. It should also be noted that there is little or no enhancement of antibody titres (such as might occur if thymectomy removed a suppressor cell population in these experiments).

IMMUNOPOTENTIATION BY ADJUVANTS IN <u>XENOPUS</u>

Studies in our laboratory on the requirements for adjuvants in antibody responses to soluble protein antigens in <u>Xenopus</u> have aimed to clarify the respective roles of phagocytes, T-lymphocytes and B-lymphocytes. To this end we have used not only Freund's complete adjuvant (which is known to evoke its effect partly through sensitized T-cells) but also <u>Corynebacterium parvum</u> which has a powerful action on B-cells (27). Both of these adjuvants potentiate antibody production to HGG in <u>Xenopus</u> but they have different effects on the lymphoid organs of this species (28). It was therefore of interest to test the activity of <u>C. parvum</u> in thymectomized animals.

Table 3 shows the results of this experiment. Operative techniques, animal material and antibody titrations were similar to those described by Turner and Manning (21). Thymectomy was performed on

TABLE 3. SERUM ANTIBODY TITRES IN XENOPUS TOADLETS THYMECTOMIZED
          EARLY IN LARVAL LIFE, AND IN SHAM-OPERATED ANIMALS,
          AFTER IMMUNIZATION WITH HGG AND C. PARVUM

Operation	Anti-HGG antibody (reciprocal log-2 passive haemagglutination titre)																
	0 (no antibody)	5	6	7	8	9	10	11	12	13	14	15	16				
Sham-oper.	-	I	I	III	I	I	I	-	I	-	-	-	I	I			
Thymectomy	IIIIIIIII	-	-	-	I*	-	-	-	-	-	-	-	-				

I = score for one animal
* this thymectomized animal had a regenerating thymus

one-week-old larvae and the animals were immunized as toadlets 5-9
months later. The adjuvant, deproteinized, delipidated cell walls
of C. parvum, was obtained from Dr. N. D. Tâm (see Turner, Tâm and
Manning (28)). It was injected via the dorsal lymph sac in a dose
of 50 μg/gm body weight together with 100 μg/gm body weight of HGG
(lyophilized human gamma globulin, Kabi, Stockholm). The animals
were killed for serum analysis 8 weeks after immunization. The thymectomized animals gave consistently negative results. This is in
contrast with the good antibody titres obtained in their sham-operated controls. Thus the experiment failed to reveal any by-pass
mechanism whereby C. parvum could elicit antibody production to HGG
in the absence of T-cells in Xenopus.

        THYMUS REMOVAL AT DIFFERENT STAGES OF DEVELOPMENT

        The recent findings of Turpen, Volpe and Cohen (4) highlight our
need for more information on the ontogeny of the thymic role in antibody production at different stages of development. Table 4 gives
some information from our laboratory on serum antibody responses to
a thymus-dependent antigen (SRBC) after removal of the thymus at
various times during histogenesis of the immune system. In these experiments the larvae were thymectomized at ages between one week and
one month (at stages 48-52 of Nieuwkoop and Faber (29)) and subsequently immunized as young toadlets as in our previous experiments.
Injections comprised 3 doses of 0.05 ml each of a 25% suspension of
SRBC (Wellcome Reagents Ltd., Beckenham, Kent) administered via the
dorsal lymph sac in 0.85% saline at 3-day intervals. The animals
were killed 4 weeks after the first injection and their serum tested
for haemolysins and haemagglutinins to SRBC by our usual methods (21).
The results (Table 4) show that thymectomy abrogates the response to
SRBC even when the operation is postponed until stage 52 of Nieuwkoop

TABLE 4.   SERUM ANTIBODY TITRES TO SHEEP ERYTHROCYTES IN <u>XENOPUS</u>
           TOADLETS THYMECTOMIZED OR SHAM-OPERATED AT DIFFERENT
           STAGES OF LARVAL DEVELOPMENT

Larval stage at time of operation, Nieuwkoop & Faber (29)		Number of animals	Anti-SRBC antibody (reciprocal log-2 haemagglutination titre)
48	Sham-operated	6	0, 2, 3, 3, 3, 4
	Thymectomized	6	No antibody production
49	Sham-operated	10	2, 3, 4, 4, 4, 5, 5, 5, 5, 5
	Thymectomized	7	No antibody production
50	Sham-operated	2	0, 4
	Thymectomized	3	No antibody production
51	Sham-operated	4	3, 3, 4, 4
	Thymectomized	4	No antibody production
52	Sham-operated	2	3, 3
	Thymectomized	2	No antibody production

and Faber (the latest stage for which we have information).

These results on the effect of larval thymectomy on antibody formation are in contrast with our findings in transplantation experiments (30).   Thus, in <u>Xenopus</u>, thymectomy impairs skin allograft responses only if it is carried out early in larval life at a stage before the peripheral lymphoid organs are fully differentiated. Similarly in urodeles (<u>Pleurodeles waltlii</u>), prolonged survival of skin allografts on thymectomized animals occurs only if thymectomy is performed at an early stage of larval development (18).   Our results are supported by the experiments of Horton, J.D., Horton, T.L., Rimmer, J. and Ruben, L.N. (personal communication) who found that thymectomy in the mid-larval stages of development in <u>Xenopus</u> (up to at least stage 54 of Nieuwkoop and Faber) suppresses the rosette-forming cell response which normally follows a single intra-peritoneal injection of 0.05 ml/gm body weight of a 10% suspension of SRBC; the formation of plaque-forming cells and of serum haemolysins was also impaired.

The fact that relatively late larval thymectomy abrogates antibody production to a thymus-dependent antigen but fails to affect graft rejection, alerts us to the possibility that there exists in amphibians a functional heterogeneity within the T-cell population: T-cells responsible for "helper" activity in antibody production may perhaps be a population which seeds to the periphery later and/or are shorter lived in extra-thymic tissues than those responsible for alloimmune reactions. There are, however, several alternative explanations. Naturally-occurring cross-reacting antigens could influence the situation for one or other type of antigen, and there remains the intriguing possibility that B-cells as well as T-cells may be spawned within the thymic environment and were being removed by larval thymectomy.

GENERAL DISCUSSION

We have shown that there exists in amphibians a part of the immune system which can respond to conventional B-cell (thymus-independent) antigens and a thymus-dependent component. If the immune reactions are brought about by lymphoid cells, the majority of which take their embryological origin from the area of the thymic rudiment, as is the case in Rana pipiens (4), we must ask: i) What is the source of cells responsible for antibody production to thymus-independent antigens in our thymectomized animals? ii) How is it that relatively normal histogenesis of the lymphoid organs can occur when larvae are thymectomized before lymphocytic differentiation in the peripheral tissues (31,32), i.e., what is the source of the lymphocytes which differentiate in the absence of the thymus? iii) What is the mechanism whereby thymectomized Xenopus eventually reject first-set skin grafts and effect second-set alloimmune reactivity?

In the experiments of Turpen et al. (4) there was a small percentage of cells in the peripheral lymphoid tissues of post-metamorphic frogs which were not thymus-derived. This could be the origin of the thymus-independent immune cells in our thymectomized animals (as well as/or a source of other haemopoietic cell lines). Alternatively these immune cells may arise as part of an embryonic exodus from the thymic rudiment (with extensive seeding early in life to account for the reactivity of our thymectomized animals). We are assuming for the purpose of this discussion that Xenopus laevis is essentially similar to Rana pipiens in these respects.

Similar explanations could account for the relatively normal lymphocytic content of the peripheral lymphoid organs; also perhaps for some of the residual alloimmune reactivity, i.e., the thymic influence in the initial establishment of the lymphocyte population may be a very early event, perhaps due to embryological migratory movements of populations of stem cells from the area of the thymic rudiment - which establish a source of morphologically recognizable lymphocytes, if not completely competent ones. However, it must be remembered that even when thymectomy is performed at 5 days post-

fertilization in <u>Xenopus</u> when the thymus comprises only some 500
cells, the animal is not totally deprived of its subsequent ability
to reject skin grafts (15). Also, although the peripheral lymphocytic
population is somewhat reduced, impressive numbers of lymphocytes
are still formed when the thymus has been absent from a very young
age. Even allowing for the fact that we are considering immature
developmental stages, this would seem to place over-heavy demands
upon stem-cell peripheralization during the short period of life up
to the time when we thymectomize the early larvae. Possibly thymic-
independent mechanisms play a part in graft rejection, or perhaps
the initial prolongation of graft survival in thymectomized animals
is due to enhancing antibodies or to early-seeded suppressor cells.

An alternative explanation is that, while the thymus is the
normal source of lymphocytes, alternative pathways of differentiation come into play in its absence. The possibility of alternative
pathways has been suggested on the basis of avian and mammalian experiments (33,34). The question at issue here is whether the
presence of a thymic epithelium, once evolved, is obligatory for
the differentiation of T-cell function or whether it merely provides a specialized microenvironment which quantitatively expands
the number of T-cells produced by the animal and/or permits a
further stage of maturation. The problem may well be resolved when
the role of possible humoral secretions by the epithelial components of the primary lymphoid organs is firmly established. Mean-
while, we should note that the question of the presence of a thymus
in agnathans (which have competent lymphocytes) remains unresolved
and that in the jawed vertebrates the thymus, although remarkably
similar in histology throughout the classes, has an embryological
origin from different pharyngeal pouches in different groups. It
could be that in the absence of the thymus from an early stage of
development, other regions of the pharyngeal epithelium can elaborate secretory products which influence lymphocytic differentiation
even though they do not provide a suitable microenvironment for the
<u>in situ</u> development of lymphoid tissue.

From this discussion it becomes apparent that new information
on the early sources of lymphocytes in amphibians has brought with
it the need to review the results of thymectomy experiments and to
reconcile the amphibian data with current views on the ontogeny of
the immune system in higher groups. Vertebrates are unlikely to
differ in anything as fundamental as the origin of their lymphoid
cells - and all vertebrate immune systems are beginning to look
basically alike now that heterogeneity of lymphocytic populations
in anurans is established and a dichotomy between thymus-dependent
and thymus-independent components in amphibians is being defined.

ACKNOWLEDGEMENTS

This study was aided in part by a Medical Research Council
project grant. One of us (MHC) was supported by a Science Research
Council studentship.

REFERENCES

1. Sailendri, K., Studies on the Development of Lymphoid Organs
   and Immune Responses in the Teleost, Tilapia mossambica
   (Peters). 128 pp. (Ph.D. Thesis, Madurai University, 1973).

2. Charlemagne, J. and Tournefier, A., J. Immunogenetics, 1:108
   (1974).

3. Cooper, E. L., Brown, B. A. and Wright, R. K., Amer. Zool. 15:
   85 (1975).

4. Turpen, J. B., Volpe, E. P. and Cohen, N., Amer. Zool. 15:51
   (1975).

5. Sailendri, K. and Muthukkaruppan, Vr., J. Exp. Zool. 191:371
   (1975).

6. Moticka, E. J., Brown, B. A. and Cooper, E. L., J. Immun. 110:
   855 (1973).

7. Emmrich, F., Richter, R. F. and Ambrosius, H., Eur. J. Immun.
   5:76 (1975).

8. Du Pasquier, L., Weiss, N. and Loor, F., Eur. J. Immun. 2:366
   (1972).

9. Collie, M. H., Turner, R. J. and Manning, M. J., Eur. J. Immun.
   (in press).

10. Goldstine, S. N. and Collins, N. H., Fed. Proc. 34:966 (1975).

11. Ruben, L. N., van der Hoven, A. and Dutton, R. W., Cell. Immun.
    6:300 (1973).

12. Cohen, N., Amer. Zool. 15:119 (1975).

13. Cooper, E. L., in Contemporary Topics in Immunobiology, 2:13
    (Plenum Press, New York and London, 1973).

14. Du Pasquier, L., Current Topics Microbiol. Immun. 61:37 (1973).

15. Horton, J. D. and Horton, T. L., Amer. Zool. 15:73 (1975).

16. Tournefier, A., J. Embryol. Exp. Morph. 29:383 (1973).

17. Charlemagne, J., Eur. J. Immun. 4:390 (1974).

18. Fache, B. and Charlemagne, J., Eur. J. Immun. 5:155 (1975).

19. Tournefier, A., C. R. Hebd. Séances Acad. Sci. D, Paris, 275:
    2443 (1972).

20. Horton, J. D., Horton, T. L. and Rimmer, J., in Cooper, E. L.
    and Du Pasquier, L., Progress in Immunology, 2, vol. 2:297
    (North Holland, Amsterdam, 1974).

21. Turner, R. J. and Manning, M. J., Eur. J. Immun. 4:343 (1974).

22. Horton, J. D. and Manning, M. J., Immunology 26:797 (1974).

23. Baculi, B. S. and Cooper, E. L., J. Exp. Zool. 183:185 (1973).

24. Wortis, H. H., Clin. Exp. Immun. 8:305 (1971).

25. Pantelouris, E. M., Immunology 20:247 (1971).

26. Crewther, P. and Warner, N. L., Aust. J. Exp. Biol. Med. Sci.
    50:625 (1972).

27. Howard, J. G., Scott, M. T. and Christie, G. H., in Ciba Foun-
    dation Symp., 18 (new series): 101 (Associated Scientific
    Publishers, Amsterdam, 1973).

28. Turner, R. J., Tâm, N. D. and Manning, M. J., J. Reticuloendo-
    thel. Soc. 16:232 (1974).

29. Nieuwkoop, P. D. and Faber, J., Normal Table of Xenopus laevis
    (Daudin), 2nd ed., 252 pp. (North Holland, Amsterdam, 1967).

30. Horton, J. D. and Manning, M. J., Transplantation 14:141 (1972).

31. Manning, M. J., J. Embryol. Exp. Morph. 26:219 (1971).

32. Horton, J. D. and Manning, M. J., J. Morph. 143:385 (1974).

33. Morris, B., in Contemporary Topics in Immunobiology 2:39
    (Plenum Press, New York and London, 1973).

34. Bryant, B. J., Progress in Immunology, 2, vol. 3:5 (North
    Holland, Amsterdam, 1974).

VERTEBRATE IMMUNOLOGY

Maturation and Modulation
of Immune Functions

PHYLOGENETIC ASPECTS OF HYPERSENSITIVITY:

IMMEDIATE HYPERSENSITIVITY REACTIONS IN FLATFISH

Brian A. Baldo and Thelma C. Fletcher*

University of Western Australia, Clinical Immunology Unit

and *Institute of Marine Biochemistry, Aberdeen

INTRODUCTION

The existence of immediate hypersensitivity reactions in poikilotherms has, for many years, been controversial. Dreyer and King[1] reported that systemic anaphylaxis was induced in goldfish, perch, rock bass and sunfish following the injection of horse serum. Later studies[2,3] failed to support this claim but anaphylaxis has recently been reported in frogs injected with *Salmonella typhosa*[4].

DEMONSTRATION OF CUTANEOUS ANAPHYLAXIS IN FLATFISH

We have studied the question of the occurrence of immediate hypersensitivity responses in poikilotherms by examining the cutaneous response of flatfish to a variety of extracts known to be allergenic in higher vertebrates. Two marine teleosts, the plaice, *Pleuronectes platessa* L., and the flounder, *Platichthys flesus* (L.) were selected for study because of their availability throughout the year, their ease of maintenance and handling and, of most importance, the clarity with which skin reactions can be seen on their non-pigmented undersurfaces.

Following the intradermal injection of certain fungal extracts, erythematous skin reactions were observed in the plaice (Fig. 1) within 5 min but not in the skin of the closely related flounder[5]. Of the extracts which produced positive reactions (*Diplococcus pneumoniae*, *Ascaris lumbricoides*, *Epidermophyton floccosum*, *Aspergillus fumigatus*, *A. flavus*, *Trichophyton mentagrophytes*, *T. rubrum*), that from the culture filtrate of the dermatophyte

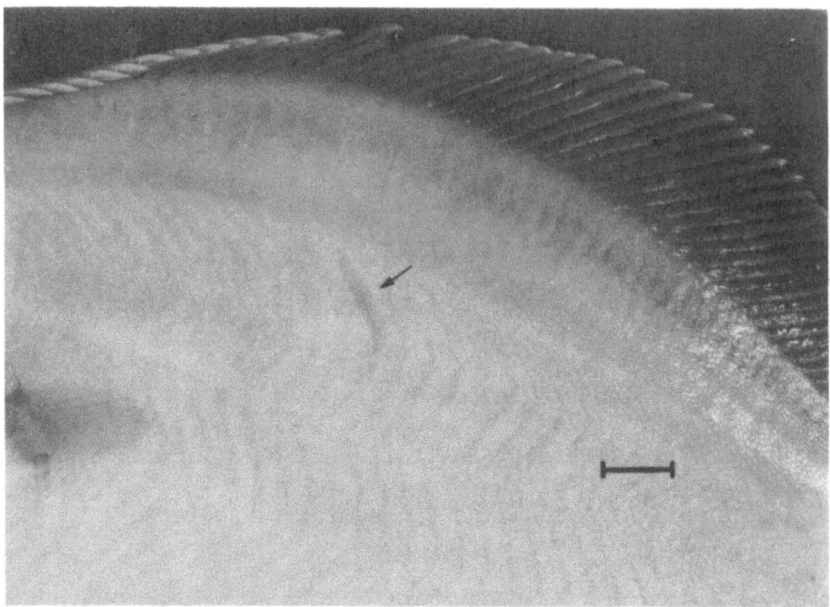

Fig. 1. Erythema reaction (arrowed) on undersurface of plaice
5 min after the intradermal injection of 0.1ml of *Epidermophyton*
floccosum extract (10 mg/ml saline). Bar=1.5cm.

E. floccosum was the most potent in producing an immediate erythema
in plaice adapted to both 4°C and 14°C. The fungal preparations
which gave positive skin tests contain a component which, in the
presence of Ca^{2+}, precipitates with human C-reactive protein (CRP)
and with most 'normal' plaice sera examined [6],[7]. For this reason
we also injected pneumococcus C-substance[8] and, as with the other
preparations, found that this polysaccharide produced an erythema
in plaice skin but no reaction in the flounder. To investigate
whether the reaction observed in plaice skin was a true immediate
hypersensitivity response, serum transfer experiments were made
between plaice and flounder (Fig. 2). Serum from plaice showing
positive skin reactions to *E. floccosum* was injected intravenously
(i.v.) into a flounder (1.5ml serum per 100 g body weight) and
after latent periods of from 3 to 48 hr the flounder was challenged
intradermally with *E. floccosum*. Clear erythema responses were
observed in the skin of such 'sensitized' flounders, demonstrating
that a transferable serum factor is involved in the flatfish
cutaneous reactions. The skin-sensitizing or tissue-fixing
properties of the plaice serum factor(s) were destroyed by heating
the serum at 56°C for 4 hr although milder treatment (56°C for 30
min) failed to destroy the activity.

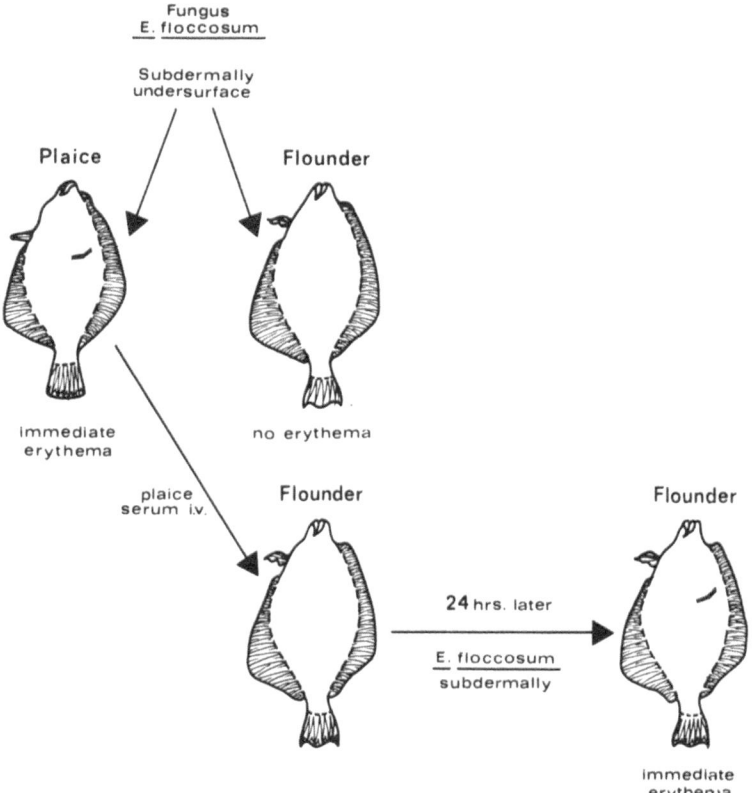

Fig. 2.   Serum transfer experiment between plaice and flounder.

NATURE OF THE FLATFISH SKIN-SENSITIZING FACTOR: POSSIBLE
INVOLVEMENT OF THE PLAICE CRP-LIKE PROTEIN IN HYPERSENSITIVITY

The extracts which produce an immediate erythema in the plaice
contain C-substance-like components which precipitate with plaice
sera. No precipitation has been observed however in the sera from
over 50 flounders. Like human CRP, the plaice fungal precipitins
have been shown to possess specificity for phosphorylcholine[9,7].
On Sephadex G-200 gel filtration of plaice serum, the fungal
precipitating and tissue-fixing activities elute in the same
fraction and this raises the possibility that the skin-sensitizing
factor(s) in plaice serum is a CRP-like protein. In man, immediate
hypersensitivity reactions are mediated via the reaginic antibody,
IgE[10,11]. Other species of higher vertebrates produce reagins[12]
but, so far, comparable antibodies have not been described in
poikilotherms. Further isolation experiments with plaice serum
will establish whether the skin-sensitizing factor(s) is the CRP-
like fungal precipitin or an antibody with tissue-sensitizing
properties.

Table I. Response of plaice to intradermal injection of 0.2ml
Epidermophyton floccosum extract (10mg/ml) after intravenous
injection of inhibitors

Inhibitor	Dose mg/100g body weight	Time before challenge	Skin erythema inhibition
Methysergide	0.04	15 min	−
Promethazine	3.00	15 min	−
Mepyramine	3.00	5 min	−
Disodium cromoglycate	16.00	1 min	+
Diethylcarbamazine	6.00	5 min	+

MEDIATORS OF IMMEDIATE HYPERSENSITIVITY

In higher vertebrates undergoing an anaphylactic reaction, the
effects seen on smooth muscle and vascular permeability are due to
a number of mediators which are released from the so-called target
cells (principally tissue mast cells and basophils). Chief among
these mediators are histamine, bradykinin, 5-hydroxytryptamine
(serotonin), slow reacting substance of anaphylaxis (SRS-A) and
the eosinophilic chemotactic factor of anaphylaxis[13-16]. Of these,
only histamine has been demonstrated in fish skin[17] and the levels
found are considerably lower than the amounts which occur in mammals[18].

We recently found[19] that intradermal injection of histamine,
serotonin and the histamine liberator, compound 48/80, produced
erythema reactions in the skin of both plaice and flounder. The
reactions were indistinguishable from those produced by the injection
of *E. floccosum* extract into plaice. In attempts to inhibit the
E. floccosum-induced skin reactions, compounds known to affect the
action of mediators were administered i.v. to plaice, prior to fungal
challenge. The results of the *in vivo* experiments shown in Table I
would suggest that histamine and serotonin are not important mediators
of the skin reaction. Diethylcarbamazine and disodium cromoglycate
have been found to affect the production of SRS-A in mammalian
systems[20,21] and it is possible that a similar mediator is implicated
in the plaice skin reaction.

Although *in vivo* experiments with inhibitors of hypersensitivity can provide valuable preliminary information, *in vitro* techniques
are likely to yield more basic information on the individual mediators.

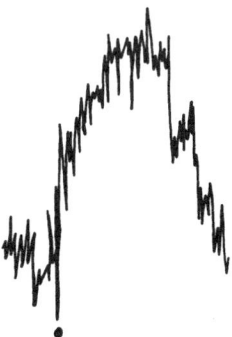

Fig. 3. Contraction of the isolated guinea pig ileum to the extract derived from plaice skin incubated for 30 min at 22°C with *E. floccosum*. Trace represents a 6 min period.

We have therefore examined plaice skin in *in vitro* experiments with *E. floccosum* extract and assayed the incubation mixture on isolated guinea pig ileum[22]. There was no release of histamine-like substances and the slow contractions of the ileum (Fig. 3) were not inhibited in the presence of 10^{-6}M mepyramine, atropine or methysergide. The release of mediators was a result of the fungal challenge of the plaice skin, since *E. floccosum* or skin alone had no effect on the guinea pig ileum. The plaice skin did not require prior sensitization with serum, and skin from any plaice showing hypersensitivity *in vivo* usually released a mediator after incubation with *E. floccosum in vitro*. Flounder skin however, did not appear to release any mediators, active on the ileum, after incubation with the fungus. Since much is now known on the mode of action of inhibitors of hypersensitivity in mammals,[15,16,23] the incorporation of inhibitors into the plaice skin *in vitro* system should provide insight into the molecular events involved in the release of mediators in poikilotherms.

PHYLOGENETIC PERSISTENCE AND POSSIBLE BENEFICIAL EFFECTS OF IMMEDIATE HYPERSENSITIVITY RESPONSES

Our studies presented here, the report of anaphylaxis in frogs[4] and the finding of similar immediate hypersensitivity responses in both marsupials and eutherians[24,12] would suggest that the immediate hypersensitivity response has primitive origins. Some would therefore conclude that this response has persisted because it possesses biological value and/or because it conferred a selective advantage in evolution[25]. Although a number of beneficial functions have been ascribed to certain components of the immediate hypersensitivity response, the conclusion that such responses are in any way beneficial to the host is open to speculation. Possible protective mechanisms may be associated with the pharmacological mediators released from the target cells. The involvement of mediators in protection against intestinal parasites is controversial[26] although Rothwell et al.,[27] have claimed that histamine and serotonin are involved in the expulsion of the nematode *Trichostrongylus colubriformis* from immune guinea pigs. A similar elimination of the cestode *Caryophyllaeus laticeps* appears to occur in the dace, *Leuciscus leuciscus*[28]. Immediate hypersensitivity may also be involved in tumour rejection[29] and defense against arthropods[30].

Recently, Steinberg et al.,[31] suggested that IgE-sensitized tissue mast cells in submucosal tissues may be triggered by specific antigen and this releases mediators which increase vascular permeability and induce translocation of serum antibodies to local sites. A similar sequence of events occurring in fish, would contribute to the defense of their mucous membranes against invasive pathogens.

CONCLUSIONS

Although we have started to examine the complex events involved in the production of the flatfish immediate hypersensitivity reactions, there are still many aspects of poikilotherm hypersensitivity responses where little information is available. For example, little is known of the cells involved in the plaice and flounder skin reactions. Circulating basophils have not been found in the plaice, although skin mast cells are present[32] and have also been demonstrated in other poikilotherms[33,34]. Recent observations with plaice suggest that eosinophilic granular cells[32] may function as target cells in this species. The cells become active and migrate from their usual basal position in the epidermis, following the intradermal injection of compound 48/80 (Fletcher and Murray, unpublished). The epidermis appears depleted of these cells in areas of cutaneous anaphylaxis, within an hour of challenge.

Work is proceeding on the isolation and characterization of the plaice tissue-fixing serum factor(s) and on the chemical mediators involved in plaice and flounder responses to *E. floccosum*, although with each of these aspects much remains to be learned. In the meantime, we would like to suggest that the cutaneous anaphylactic reactions which we have described in the teleost order Heterosomata, will provide a useful model for the more detailed analysis of the cellular and molecular events involved in immediate hypersensitivity responses in poikilotherms.

REFERENCES

1. Dreyer, N.B. and King, J.W., J. Immun., 60: 277 (1948).

2. Lukyanenko, V.I., Izv. Akad. Nauk SSSR, 3: 426 (1967).

3. Clem, L.W. and Leslie, G.A., in Immunology and Development, M. Adinolfi, Ed. 62 (Spastics International Medical Publications, London, 1969).

4. Cohen, S.G., Sapp, T.M. and Shaskas, J.R., J. Allergy Clin. Immunol., 47: 121 (1971).

5. Fletcher, T.C. and Baldo, B.A., Science, 185: 360 (1974).

6. Longbottom, J.L. and Pepys, J., J. Path. Bact., 88: 141 (1964).

7. Baldo, B.A. and Fletcher, T.C., Nature, 246: 145 (1973).

8. Tillett, W.S. and Francis, T., J. exp. Med., 52: 561 (1930).

9. Volanakis, J.E. and Kaplan M.H., Proc. Soc. exp. Biol. Med., 136: 612 (1971).

10. Ishizaka, K. and Ishizaka, T., J. Immun., 99: 1187 (1967).

11. Ishizaka, K. and Ishizaka, T., Clin. Exp. Immunol., 6: 25 (1970).

12. Bloch, K.J. and Ohman, J.L., in Biochemistry of the Acute Allergic Reactions, K.F. Austen and E. L. Becker, Eds, 45 (Blackwell, Oxford, 1971).

13. Kay, A.B., Stechschulte, D.J. and Austen, K.F., J. exp. Med., 133: 602 (1971).

14. Orange, R.P., Kaliner, M.A. and Austen, K.F., in Biochemistry of the Acute Allergic Reactions, K.F. Austen and E. L. Becker, Eds, 189 (Blackwell, Oxford, 1971).

15. Orange, R.P., in Progress in Immunology II, L. Brent and J. Holborow, Eds, 4: 29 (North-Holland, Amsterdam, 1974).

16. Piper, P.J., Ibid., p.51.

17. Lorenz, W., Matejka, E., Schmal, A., Seidel, W., Reimann, H.-J., Uhlig, R. and Mann, G., Comp. Gen. Pharmac., 4: 229 (1973).

18. Reite, O.B., Physiol. Rev., 52: 778 (1972).

19. Baldo, B.A. and Fletcher, T.C., Experientia, 31: 495 (1975).

20. Orange, R.P., Valentine, M.D. and Austen, K.F., Proc. Soc. exp. Biol. Med., 127: 127 (1968).

21. Dawson, W. and Tomlinson, R., Br. J. Pharmac., 52: 107P (1974).

22. Kuritzky, B. and Goodfriend, L., Int. Archs Allergy appl.
     Immun., 46: 552 (1974).

23. Kaliner, M. and Austen, K.F., Biochem. Pharmac., 23: 763 (1974).

24. Lynch, N.R. and Turner, K.J., Aust. J. exp. Biol med. Sci.,
     52: 425 (1974).

25. Thomas, L., in Immunopathology of Inflammation, B.K. Forscher
     and J.C. Houck, Eds, 1 (Excepta Med. Foundation, Amsterdam,
     1971).

26. Ogilvie, B.M. and Jones, V.E., Prog. Allergy, 17: 93 (1973).

27. Rothwell, T.L.W., Pritchard, R.K. and Love, R.J., Int. Archs
     Allergy appl. Immun., 46: 1 (1974).

28. Kennedy, C.R. and Walker, P.J, J. Parasit., 55: 579 (1969).

29. Bartholomaeus W.N. and Keast, D. Nature: New Biology, 239:
     206 (1972).

30. Stebbings, J.H., Perspect. Biol. Med., 17: 233 (1974).

31. Steinberg, P., Ishizaka, K. and Norman, P.S., J. Allergy Clin.
     Immunol. 54: 359 (1974).

32. Roberts, R.J., Young, H. and Milne, J.A., J. Fish Biol., 4:
     87 (1972).

33. Veil, C., Acta physiol. pharmac. néerl., 6: 386 (1957).

34. Kapa, E. and Csaba, G., Acta biol. hung., 24: 19 (1973).

IMMUNITY IN THE DEVELOPING AMPHIBIAN

Susan H. Pross and David T. Rowlands, Jr.

Departments of Biology and Pathology

University of Pennsylvania, Phila., Pennsylvania 19174

Studies of immunologic development require animal models in which the effects of antigenic stimulation can be measured accurately with regard to various states of lymphoid development (1). Anuran amphibia represent one such group of animals. From an evolutionary perspective, adult amphibia are the first animals to possess a bone marrow which is similar to that of mammals, tissues resembling mammalian lymph nodes, and an "IgG"-like immunoglobulin (2-4). Similarly, the two life forms of amphibian tadpoles and frogs invite ontogenetic studies of the immune system as it relates to development of lymphoid tissues.

The central themes of this paper will be to relate the effector elements of the immune system to the structures of the lymphoid system and to compare the immune system of tadpoles with that of adult frogs. We will conclude that the humoral immune responses of adults and tadpoles are qualitatively similar but differ quantitatively. This conclusion implies that a wide range of immunologic diversity is generated relatively early in the maturation of amphibia.

MORPHOLOGICAL DEVELOPMENT OF THE LYMPHOID SYSTEM

As is the case in other animals, the thymus is the first organ to be populated by lymphocytes in Rana catesbiana tadpoles (5). This organ enlarges throughout the larval period. After metamorphosis, the thymus consists of distinct cortical and medullary areas surrounded by a connective tissue capsule.

373

In contrast to structural similarities between the thymus of adult amphibia and mammals, thymocytes of amphibia and mammals are functionally dissimilar in certain respects. For example, immunoglobulins have been detected on the surfaces of thymic lymphocytes in Xenopus laevis (6), but only a very small minority of thymocytes from mammals can be shown with similar ease, to have surface immunoglobulins. During larval life, the numbers of immunoglobulin positive lymphocytes remains constant (60 - 80%), but the percentage of thymocytes with detectable surface immunoglobulins decreases markedly to 9% in adult amphibia.

Larval R. catesbiana have primitive lymph glands located between the 3rd aortic arch and the anterior cardinal vein. As is the case in similar structures found in the adult, no lymphatics are associated with these lymph glands but, in both cases, vascular connections are present. Apparently, during metamorphosis, the lymph glands of larvae disappear and are replaced by "jugular bodies" which resemble mammalian lymph nodes (5). These organs, although devoid of lymphatic connections, phagocytized india ink readily (2). Jugular bodies differ from mammalian lymph nodes in having no true capsule so that they are bathed directly in tissue fluids. It should be pointed out that lymph glands and jugular bodies have not been found in all anurans. Baculi and Cooper (2), failed to identify lymphoid organs in Kassina senegalensis, Bufo boreas, or Bufo powerii.

Cooper (7) found that bilateral extirpation of the lymph glands of the tadpole of R. catesbiana led to a depressed immune response to bovine serum albumin. On the other hand, allografts were rejected by these animals in the same manner as in unmodified hosts. These results are interesting in terms of earlier work demonstrating that thymectomy in larval amphibia resulted in prolongation of skin graft rejection (8). The results of these studies taken together suggest that the lymphoid system of larval amphibia is similar to that of mammals (9). There may be two distinct compartments with the thymus being responsible for cellular immunity and the lymph glands regulating antibody production.

IMMUNOGLOBULIN DEVELOPMENT

Marchalonis and Edelman (10), demonstrated that R. catesbiana adult frogs synthesize two classes of immunoglobulins, IgM and "IgG". Since the lower molecular weight immunoglobulin of these frogs differ in electrophoretic mobility and molecular weight from mammalian IgG, Marchalonis and Cone (11) were cautious in concluding that this immunoglobulin class was a direct ancestor of mammalian IgG.

Until very recently, it was thought that Rana catesbiana tadpoles could synthesize only IgM immunoglobulins, the production of IgG occurring after metamorphosis (12). Immunochemical studies employing polyacrilamide gel analyses have now indicated that R. catesbiana tadpoles do, in fact, synthesize both IgM and IgG immunoglobulins (13). Marchalonis' work with R. pipiens tadpoles has shown that at stage #25 (a premetamorphic stage) there is little protein migrating with gamma mobility (14). During metamorphosis (stages #29-32), proteins appeared that resembled IgM and, perhaps, IgA. The size and mobility of this second protein was intermediate between IgM and IgG. Although the amount of protein was too small to permit isolation and characterization of this embryonic material, Marchalonis felt that its ability to precipitate with antisera to IgM, and its characteristic molecular weight and mobility, were suggestive of its immunologic significance.

ANTIBODY RESPONSE IN FROGS AND TADPOLES

In order to expand the information available on immune responses in amphibia, we immunized frogs and tadpoles of R. catesbiana with a variety of antigens. In this study we were especially interested in the range of antigens to which these animals responded and the characteristics of the antibodies produced.

Previous studies by other investigators showed that adult R. catesbiana responded to immunization with a variety of antigens including bacteriophage (10) and hapten-carrier conjugates (15). In order to establish a base for comparison with tadpoles we extended these observations to include immunization of adult frogs with 3 bacteriophage (f2, ØX-174, and T4) and the 2 haptens, 2,4 dinitrophenyl (DNP) and fluorescein isothiocyanate (FTC) on 3 different carriers, bovine serum albumin (BSA), bovine gamma globulin (BGG), and horseshoe crab hemocyanin (Hycn). These antigens were emulsified in Freund's complete adjuvant (FCA) before immunization. In each case an immune response was generated slowly, requiring as long as 24 weeks for peak antibody levels to be reached. In most instances, however, antibodies could be detected in sera of these animals at the first bleeding, 3 weeks after immunization.

R. catesbiana tadpoles (stages 26 to 31) were immunized with 0.1 ml containing 5×10^{10} of each bacteriophage emulsified 1:1 in Freund's complete adjuvant (FCA). These animals were then bled at 3 week intervals. In tadpoles at each stage of development (16) antibody activities appeared throughout the entire 12 weeks of the study. In the case of bacteriophage ØX-174 a peak antibody response was achieved at 6 weeks but the peak was reached later when either bacteriophage f2 or T4 served as the immunogen. The most striking observation is that tadpoles and frogs responded to the same battery of antigens. In both groups, immunization with ØX-174 bacteriophage resulted in higher antibody titers than did immunization with the other bacteriophage. There was no measurable difference in the immune responses of the tadpoles at any of the 6 stages of larval development tested. No apparent difference was noted in immune responses of similar groups of tadpoles tested with 10 fold greater or 10 fold lesser amounts of these antigens.

A similar pattern of immune response emerged when tadpoles at stages 26 to 30 were immunized with either the hapten DNP or FTC complexed to BSA, BGG, or Hycn. In these cases antibody activity could not be identified 3 weeks after immunization but could be readily identified by 6 weeks. As was the case with bacteriophage, the immune response appeared to be independent of the stage of larval development at the time of immunization.

CHARACTERIZATION OF ANTIBODIES IN TADPOLES

The antibodies formed in tadpoles were analyzed by sucrose gradient centrifugation to define the antibodies formed with regard to their molecular sizes and by isoelectrofocusing with respect to the heterogeneity of these antibodies. Preliminary studies of sera obtained from adult R. catesbiana indicated that although most antibody activity was in a heavy fraction, a lesser amount appeared in a lighter fraction as early as 9 weeks after primary stimulation with bacteriophage f2 and ØX-174 and with the haptens DNP and FTC.

Our analyses of tadpole antibodies were carried out using bacteriophage neutralization, which approaches radioimmunoassay in sensitivity (17). The results of our studies are illustrated in Fig. 1. Serum recovered 9 weeks after primary immunization of tadpoles with FTC-Hycn was applied to a linear sucrose gradient (10-37%) and centrifuged for 16 hours at 37,000 rpm in an SW 50 swinging bucket rotor. Fractions were collected by puncturing the bottoms of the centrifuge tubes. In this case antibody activities of the various fractions were measured by incubating aliquots with a conjugate of FTC-T4 for one hour at $37^{\circ}C$. Neutralization of the bacterial lytic properties of this bacteriophage preparation was taken as a measure of antibody activity (18). As can be clearly seen, a major portion of the antibody activity in this serum was associated with the heavy (19S) fractions but a significant level of serum antibody was also found in a lighter (7S) fraction.

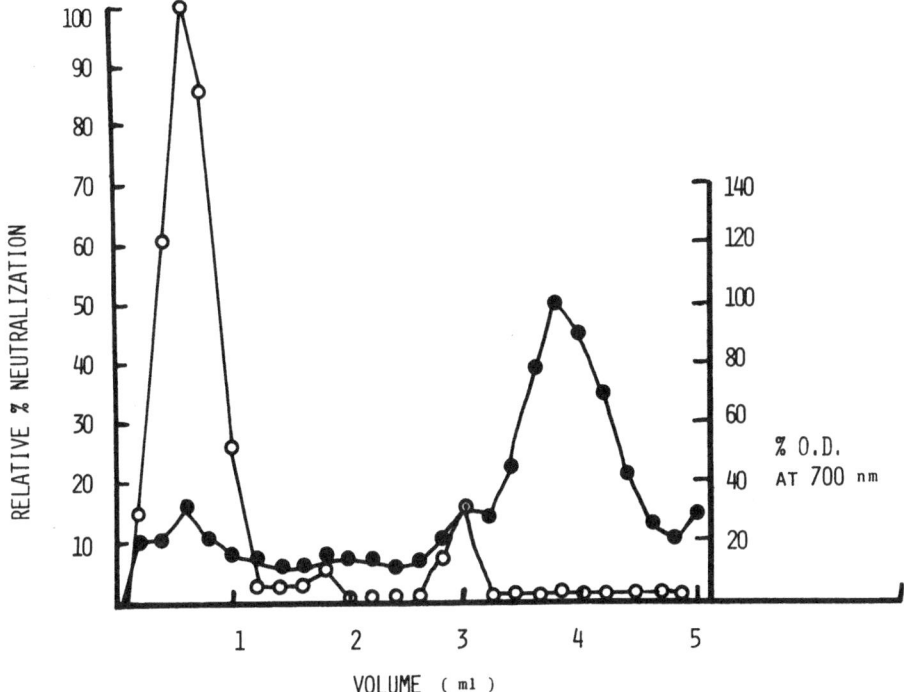

Figure 1. Sucrose density gradient of serum from R.
catesbiana tadpoles immunized with FTC-Hycn. Closed circles
represent the protein in each fraction. The open circles
represent the antibody activity in each fraction and are plotted
relative to the fraction having maximum antibody activity.

        Earlier studies (12) suggested that tadpoles produced only
IgM antibodies but Green et al (19) reported that tadpoles did,
in fact, have IgG antibodies. It seems likely that the difference in these observations lies in the sensitivities of the assay
systems used. Those who have not been able to demonstrate IgG
antibodies used an agglutination system to detect antibodies for
sheep red blood cells while Green et al (19) used a more sensitive radioimmunoassay.

        A second measure of maturity of development of the immune
system in embryos is the degree of heterogeneity of antibodies
as compared with similar studies of adults of the same species.
Using isoelectricfocusing as an index, Montgomery and Williamson
(20) concluded that the immune response of neonatal rabbits to

the hapten DNP was restricted as compared to similar immune responses in adult rabbits. In contrast, Silverstein (21) reported that once a lamb can respond to an antigen, the heterogeneity of its response is as complex as that of the adult sheep.

We compared the isoelectricfocusing characteristics of antibodies of frogs and tadpoles. Fig. 2 is a representative study. In this case both adults and tadpoles had been immunized with the bacteriophage ØX-174. The antibody activities in both adults and tadpoles extend over several pH units suggesting that premetamorphic and mature anura are capable of manifesting a heterogeneous humoral response.

RESPONSE OF BLOOD CELLS TO MITOGEN

Lymphocytes of lower vertebrates have been thought generally to respond poorly to the mitogen, phytohemagglutinin (PHA) (22, 25). Recently reported studies of Goldshein and Cohen (24) have shown that peripheral blood lymphocytes of the toad, Bufo marinus, can proliferate as a result of mixed lymphocyte interaction as well as in response to PHA. DuPasquier and Weiss (25) made similar observations in Xenopus laevis.

In experiments carried out in collaboration with Dr. Peter Nowell, we were able to show that the peripheral lymphocytes of both tadpole and adult R. catesbiana proliferate when exposed in vitro to PHA. Cytological evaluations of mitoses was used to define proliferation. Figure 3 illustrates the results of a study in which 0.1 ml of blood from tadpoles was cultured with 400 µg of PHA-M for varying times before harvesting. As can be seen, the peak proliferative response was not evident until 90 hours after stimulation. A similar study using frog blood indicated that the peak proliferative response in the adult was reached between 60 to 90 hours after stimulation.

In the course of these studies, an interesting distinction between red blood cells in tadpoles and adult frogs was observed. Red blood cell mitoses were readily detectable in cultures of tadpole blood. PHA did not stimulate red cells to divide. In fact, PHA seems to inhibit the division of nucleated red blood cells in the tadpole.

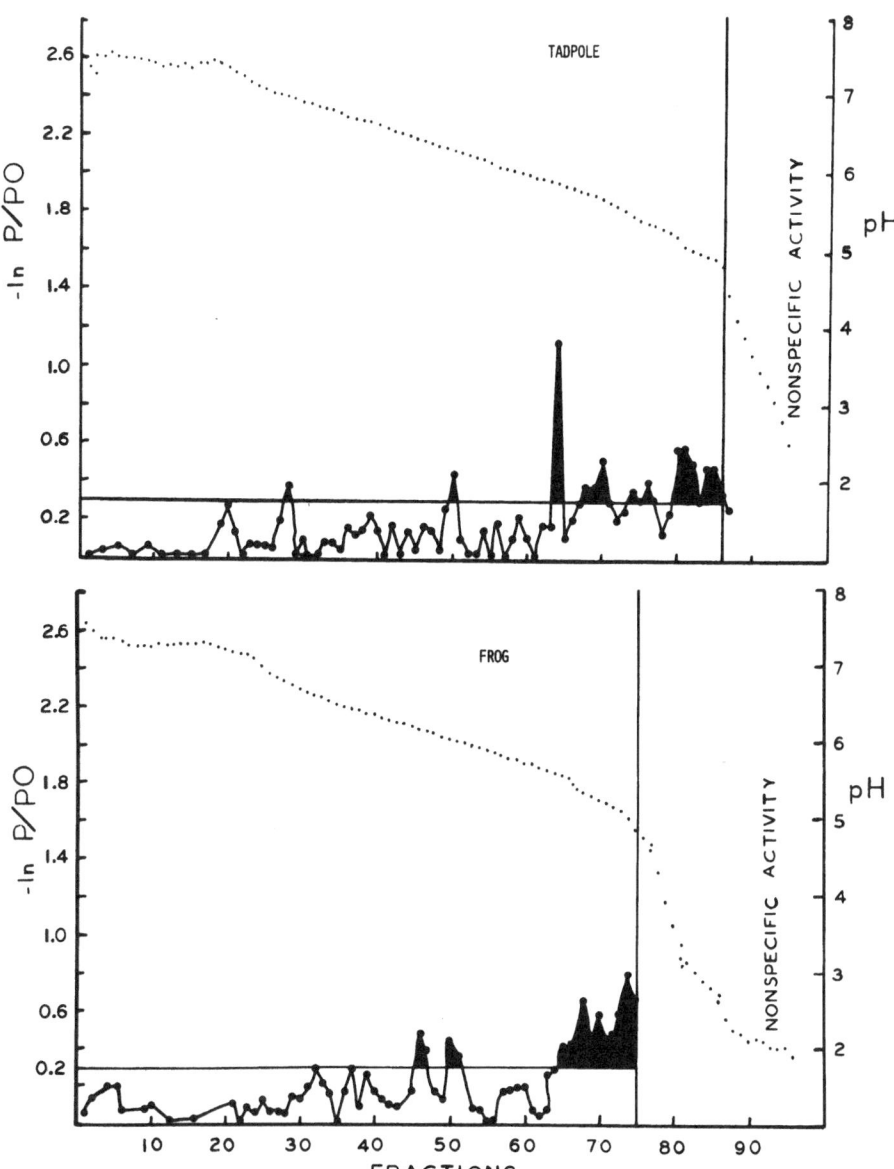

Figure 2. Isoelectric focusing of tadpole and frog anti-ØX-174 serum. 8 µl of tadpole serum and 2 µl of frog serum of animals immunized 6 weeks previously were focused in a sucrose density gradient. The pH of each fraction is represented by dotted line. The darkened areas represent fractions with significant antibody activity to ØX-174 (P/Po ≤ 0.75).

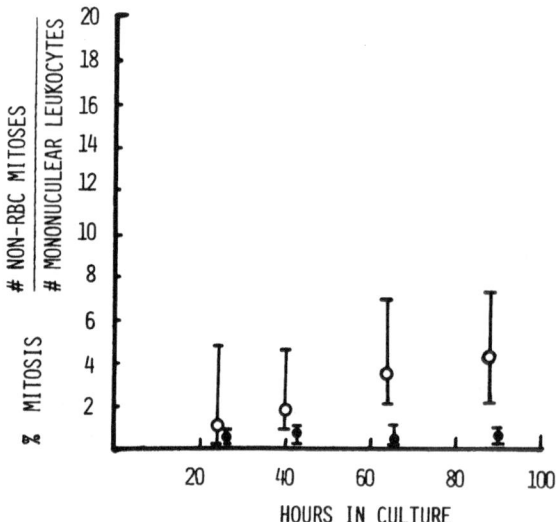

Figure 3. Mitotic response of tadpole peripheral blood leukocytes to PHA. Open circles represent the averages of 3 or 4 studies of tadpole peripheral blood leukocytes stimulated with PHA. Closed circles represent the responses of tadpole leukocytes which were not exposed to PHA.

DISCUSSION

The experiments of Silverstein et al (26) with sheep, and the more recent studies of Rowlands et al (27) and Sherwin and Rowlands (1) with opossums and irradiated-reconstituted mice have suggested that embryos display a distinct hierarchy with respect to the development of their ability to respond to various antigens. Although it may be that less well developed tadpoles would display such a hierarchy, our studies, as well as those of other investigators (28), indicate that tadpoles differ from the other animals mentioned above in having lymphoid responses which more nearly approach the sophistication of adults of the species. Tadpoles of R. catesbiana respond to the same diverse group of antigens as do adults and both tadpoles and adults are apparently able to produce both IgM and "IgG" antibodies. In addition, antibodies of tadpoles and adults appear heterogeneous when measured by isoelectricfocusing. Haimovich and DuPasquier (29) have recognized the broad immune capabilities of the tadpole in contrast to the relatively small numbers of immunologically reactive cells they possess. They reconcile this disparity by postulating a possible multispecificity in the tadpole immunocompetent cells. It may, therefore, be that a significant step in development of these animals as they move through metamorphosis is restriction of specificity of individual populations of cells.

The relationships between various lymphoid tissues of amphibia may also differ from what is commonly found in mammals. We have found that both R. catesbiana frogs and tadpoles have lymphocytes which respond to PHA, and other investigators (24,25) have demonstrated that lymphocytes of amphibia can respond by proliferation in a mixed lymphocyte culture. Both of these observations suggest that amphibia have a subpopulation of lymphocytes which resemble T cells of mammals. However, there are observations which make such an analogy difficult to accept. Turpen et al (30), for example, suggest that lymphocytes of R. pipiens are derived directly from the thymus. Other studies have also suggested that the thymus of amphibia differs anatomically and functionally from mammals. As mentioned previously (25) readily detectable immunoglobulins have been reported on the surfaces of thymic cells of Xenopus laevis. Turner (31) noted that thymectomy obliterates both the IgM and IgG antibody responses in Xenopus laevis tadpoles.

It would seem, therefore, that more thorough and systematic analysis of the immune system of amphibia, including its development, would be rewarding in expanding our knowledge of the mechanism of differentiation.

References

1. Sherwin, W.K., and Rowlands, D.T. Jr. J. Immunol., 113:1353 (1974)
2. Baculi, B.B., Cooper, E.L. and Brown, B.A. J. Morph., 131: 315 (1970)
3. Diener, E., and Nossal, G.J.V. Immunol. 10:535 (1966)
4. Marchalonis, J.J., and Cone, R.E. Aust. J. Exp. Med. 51:461 (1973)
5. Cooper, E.L. J. Morph. 122:381 (1967)
6. DuPasquier, L., Weiss, L., and Loor, F. Eur. J. Immunol. 2:366 (1972)
7. Cooper, E.L. Anat. Rec. 162:453 (1968)
8. Cooper, E.L., and Hildemann, W.H. Ann. N.Y. Acad. Sci. 126:647 (1965)
9. Raff, M.C. Transplant. Rev. 6:52 (1971)
10. Marchalonis, J.J. and Edelman, G.M. J. Exp. Med. 124:901 (1966)
11. Marchalonis, J.J. and Cone, R.E. Aust. J. Exp. Biol. and Med. Sci. 51:461 (1973)
12. Moticka, E.J., Brown, B.A., and Cooper, E.L. J. Immunol. 110:855 (1974)
13. Geczy, C.L., Green, P.C., and Steiner, L.A. J. Immunol. 111: 1261 (1973)

14. Marchalonis, J.J. Dev. Biol. 25:479 (1971)
15. Rosenquist, G.L., and Hoffman, R.Z. J. Immunol., 108:1499 (1972)
16. Witschi, E. Development of Vertebrates (Saunders, Phil., 1956)
17. Blakeslee, D., Antczak, D.F., and Rowlands, D.T. Jr. Immunochem. 10: 61 (1973)
18. Adams, M.H. Bacteriophage (Interscience, New York 1959)
19. Green, P.C., Epstein, S.M., Epstein, K.A., and Steiner, L.A. Fed. Proc. 33:735 (1974)
20. Montgomery, P.C., and Williamson, A.R. Nature 228:1307 (1970)
21. Silverstein, A.M. Ontogeny of Acquired Immunity (Elsvier, Excerpta, Medica, North Hall and Associated Scientific Publishers, 1972)
22. Smith, R.T. Developmental Aspects of Antibody Formation and Structure (Academia Publishing House of the Czechoslovak Academy of Science 1 Prague, 1970)
23. Cooper, A.J. Proceedings of the Fourth Annual Leukocyte Culture Conference (Appleton-Centry-Crofts, New York, 1971)
24. Goldshein, S.J., and Cohen, N. J. Immunol. 108:1025 (1972)
25. DuPasquier, L. and Weiss, L. Eur. J. Immunol. 3:773 (1973)
26. Silverstein, A.M., Uhr, J.W., and Kramer, K.H. J. Exp. Med. 124:799 (1966)
27. Rowlands, D.T. Jr., Blakeslee, D., and Angala, E. J. Immunol. 112:2148 (1974)
28. DuPasquier, L. Curr. Topics in Micro and Immuno. 61:37 (1973)
29. Haimovich, J. and DuPasquier, L. Proc. Nat. Acad. Sci. 70:1898 (1973)
30. Turpen, J.B., Volpe, E.P., and Cohen, N. Science 182:931 (1973)
31. Turner, R.J. and Manning, M.J. Eur. J. Immunol. 4:343 (1974)
32. This work was supported in part by USPHS Grants HL-15061 and CA-15822

DEMONSTRATION OF AN INVERSE RELATIONSHIP BETWEEN REGENERATIVE

CAPACITY AND ONCOGENESIS IN THE ADULT FROG, RANA PIPIENS

Outzen, H. C., Custer, R. P., and Prehn, R. T.

The Institute for Cancer Research

The Fox Chase Cancer Center, Phila., Pa. 19111

SUMMARY

In a series of 105 adult frogs (Rana pipiens) 19 sarcomas were induced at the implantation site of 3-methylcholanthrene pellets. Two tumors arose first in the control forelimbs, whereas 13 tumors arose first in the denervated forelimb. The remaining tumors occurred in a previously tumor-bearing frog. Ten months was the average latent period required until tumor formation occurred.

INTRODUCTION

The relationship linking regeneration and neoplasia is an old hypothesis. Waddington [1] and others [2, 3] proposed that formation of tumors may occur when an animal has a defective or incomplete regenerative response. More recently it has been suggested that a tumor formation is actually an abortive attempt at blastema formation in an animal whose regenerative response is defective [3].

Increasing or decreasing the nerve supply to the forelimbs of R. pipiens has been demonstrated to respectively increase [4] or decrease [5] the regenerative capacity of those limbs. In using these surgical techniques to manipulate the regenerative capacity in the forelimbs, we could observe whether or not these relative differences in regenerative capacity would correlate with the induction of tumors by a chemical oncogen.

MATERIALS AND METHODS

Adult Rana pipiens were obtained from the J. M. Hazen, Co.,
Alburg, Vermont. These frogs were housed in plastic aquaria that
had chlorinated city water held at 25 C constantly flowing through
them at a depth of 1-2 inches. Wooden blocks were placed in the
aquaria to provide an out of water perch for the frogs. Light was
provided by Fluorescent Vitalites (Durotest Corp., North Bergen,
N. J.) and was regulated to provide a normal light cycle. The
frogs were force fed 2-5 day old baby mice twice a week. Vitamin
supplementation was provided by placing a drop of a multivitamin
preparation on the mice.

The frogs were anesthesized with tricaine methanesulfonate;
one forelimb was denervated, and the other was either sham-denervated
or sham-denervated and nerve-supplemented using a method similar
to that described by Singer (4, 5). Twenty percent 3-methylchol-
anthrene pellets were prepared in a manner similar to that described by Bartlett (6) and were implanted intramuscularly in the
forelimb of the frogs. Paraffin control pellets were prepared in
the same manner.

RESULTS

Nineteen sarcomas arose at the implantation site of the 20%
MCA pellets in a total of 105 treated frogs. The time from
carcinogen treatment until tumor arisal ranged from 2.2 months to
24.8 months. All tumors were confirmed histologically at the time
of death. The average latent period was 10.2 months after
carcinogen application. Frogs treated with control paraffin pellets
have remained free of tumor over an average observation period of 10
months, with several in excess of 16 months.

Since each individual frog received an experimental treatment
and a concomitant control treatment, it was possible to consider
each frog as a separate experiment. The first appearance of a
tumor in these frogs occurred earlier in the denervated limbs
than in the control limbs. Sixteen frogs developed tumors in their
forelimbs, 13 arose first in the denervated forelimbs and only 2
arose first in the control limbs. The probability of this distribution occurring by chance was 0.004 using the Sign Test. Two other
tumors developed secondarily in the control forelimbs and one frog
developed tumors in both its forelimbs within the same observation
period.

The tumors were readily detectable grossly in that they formed
a hemispherical cap over the implanted MCA pellet. In general, they
expanded locally but occassionally they would infiltrate the entire
limb. During the period of observation none of these tumors

metastasized.

The same basic histologic pattern was found in each case; the tumors were composed of wavy spindled cells usually arranged in interlacing fasciculi to form short radial whorls, palisades, and herring-bone stripes. The aggressive invasiveness of one of these tumors was demonstrated by the voluntary muscle fibers being pushed widely apart by the infiltrative growth.

DISCUSSION

Reports of successful induction of malignant mesencymal cell tumors in amphibia have been very limited (7). Briggs (8) observed 3 tumors, only one of which was apparently malignant, in 154 R. pipiens tadpoles treated with MCA. Breedis (9) and Ingram (10) noted the development of sarcomas in 2 of 500 newts and 1 of 200 newts, respectively, that were treated with various hydrocarbon oncogens. Thus our report on the induction of 19 MCA-induced sarcomas in adult frogs is unusual.

The hypothesis linking oncogenesis inversely to regenerative capacity is old (1-3) and it has been approached experimentally in the past without much success (7). The correlation between denervation of a limb and the resultant depression of its regenerative capacity (5) was the means we employed to test the Waddington hypothesis (1).

This inverse relationship between regenerative capacity and tumor arisal has been championed by Seilern-Aspang and Kratochwil (11). Their report that increased incidence of epithelial tumors arose in the less regenerative areas of newts has, however, been questioned by Balls and Ruben (7).

The hypothesis that we wish to reconsider and which our data support, is the existance of a relationship between regenerative capacity and tumor formation following treatment with a chemical carcinogen.

Whether or not the increased incidence of tumor formation seen in the denervated forelimbs is directly related to the inability of these limbs to regenerate or is influenced by the absence of a normal nerve supply in some other way cannot yet be determined. The increased number of tumors arising in the denervated limbs suggests that an intact nerve supply is an adequate anti-tumor defense in the frog. The mechanism of tumor resistance in the normal limbs is not understood, but we have shown that it is under the influence of the nervous system. Since the regeneration field is also influenced by the nerve supply, the hypothesis that there may be a relationship between regenerative capacity and oncogenesis has been rendered more attractive.

REFERENCES

1.   Waddington, C. H., Nature, 135: 606-608 (1935).
2.   Needham, J., Proc. Royal Soc. Med., 29: 1577-1626 (1936).
3.   Prehn, R. T. Prog. Exp. Tumor Res., 14: 1-24 (1971).
4.   Singer, M., J. Exp. Zool., 126: 419-471 (1954).
5.   Singer, M., Kamrin, R. P., and Ashbaugh, A., J. Exp. Zool., 136: 35-51 (1957).
6.   Bartlett, G. L., J. Natl. Cancer Inst. 49: 493 (1972).
7.   Balls, M. and Ruben, L. N., Experientia, 15: 241-296 (1964).
8.   Briggs, R. W., Nature, 146: 29 (1940).
9.   Breedis, C., Can. Res., 12: 861-873 (1952).
10. Ingram, A. J., J. Embryol. and Exp. Morph. 26: 425-441 (1971).
11. Seilern-Aspang, F. and Kratochwil, K., J. Embryol. and Exp. Morph., 10: 337-363 (1962).

POLYFUNCTIONAL ANTIGEN-BINDING SPECIFICITY IN HAPTEN-CARRIER RESPONSES OF THE NEWT, TRITURUS VIRIDESCENS [1]

Laurens N. Ruben and Eric U. Selker[2]

Department of Biology, Reed College

Portland, Oregon 97202

INTRODUCTION

Carrier specific enhancement of an anti-hapten response has been reported for spleen cells of the newt, Triturus viridescens (1). The response was monitored by using immunocytoadherence (ICA). Pooled chicken or toad (Bufo marinus) erythrocytes (CRBC or TRBC) were conjugated with 2,4,6 trinitrophenyl (TNP) as previously described. TNP-TRBC were injected intraperitoneally (i.p.) and after 8 days sensitized spleen cells from 4 adult newts were mechanically dissociated, pooled, washed, counted and incubated 12-16 hours at $4^{\circ}C$ with either horse erythrocytes (HRBC) or TNP-HRBC. Spleen cells previously sensitized to test immunogens will bind them on their surface. After the incubation, the numbers of antigen binding cells (ABC) in each incubation mixture were counted in hemacytometer chambers. In the absence of carrier immunization or with immunization by injection of an erythrocyte species other than the one used as carrier, a consistently small proportion of the spleen cells bound either antigen. This low degree of binding, which exceeded that found

---

[1] This research was partially supported by grants from the National Science Foundation (GB-38480), the National Institutes of Health (AI-611-75), Washington, D.C. and from the Zlinkoff Fund for Medical Research and Education Inc., N.Y.C., N.Y.

[2] Present address: Department of Biological Sciences, Stanford University, Stanford, California. Supported by an U.R.P.P. Grant from the National Science Foundation, Washington. D.C. to the Department of Biology, Reed College.

when no prior immunization was effected, served as a measure of cross reactivity between the two erythrocyte species used. However, when the newt spleen cells had been sensitized with the carrier species of erythrocytes within 4 days prior to hapten presentation, a substantial enhancement in the number of cells binding TNP-HRBC over those binding HRBC was observed. The number of cells binding due to cross reactivity between the carrier and HRBC, which was itself enhanced by immunization, can be subtracted from the average number of TNP-HRBC ABC in order to arrive at the number of TNP specific ABC. That these were indeed TNP specific was shown by pre-incubating the sensitized spleen cells with TNP-human serum albumin (HSA) prior to performing the binding assay. Only TNP-HRBC ABC were blocked, those remaining reflecting the degree of cross reactivity with HRBC. Because similar results obtained with other animals (e.g. the rodent) were shown to reflect cell cooperation between carrier specific "helper" and antibody producing cell (APC) subpopulations (2, 3, 4), it was suggested the cell cooperation was also required for hapten responses in the newt. This assumption was strengthened by further studies (5) which showed that, as in the rodent (6), low immunogen doses (0.0025% RBC) enhance "helper" activity, even when they do not stimulate antibody synthesis. It was found that low and high immunogen dose-initiated antigen binding responses exhibit very different kinetics. Low dosages stimulate maximum ABC activity by 2 days, while high doses generated a much higher number of ABC, but this activity did not reach a maximum until 8 days post-primary challenge. While we cannot yet be certain, this difference is at least consistent with the hypothesis that two populations of spleen cells can be visualized by ICA and that they are involved in anti-hapten responses in the newt.

In the experiments reported below, "helper" activity was maximized by immunization with low doses (0.0025%) of the carrier RBC 2 days before high dose (10%) hapten-carrier presentation. The spleen cells were assayed 8 days following the second injection, a time corresponding to maximum ABC response. The assay protocols were essentially as described previously (1) although a few modifications have been used. In each case where preincubation treatment was used, the volumes placed into the 10 x 75 mm assay tubes were as follows: 50 µl of $2 - 5 \times 10^5$ newt spleen cells in 7:2 (Leibovitz-L-15 medium - GIBCO : twice glass distilled water); 10 µl of the preincubating medium or cell population and 5 hours later, 20 µl of 1% RBC for binding. The preincubations were always carried out at 4°C for 5 hours, a time previously determined to be required for stabilization of the number of ABC (7). All preincubation mixtures which did not involve RBC or TNP-RBC, were swirled thoroughly every hour. In those few series where the spleen cells are preincubated with 1% RBC or TNP-RBC, no swirling took place, although gentle re-suspension was effected so as to mix, but not break off bound RBC from the ABC just before addition of the test erythrocytes for incu-bation. Finally, in all cases, consistent, gentle resuspension before counting ABC in hemacytometer chambers was brought about by inserting the coded incubation tube into an appropriately sized short piece of tubing which was attached to a teflon stirring rod inserted into a power stirrer (Polyscience Corp.) which in combination with a "Powerstat" (I. Sorvall Co.) revolved at about 20 r.p.m. The incubation mixture tube revolved slowly in ice at an angle of 45°. Fifteen to 20 minutes was sufficient to provide an even distribution of cells to be dispersed into the counting chambers. This innovation, suggested by Mr. Marc Halperin in this laboratory, provides consistency and reduces the time required for assays by one-half. The numbers of ABC in two hemacytometer chambers were averaged with those counted from a duplicate incubation mixture, and since the number of spleen cells per unit volume was known, the ABC were expressed as a number per 10^6 spleen cells.

"HELPER" SPECIFICITY

In order to test the specificity of "helper" function in the newt, low dosages (0.0025%) of TNP-sheep erythrocytes (SRBC) were injected i.p. 2 days prior to high dose (10%) challenge by TNP-CRBC. As in all prior experiments, 0.2 ml RBC was used. After 8 days, the sensitized spleen cells were assayed for binding activity with HRBC or TNP-HRBC. The data are presented in Table 1 Schedule A (lines 1 and 2) and clearly show that in spite of having received 2 exposures to the hapten, no anti-hapten response could be demonstrated. No hapten specific "helper" activity was generated by presentation of TNP on heterologous RBC during immunization. The necessity for a carrier sensitive cell population capable of providing carrier specific enhancement of the anti-hapten response has been confirmed. Cross-reactivity alone between heterologous species of erythrocytes cannot account for the presence of the TNP specific binding cells described in the original report (1).

A QUESTION ABOUT ABC SPECIFICITY

The first indication that the analogy with mammalian species might not be totally applicable to the newt came from blocking experiments with RBC. Preliminary experiments, not reported here, showed that the binding of TNP-RBC to newt spleen cells sensitized to carrier (either CRBC or SRBC) and TNP-carrier, could be blocked by preincubation with the carrier RBC. It was concluded that these blocking carrier RBC physically prevented the TNP-conjugated RBC from gaining access to the TNP sites on the immunocyte surface or in some other way prevented firm attachment between the hapten and its receptors. This suggested that TNP-specific spleen cells have carrier specific binding sites. This possibility was examined further as shown in Schedule B, Table 1. Spleen cells which had been immunized to CRBC and TNP-CRBC were mixed with HRBC or TNP-HRBC for 5 hours prior to

the addition of CRBC. The reciprocal experiment in which HRBC was
used as the carrier was also done. The results clearly show that
TNP-heterologous-carrier RBC preincubation severely blocked binding
to the homologous carrier erythrocyte species. These results
suggested that at least some newt immunocytes have the capacity to
bind both carrier and hapten. Since erythrocytes are likely to have
many antigenic determinants and represent gross binding entities
which might cover different but neighboring binding sites, we performed a series of experiments to determine whether pre-incubation
of newt spleen cells with a small molecular conjugate of TNP, e.g.
TNP-glycine, could be used to block TNP binding sites selectively.

TNP-GLYCINE INHIBITION OF ABC

Spleens which had been sensitized with CRBC and TNP-CRBC were
preincubated with either TNP-glycine or glycine (N. B. Co.) before
being tested for ABC with HRBC or TNP-HRBC. Log dilutions of from
10^{-3}M to 10^{-8}M TNP-glycine were tested. Concentrations of 10^{-3}M
through 10^{-5}M TNP-glycine were found to increase the number of ABC
against both HRBC and TNP-HRBC, suggesting that the compound was
unspecifically affecting immunocyte membranes. Concentrations of
10^{-6}M - 10^{-8}M TNP-glycine, however, blocked the number of cells binding TNP-HRBC specifically. The data in Schedule C, Table 1 show the
effect of 10^{-7}M TNP-glycine and glycine pretreatment, the concentration chosen for the experiments described below. Similar results
were also obtained for the reciprocal experiment as well, that is,
HRBC, and TNP-HRBC sensitized spleen cells assayed against CRBC or
TNP-CRBC. As an additional control, spleen cells previously immunized against two comparable injections of HRBC only were tested with
glycine and TNP-glycine to determine whether either preincubation
treatment altered binding to HRBC. They did not. A comparison of
lines 2 and 3 led us to conclude that TNP-glycine can be used to
selectively block TNP binding and that 50% of the ABC are TNP specific.

POLYFUNCTIONAL BINDING BY NEWT ABC

In the following experiments, designed to measure the degree of
antigen-binding specificity exhibited by newt spleen cells, the RBC
species used as immunogen and carrier were the same as that employed
in the assay. Spleen cells sensitized to carrier and then TNP-carrier
were preincubated with either 10^{-7}M glycine or 10^{-7}M TNP-glycine
prior to assaying their ability to bind carrier and TNP-carrier.
The results of these experiments, which are presented in Schedules
A and B, Table 2 established the following: First, regardless of
whether the spleen cells had been immunized with CRBC and TNP-CRBC
or with HRBC as immunogen and hapten-carrier, newt spleen cells,
preincubated with 10^{-7}M glycine, bound carrier RBC or TNP-carrier
RBC equally well (lines 1 and 2). This confirmed the suggestion

TABLE 1. Antigen binding in hapten-carrier responses by adult spleen cells of the newt, _Triturus viridescens_. All injections were 0.2 ml., i.p. All priming doses were 0.0025% RBC; hapten-carrier, given 2 days later, was 10% RBC. All preincubation treatments were for 5 hours at $4^{o}C$ before the sensitized spleen cells were incubated overnight at $4^{o}C$ with the test RBC (1%) for binding. All binding assays were made 8 days after hapten (TNP-) challenge. (See text for details.)

IMMUNIZATION SCHEDULE	PREINCUBATION TREATMENT	TEST RBC	ABC/10^6 SPLEEN CELLS	AVERAGE % INCREASE OR DECREASE
A.1.TNP-SRBC,TNP-CRBC	NONE	HRBC	2370 ± 1321[a]	----
2. " " " "	"	TNP-HRBC	1668 ± 722	N.S.C.[b]
B.1. CRBC, TNP-CRBC	1% HRBC	CRBC	7985 ± 792	----
2. " " "	1% TNP-HRBC	"	4906 ± 473	-38
3. HRBC, TNP-HRBC	1% CRBC	HRBC	6736 ± 883	----
4. " " "	1% TNP-CRBC	"	3483 ± 772	-48
C.1. CRBC, TNP-CRBC	10^{-7}M glycine	HRBC	2493 ± 185	----
2. " " "	" "	TNP HRBC	5433 ± 612	+118
3. " " "	10^{-7}M TNP-glycine	HRBC	2582 ± 376	N.S.C.
4. " " "	10^{-7}M TNP-glycine	TNP-HRBC	2662 ± 820	-51

a Standard deviations reflect variation among 3 populations of spleen cells, each pooled from 4 different adult newts injected from different RBC pools.
b No significant change in average total number of ABC ± S.D.

that at least some individual newt spleen cells can bind to carrier or the hapten. The magnitudes of these responses suggest that the "dual specific" cells had been stimulated by the sensitizing injections. This thesis was further strengthened by accompanying data, derived simultaneously from the same pools of spleen cells, which showed that preincubation of the immunized spleen cells with TNP-glycine blocked newt spleen cell binding to carrier and hapten

TABLE 2. Polyfunctional antigen binding in carrier-hapten responses by adult spleen cells of the newt, <u>Triturus viridescens</u>. See the description and footnotes with Table 1 and the text for details.

IMMUNIZATION SCHEDULE	PREINCUBATION TREATMENT	TEST RBC	ABC/10^6 SPLEEN CELLS	AVERAGE % INCREASE OR DECREASE
A.1.CRBC,TNP-CRBC	10^{-7}M glycine	CRBC	14,416 ± 2635	----
2. " " "	" "	TNP-CRBC	12,012 ± 691	N.S.C.
3. " " "	10^{-7}M TNP-glycine	CRBC	5,635 ± 985	-60
4. " " "	10^{-7}M TNP-glycine	TNP-CRBC	4,810 ± 400	-60
B.1.HRBC,TNP-HRBC	10^{-7}M glycine	HRBC	10,786 ± 253	----
2. " " "	" "	TNP-HRBC	11,336 ± 1350	N.S.C.
3. " " "	10^{-7}M TNP-glycine	HRBC	6,135 ± 611	-43
4. " " "	10^{-7}M TNP-glycine	TNP-HRBC	5,106 ± 397	-54
C.1.HRBC,TNP-HRBC	10^{-7}M DNP-glycine	HRBC	2,815 ± 52	-54[a]
2. " " "	10^{-7}M DNP-glycine	TNP-HRBC	2,972 ± 378	-33

a The internal control values are not shown.

<u>equally</u> (lines 3 and 4). The degree of inhibition in each case leads us to the conclusion that <u>nearly 50% of all the ABC share this duality</u>.

     Finally, to test the specificity of this binding inhibition by hapten preincubation, DNP-glycine was used instead of TNP-glycine (Table 2, Schedule C). Spleen cells, previously sensitized to HRBC and TNP-HRBC and pretreated with DNP-glycine, were tested with respect to their binding capacity to either the carrier or haptenated-carrier. It was found that binding in each instance was equally and effectively blocked. That both DNP- and TNP-glycine successfully block binding of carrier or haptenated carrier to TNP-carrier sensitized spleen cells suggests that the hapten binding sites on newt immunocytes are not highly specific. That DNP-lysine could suppress an anti-TNP response has previously been shown for larval _Xenopus_ _laevis,_ the South African clawed toad (8) and the rodent (9).

DISCUSSION

In the newt _Triturus_ _viridescens,_ both carrier and hapten-carrier recognizing splenic cells are generated in response to injections of carrier followed by hapten-carrier. While we cannot be certain, the data strongly suggest that no spleen cells appear to be generated which are restricted to binding the hapten alone.

The polyfunctional specificity of newt antigen binding cells may be a clue to the immunologic mechanism employed by primitive and modern vertebrates having relatively small numbers of immunocytes, and yet capable of contending with a myriad of potential immunogens. It has been estimated that mammals can produce antibodies to provide for at least 10^6 different specificities (10, 11). If one assumes absolute phenotypic restriction for each ABC, then the diversity of the organismal response requires at least this number, if one sensitive cell were to be set aside for each potential antigenic determinant. Estimates place the number of antibody producing cells at between 10^6 and 10^8 for the mouse (12). While large numbers of antigen specific cells are not required to provide a pool capable of clonal expansion, thereby amplifying the response, it is difficult to imagine how adult vertebrates such as the newt, with between 1 - 2.5×10^6 spleen immunocytes, and more especially amphibian immuno-competent _larvae_ which live in a hostile environment and utilize 2×10^4 or fewer spleen cells to generate specific adaptive responses (7, 13), can provide this degree of functional diversity. Some possible explanations which seem to be available for consideration include: (A) They simply do not clear and therefore ignore a large number of potential antigenic determinants, especially those to which they are not usually exposed in their natural environment. (B) They may clear many foreign materials by more primitive and non-immunogenic mechanisms, e.g. unspecific phagocytosis. (C) Individual immunocytes might be phenotypically restricted to a particular antigenic determinant, but this specificity might vary during the lifetime of each cell, thereby providing greater immunologic diversity to the organism as a whole (8). (D) Polyfunctional immunocytes may be responsible for the observed high degree of diversity. It should be noted that this last possibility is not in conflict with the characteristic high specificity of immune responses. A number of antibodies, each having a partial fit for a given antigen, can produce an antiserum having a high degree of specificity (14).

As noted above, the finding that many newt spleen cells

sensitized to carrier and hapten-carrier can bind either the hapten
or carrier suggests that the newt may employ polyfunctional receptor
sites which may be immunoglobulin. In this context it is interesting
that polyfunctionality of some daughter cells of RBC cloned mammalian
cells has recently been suggested (15), and others (16) have shown
that a portion of a population of antigen binding cells of mouse,
rabbit and chick embryos may bind two antigens non-competitively when
both are available in the medium. But most importantly, the polyfunctionality of mammalian immunoglobulin itself has been suggested
(14). The lack of restriction of adult antigen binding cells of the
newt would seem to be of potential import in understanding the phylogeny of the immune response. For example, the possibility that the
newt routinely employs polyfunctional cell surface receptors and
serum immunoglobulin suggests a simple model to explain the observed
carrier induced enhancement of the newt's anti-hapten response
without postulating cell cooperation. It seems possible that the
initial injection of carrier stimulates the proliferation of all
immunocytes with receptor molecules recognizing the carrier. The
subsequent injection of hapten-carrier could cause a secondary amplification primarily of those immunocytes with polyfunctional sites
which recognize both the carrier and the hapten. Polyfunctional
recognition provides for a higher energy of interaction, which in
turn ensures a higher avidity for antigen-cell surface binding, leading to preferential stimulation and clonal expansion. The failure
of TNP-SRBC followed by TNP-CRBC to produce an anti-hapten response,
can then be explained on these grounds, as well as in terms of cell
collaboration. No secondary amplification of a measurable amount
would be developed without the aid of dual binding identity, since
many fewer cells might be expected to recognize the single determinant, TNP, than those able to respond to a RBC or a soluble protein.
In the absence of secondary amplification, no ABC generated by the
initial low immunizing dose would be recoverable from the newt spleen
by 10 days after injection (5).

While this represents a thought model which is attractive because
of its simplicity, the information available at this time does not
allow us to eliminate the cell cooperation analogy which requires an
interaction between at least two populations of immunocytes, one
carrier sensitive, the other hapten-carrier sensitive. Indeed, it
would seem reasonable to suppose that those ABC which bind carrier
only may be "helper", while those possessive of dual binding capacity
are in the process of generating polyfunctional antibody which will
eventually be found in the serum. Future experiments should allow
us to distinguish more effectively between these two possibilities.
Regardless of their outcome, however, it should be noted that both
schemes involve the generation of cells which share hapten and
carrier binding specificities and therefore may properly be defined
as polyfunctional.

ACKNOWLEDGEMENTS

The authors wish to take note of the excellent technical assistance provided by Ms. Judith Ruben during the course of this research. We also wish to thank Dr. Marvin Rittenberg, of the University of Oregon Health Sciences Center, for his suggestion to use TNP-glycine and for his helpful comments during the course of this work.

REFERENCES

1. Ruben, L. N., Vander Hoven, A., and Dutton, R. W. Cell. Immunol. 6:300 (1973).
2. Claman, H. N. and Chaperon, E. A. Transplantation Rev. 1:92 (1969).
3. Rajewski, K., Schirrmacher, V., Nase, S., and Jerne, N. K. J. Exp. Med. 129:1131 (1969).
4. Mitchison, N. A., Taylor, R., and Rajewski, K., in Developmental Aspects of Antibody Formation and Structure. Ed. J. Sterzl, p.547 (Publ. House Czech. Acad. Sci., Prague, 1970).
5. Ruben, L. N. Amer. Zool. 15:93 (1975).
6. Playfair, J. H. L. Clin. Exp. Immunol. 8:839 (1971).
7. Kidder, G. M., Ruben, L. N., and Stevens, J. M. J. Embryol. Exp. Morphol. 29:73 (1973).
8. Haimovich, J., and Du Pasquier, L. Proc. Nat. Acad. Sci. (U.S.A.) 70:1898 (1973).
9. Little, J. R., and Eisen, H. N. J. Exp. Med. 129:247 (1967).
10. Jerne, N. K. Proc. Nat. Acad. Sci. (U.S.A.) 41:849 (1955).
11. Haurowitz, F. Cold Spring Harbor Symp. Quant. Biol. 32:559 (1967).
12. Eisen, H. N. in Progress in Immunology, p.243 (Academic Press, N.Y., 1971).
13. Du Pasquier, L. Immunol. 19:353 (1970).
14. Richards, F. F., Konigsberg, W. H., Rosenstein, R. W. and Varga, J. M. Science 187:130 (1975).
15. Cunningham, A. J. and Fordham, S. A. Nature (Lond.) 250:669 (1974).
16. Decker, J. M., Clarke, J., Bradley, L. M., Miller, A. and Sercarz, E. E. J. Immunol. 113:1823 (1974).

SURFACE CHARACTERISTICS OF SPLEEN CELL-ERYTHROCYTE ROSETTE FORMATION IN THE GRASS FROG RANA PIPIENS

B. F. Edwards[1], L. N. Ruben[2], J. J. Marchalonis[3] and
C. Hylton
Department of Biology, Reed College, Portland, Oregon 97202
and The Walter and Eliza Hall Institute for Medical
Research, P.O. Royal Melbourne Hospital, Victoria, 3050,
Australia.

INTRODUCTION

Recent evidence indicates that cooperative cellular interactions may occur in amphibia in response to heterologous erythrocytes (RBC) or hapten-carrier (TNP-RBC) conjugates (1). In addition, the immune armament of the amphibia consists of a variety of cell types distinguishable by their location (2), by differences in their surface immunoglobulin (Ig) (3), their response to mitogens (4), and differences in bouyant density and size (5). Thus there is both functional and physical evidence for the involvement of a spectrum of cell types analogous to those found in mammalian systems. Since cell-cell cooperation has been shown to play a key role in the immune response of birds (6) and mammals (7) it is likely that further study of this phenomenon in lower vertebrates will aid in understanding the ontogeny and phylogeny of this important interaction. Fundamental to this understanding is the necessity for a clear definition of the participating cell types.

Immunocytoadherence (ICA) has been used to quantitate the early stages of a primary immune response to foreign RBC by monitoring

[1] Postdoctoral Fellow of the Sloan Foundation.

[2] This research was partially supported by grants from the National Science Foundation (GB-38480) and from the National Institutes of Health (AI-611-75) Washington, D.C., U.S.A.

[3] Supported by a grant from the National Institutes of Health (AI-12565), Washington, D.C., U.S.A.

increases in the number of lymphocytes capable of recognizing and binding antigen in a lymphoid organ such as the spleen. For example, in Rana pipiens a maximum number of splenic rosette forming cells (RFC) is seen two days after a priming low dose (0.0025%) of sheep erythrocytes (SRBC) whereas, a high dose (25% SRBC) generates a peak response by eight days (8). A feature of the amphibian system provides, what may be, a unique advantage for the study of the cell populations involved in a cooperative response. When lymphocytes from an immune animal are incubated at $4^{\circ}C$ with the same species of RBC used as antigen, relatively stable rosettes of two distinct morphologies result. Secretory (S+) RFC are those sensitized spleen cells which bind more than one layer of adherent red cells on to their surfaces. Non-secretory (S-) RFC bind only a single layer of red cells. This distinction has been made before for other systems (9) but the important point here is that, because S+RFC can form at $4^{\circ}C$ in ICA assays with amphibia, S- and S+RFC may represent two distinct populations of immune cells which can be visualized at the same time in a single assay. The generation of S+RFC in mammals requires $37^{\circ}C$, while S-RFC are best demonstrated at $4^{\circ}C$ (10). The relative proportion of S- to S+RFC during the progressive primary anti-erythrocyte response depends on the time between injection and assay and is characteristic of the source of the lymphocytes assayed (thymus vs spleen). Different immunogen doses affect different RFC kinetics.

When the above parameters are taken into consideration, an argument can be made for relating S-RFC and S+RFC to specific functional roles in the cooperative response (8). Since low concentrations of immunogen stimulate high numbers of S-RFC in two days when "helper" activity is maximized, S-RFC may represent the carrier-primed helper cells in a hapten-carrier response. On the other hand, the timing and conditions under which the proportion of S+RFC is maximized suggest that these represent antigen-producing cells (APC). It is with these analogies with the rodent (11) system in mind, that further attempts have been made to investigate the parameters of rosette formation and to determine whether or not S- and S+RFC represent two physiologically different populations of responding cells.

MATERIALS AND METHODS

Since there are a large number of variables inherent in the ICA technique, consistently reproducible results can only be obtained by careful regulation of as many parameters as possible. For this reason, the assay procedure used in these studies will be described in some detail.

Immunization procedures and preparation of lymphocyte suspensions from thymus and spleen of Rana pipiens have been described previously

(8). In order to obtain consistently high yields of undamaged
lymphocytes certain precautions must be taken in the preparation and
handling of these cells. Failure to do so leads to cell clumping
and generation of "false rosettes" due to cell membrane damage. All
glassware was cleaned with a detergent especially formulated for
tissue culture work (7X, Linbro Chem. Co.), then rinsed exhaustively
in tap and glass distilled water before autoclaving. Lymphoid organs
were initially dissociated in a volume (1.5 ml/organ) of ice cold
medium (5 parts GIBCO L-15 : 4 parts 2x glass-distilled water : 1
part decomplemented fetal calf serum) sufficient to prevent cell
surface damage by lytic enzymes and all succeeding manipulations were
performed at 4°C. The L-15 medium and all other reagents which cells
were exposed to were made up with 2x glass-distilled water to mini-
mize deleterious heavy metal ions. The introduction of air bubbles
into cell suspensions during pipetting must be avoided to prevent
damage of cells at air-water interfaces.

The dissociated immunocyte concentration was adjusted to 4-6
$\times$ 10^6 cells/ml and 50 µl combined with 10 µl of a 1% suspension of
SRBC (10^6 cells) in a 10 $\times$ 75 mm glass tube on ice. Duplicate assay
tubes were coded, covered and stored upright at 4°C for 16-20 h.
Cells were allowed to settle at 1 $\times$ g and no fixatives were used.
The resultant pellet was resuspended on ice by gentle rotation (20
RPM) of the tube by a mechanical stirrer set at a 45° angle. Following 10 min of resuspension, duplicate samples were gently pipetted
into the dual chambers of an Improved Neubauer hemacytometer and
antigen-binding cells were counted throughout the entire grid area
at 250x. With the lymphocyte concentrations used in the initial set
up, approximately 2-4 $\times$ 10^3 lymphocytes were scanned per chamber.
Only undamaged lymphocytes with three or more SRBC adhering tightly
to their surfaces were scored as RFC. Macrophages with adherent RBC
are easily distinguishable by their irregular cellular outlines from
lymphocytes and were not included in the cell count or scored as RFC.
All experiments were internally controlled by including an assay
against a species of RBC other than that used as immunogen. Whenever
possible, blood from the same stock pool was used for both immunization and assay. The ratio of RBC to lymphocytes was always adjusted
to ca. 30:1 in these assays since the number of RFC/10^6 lymphocytes
can vary with the relative concentration of RBC (12).

Stock solutions of colchicine (NBC), cytochalasin B (Cal Biochem)
and emetine-HCl (Sigma) were made up no more than 24 hours prior to
use. Rabbit antibody against Rana pipiens IgM (RARP) and Rana pipiens
IgM were prepared according to Marchalonis (13).

TREATMENT OF ICA DATA

Table 1 summarizes the data obtained from three separate experiments in which three groups of adult northern Rana pipiens (2 animals

Table 1. Variation in the anti-SRBC response among different animal populations. In all cases immunization was with 25% SRBC and assays were 8 days post-injection.

ANIMAL GROUP#	RFC/10^6 CELLS SAMPLE[a]				X ± σ
	A	B	C	D	
1	6875	7105	6415	6630	6750 ± 175
	(45)[b]	(41)	(44)	(40)	(42.5 ± 2.5)
2	7685	7950	8050	8260	7985 ± 235
	(51)	(47)	(43)	(47)	(47 ± 3.5)
3	5525	5375	5475	5290	5415 ± 105
	(56)	(50)	(51)	(46)	(50.5 ± 4.5)
	POOLED DATA FROM THREE ANIMAL GROUPS:				6715 ± 1795

[a] two samples each from duplicate assay tubes

[b] % of S-RFC

per group) were immunized with 25% SRBC and their splenic lymphocytes assayed by ICA after eight days. Animals comprising groups #1 and #2 were taken from a different shipment than group #3 animals. Each pair of animals was immunized/assayed with a pool of SRBC obtained from different shipments (Colorado Serum Co.). Calculation of standard deviations for each experiment indicates that variation among samples from a single assay is less than 10% for total RFC counts/10^6 spleen cells and less than 5% for the percentage of S- or S+RFC. The results show considerably greater variation (20-25%) when data are pooled from separate experiments involving different animal populations and sources of blood. These results have obvious implications with regard to experimental design and the manner in which the resulting data should be treated. It is the relative differences between the experimentals and controls within an experiment that are important. The absolute numbers are subject to variation through the genetic and physiological heterogeneity of animal populations as well as experimental technique.

Table 2. All data are for lymphocytes from adult <u>Rana pipiens</u> assayed against 1% SRBC. The numbers in parentheses indicate the number of days elapsed between immunization and assay. See text for additional details.

IMMUNIZING DOSE (%SRBC)	ORGAN	TOTAL RFC/ 10^6 CELLS	%S-	%S+
NONE	SPLEEN(8)	370 ± 30	100	0
0.0025	THYMUS(2)[a]	2615 ± 624	100	0
0.0025	THYMUS(8)	896 ± 115	100	0
25	THYMUS(2)	3016 ± 1092	100	0
25	THYMUS(8)	1350 ± 474	100	0
0.0025	SPLEEN(2)	3875 ± 619	81	19
0.0025	SPLEEN(8)	1140 ± 481	76	24
25	SPLEEN(2)	1035 ± 265	77	23
25	SPLEEN(8)	7550 ± 1735	45	55
SRBC/10% TNP-SRBC	SPLEEN(10)	8273 ± 1100	39	61

[a] Values for thymus cells were taken from P. Levin (12)

SIGNIFICANCE OF S- AND S+RFC

The circumstantial evidence that S-RFC and S+RFC reflect the presence of two related populations of immune cells is summarized in Table 2. ICA assay of <u>R. pipiens</u> thymocytes invariably yields only S-RFC regardless of the immunizing dose (none, 0.0025%, or 25%) or time of assay (two or eight days post-injection). In addition, only S-RFC are found in the spleens of non-immunized animals. Non-secretory rosettes also predominate (10-80%) in the spleens of animals two days after low or high dose injections. Secretory rosettes begin to increase in number however, and constitute 45-60% of the total RFC population in the spleen by day eight, the time when the maximum total number of RFC is found. The results presented in Table 2 also indicate that maximum contribution by S+RFC is generated by an anti-hapten (TNP) response measured 10 days after a priming injection of carrier SRBC. That is, the enhancement in RFC number generated after carrier-specific priming which binds the hapten, can be almost entirely accounted for by S+RFC. In cooperative responses

in the mammal, one would expect all cells committed to anti-hapten
responses to be antibody producing cells since hapten-specific helper
cells have not been demonstrated.

Considered as a whole, the data strongly suggest a correlation
between S-RFC and "helper" cell function and between S+RFC and antibody-producing cells. The significance of the absolute number of each
rosette type is difficult to assess because a number of cells scored
as S-RFC may represent potential S+RFC or S+RFC that have lost their
multiple layers of RBC due to mechanical shear. Furthermore, there
is as yet no direct correlation between S+RFC and plaque-forming
cells in this system, though there is some evidence from other
systems (14) that they may be related.

MEMBRANE PROPERTIES AND ROSETTE FORMATION

In order to identify those properties of the cell surface which
are involved in the binding of SRBC and in an attempt to clarify the
difference between S- and S+RFC, sensitized frog splenic lymphocytes
were treated with metabolic inhibitors and agents known to affect
mammalian cell surface properties. All immunizations were with 25%
SRBC and ICA assays were performed eight days post-immunization,
when the ratio of S-:S+ approaches 50:50. Pre-incubation of cells
with agents being tested were for 6 h at 4°C with periodic agitation.
In those cases where reversibility of the treatment was investigated,
pre-incubations were for 5 h at 4°C followed by two washes and re-
suspension in fresh medium for 1 h before addition of 10 μl of 1%
SRBC.

The idea that an IgM-like surface molecule is involved in rosette
formation and the possibility that S- and S+RBC may be distinguished
by the number or arrangement of these molecules was tested by pre-
incubating lymphocytes with rabbit anti-Rana pipiens IgM (RARP) before
addition of test antigen. At an effective concentration of 0.7 mg/ml,
RARP greatly reduced the total number of RFC, showing a slight but
reproducible preference for blocking RFC of the S- variety. Lower
concentrations failed to block RFC. Pre-incubation with normal
rabbit serum showed no such reduction and the blockage by anti-IgM
could be relieved by including purified R. pipiens IgM in the preincubation mixture. These results suggest that an IgM-like molecule
is involved in the specific recognition and binding of RBC antigen.
An indirect effect of anti-IgM binding can't be ruled out, however,
since formation of IgM-anti-IgM complexes at the cell surface may
block a non-IgM SRBC receptor by steric hindrance.

Pre-treatment of cells with 10^{-3}M NaN$_3$ yields a similar overall
effect, in that there is a general reduction of RFC. However, in
contrast to anti-IgM, NaN$_3$ inhibition is more selective for S+RFC.

Hammerling and McDevitt (15) have described the inhibition of antigen binding in mouse peripheral T cells with similar concentrations of NaN$_3$. They describe a complex effect in that NaN$_3$ inhibited antigen binding by T cells when the temperature was raised to 37°C in the presence of antigen, but once receptors had appeared on the cell surface they were "frozen" there by the NaN$_3$. NaN$_3$ at 10^{-1}M or DNP at 10^{-3}M have also been shown to inhibit cap formation in mouse spleen cells treated with fluoresceinated anti-Ig (16). The inhibition of normal membrane function by NaN$_3$ suggests that metabolic activity is necessary for the normal appearance and distribution of antigen receptor sites on the cell surface and for secretion by potential S+RFC. As will be discussed later, the lateral mobility of receptors such as in cap formation is not a prerequisite for the binding of a single layer of SRBC by amphibian lymphocytes.

The role of cell metabolism in rosette formation was investigated further with emetine-HCl and cycloheximide, inhibitors of protein synthesis (17). The inhibitory effect of emetine-HCl on normal R. pipiens splenic lymphocytes was tested by pre-incubating a cell suspension in the drug for 1 hour. At 10^{-4}M, the drug reduced incorporation of tritiated amino acids into TCA-precipitable material to less than half that of controls. The results shown in Table 3 clearly indicate that emetine-HCl interferes either directly with the synthesis of receptor molecules or indirectly at some point in the secretory process. While the total number of RFC is reduced slightly, the predominant effect is on the S+RFC which are reduced by 54%. Apparently, the turnover rate of cell surface molecules is slow enough at 4°C that inhibition of new protein synthesis does not decrease the number of S-RFC.

Both colchicine (10^{-4}M) and cytochalasin B (2.5 µg/ml) caused a slight (10%) reduction of RFC, primarily accounted for by decreases in the S+ category. A more dramatic inhibition resulted when colchicine and cytochalasin B were applied together. The total number of RFC was cut by 50%, as S+RFC suffered a 74% decrease. This effect was largely reversible by a 1 h wash in drug-free medium. Since the medium used has galactose as the major sugar source, the cytochalasin B effect is not attributable to interference with glucose transport (18).

Recent studies from several laboratories (19,20) implicate microtubular proteins as having some influence on events at the cell surface, including anti-Ig induced capping of murine lymphocytes (21). Unanue and Karnovsky (22) have reported a synergistic negative effect of colchicine with cytochalasin B on cap formation. Presumably the two agents act together to interrupt both the movement of receptors within the cell membrane and translational movement of the cell itself. The firm binding of a ligand as large as SRBC to a lymphocyte surface may require the cooperation or aggregation of several receptor molecules at the cell surface. The inhibition of rosette formation

Table 3. Effects of various agents on rosette formation and on the relative proportion of S- and S+RFC. The percentages are given as the average for three experiments, except for anti-IgM/IgM, where only one trial was run. CB = cytochalasin B.

PRE-INCUBATION	TOTAL RFC/ 10^6 CELLS	%S-	%S+	% CHANGE S-	S+
CONTROL	5590 ± 635	46	54	–	–
ANTI-IgM(0.7 mg/ml)	1375 ± 157	7	93	-96	-59
ANTI-IgM IgM(0.4 mg/ml)	2552	70	30	-32	-75
CONTROL	4080 ± 1110	68	32	–	–
10^{-3}M NaN$_3$	780 ± 280	91	9	-75	-95
CONTROL	7340 ± 1290	41	59	–	–
10^{-4}M EMETINE	6220 ± 815	68	32	+27	-54
CONTROL	6980 ± 1040	42	58	–	–
10^{-4}M COLCHICINE 2.5 µg/ml CB	3571 ± 680	63	37	-31	-74
1 HOUR WASH	5229 ± 900	57	43	+2	-55
CONTROL	6418 ± 1112	49	51	–	–
1% PARA-FORMALDEHYDE	6495 ± 980	91	9	+55	-79

by this combination of drugs may occur because normal receptor mobility is inhibited. Parkhouse and Allison (23) have reported that colchicine and cytochalasin B do not interfere with the actual secretion of Ig from mouse plasmocytoma cells. An additional observation that may bear on this point arises from electron microscope studies on rosette forming cells (24). Lin and Wallach have found that contact and rosette formation between SRBC and a human leukemic cell line induces the formation of microvilli from the lymphocyte surface and that these microvilli arise only near sites of contact with SRBC. It is likely that the membrane distortions forming these microvilli are dependent on the presence of cytochalasin B sensitive contractile

filaments. If the microvilli are instrumental in maintaining a firm
attachment between SRBC and lymphocyte, this would provide an alternate explanation for the inhibitory effect of cytochalasin B on
rosette formation.

    The role of cell surface components and in particular, the pos-
sibility that mobility of membrane receptors is necessary for SRBC
binding was further investigated by testing paraformaldehyde fixed
cells for their ability to bind SRBC. Splenic lymphocytes from R.
pipiens immunized with 25% SRBC were suspended in 1 ml of medium at
0°C and 5 ml of 1% paraformaldehyde in amphibian Ringer's was added
slowly with stirring. Fixation was allowed to proceed for 1 h at
0°C. The cells were washed twice with fresh medium and subjected to
the standard ICA assay. While the total number of RFC is unaffected,
paraformaldehyde treatment virtually eliminates the S+ category.
Experiments with cells from spleens of unimmunized animals verified
that paraformaldehyde fixation does not create "false rosettes". The
fixation process seems to freeze the cell membrane and prevent the
release of antigen binding molecules which give rise to S+RFC. Since
the total number of RFC is not reduced the potential S+RFC appear as
S-RFC, i.e., they possess the receptor molecules on their surface but
do not secrete them into the medium. With regard to the mobility of
receptors, either laterally in the plane of the cell membrane or
movement in and out of the membrane, it is apparent from these results
with fixed cells, that this mobility is not a prerequisite for binding
of SRBC.

    Electron microscope examination of ferritin labeled mouse spleen
cells has shown that paraformaldehyde fixation does not cause a gross
rearrangement of surface receptors (25). In a finding relevant to
the results reported here, they also report that mouse cell membranes
fixed with paraformaldehyde were able to bind anti-H-2 antibodies to
the same extent as fresh membranes.

DISCUSSION

    Immunocytoadherence is a useful technique for quantitating the
early stages of a humoral immune response when the appropriate variables are controlled for. It is essential that each experiment be
internally controlled and that the emphasis be placed on the relative
numerical differences between experimental and control results. The
variability inherent among different cellular pools and in different
batches of RBC may be controlled by resorting to syngeneic animals
and a stable (e.g. glutaraldehyde-fixed) stock of blood for immunization and assay.

    Binding of SRBC involves lymphocyte metabolic activity partic-
ularly with respect to the formation of S+RFC. Inhibition of roset-
ting by NaN_3 and emetine-HCl is probably due in part to inhibition of

the normal secretory process, and hence the reduction of multi-
layered rosettes. It should also be noted that raising the temperature of the assay for 1-2 h prior to incubation at 4°C preferentially
increases the number of secretory RFC (8).

Colchicine and cytochalasin B act synergistically to inhibit
binding of SRBC, presumably through interference with the conformation of the cell membrane or arrangement of receptor molecules at
the surface. The reversibility of the effect indicates that it is
not one of general toxicity. Mobility of receptors once they appear
on sensitized cells is not necessary for binding, since fixed cells
bind a single layer of SRBC perfectly well.

Antibody against R. pipiens IgM blocks binding of SRBC to lymphocytes and suggests that an IgM-like molecule may function as the antigen receptor. This is an interesting result in that both S- and S+
RFC are affected (S- more so than S+) by anti-IgM. This means that
if S- and S+RFC do in fact represent distinct cell populations, they
at least share the feature of the surface IgM. It should be noted
that two molecular weight classes of Ig have been described for the
adult anura (13). We cannot exclude the possibility that anti-IgM
used in these studies may be interacting to some extent with the
lower molecular weight class of Ig if there is light chain sharing
between the two classes. The difference in susceptibility of the
two rosette types to anti-IgM blockage (96% suppression of S- vs 59%
suppression of S+) may mean that the arrangement or density of surface
IgM is different between the two. Hammerling and McDevitt (15) have
reported that antigen-binding B cells bind five times more antigen
than do T cells and speculate that these B cells are endowed with a
greater number of receptors. Alternatively, it could be that potential S- and S+RFC blocked by anti-IgM are not significantly different
and that it is only the residual unblocked S-RFC and S+RFC that are
truly different.

The results obtained to date have not been able to establish a
clear distinction between S- and S+RFC. The formation of S+RFC seems
to be dependent on a physiologically active cell with intact membrane
functions. A single assay involves a population of cells from a
single organ (e.g. spleen) at a single particular moment during the
immune response. It is possible that S-RFC and S+RFC represent
essentially identical cell types caught at different stages of maturation or differentiation. For example, the fact that only S-RFC
are seen in the thymus and S-RFC predominate in low dose stimulated
spleens does not exclude the possibility that these S- cells migrate
to other regions and become APC, or that a second exposure to antigen may convert them to S+RFC.

ACKNOWLEDGEMENTS

The authors wish to thank Ms. Judith Ruben for her excellent technical assistance during the course of this research.

REFERENCES

1. Ruben, L. N., Vander Hoven, A. and Dutton, R. W. Cell. Immunol., 6:300 (1973).
2. Cohen, N. Am. Zool., 15:119 (1975).
3. DuPasquier, L., Weiss, N. and Loor, F. Eur. J. Immunol., 2:366 (1972).
4. Goldstine, S. N. and Collins, N. H. Fed. Proc., 34:966 (1975).
5. Kraft, N. and Shortman, K. J. Cell Biol., 52:438 (1972).
6. Warner, N. L., Szenberg, A. and Burnet, F. M. Aust. J. Exp. Biol. Med. Sci., 40:373 (1962).
7. Claman, H. N. and Chaperon, E. A. Transplant. Rev., 1:92 (1969).
8. Ruben, L. N. Am. Zool., 15:93 (1975).
9. Greaves, M. F., Moller, E. and Moller, G. Cell. Immunol., 1:386 (1970).
10. Elson, C. J., Allan, D., Elson, J. and Duffus, W. H. P. Immunol., 22:291 (1972).
11. Playfair, J. H. L. Clin. Exp. Immunol., 8:839 (1971).
12. Levin, P. R. Thesis (1973).
13. Marchalonis, J. J. Dev. Biol., 25:479 (1971).
14. McConnell, I. Nat. New Biol., 233:177 (1971).
15. Hammerling, G. J. and McDevitt, H. O. J. Immunol. 112:1726 (1974).
16. Taylor, R. B., Duffus, W. H. P., Raff, M. C. and dePetris, S. Nat. New Biol., 233:255 (1971).
17. Grollman, A. P. Proc. Nat. Acad. Sci. (U.S.A.), 56:1867 (1966).
18. Yamada, K. M. and Wessells, N. K. Dev. Biol., 31:413 (1973).
19. Berlin, R. D., Oliver, J. M., Ukena, T. E. and Yin, H. H. Nat. (Lond.), 247:45 (1974).
20. Edelman, G. M., Yahara, I. and Wang, J. L. Proc. Nat. Acad. Sci. (U.S.A.), 70:1442 (1973).
21. dePetris, S. Nat. (Lond.), 250:54 (1974).
22. Unanue, E. R. and Karnovsky, M. J. J. Exp. Med., 140:1207 (1974).
23. Parkhouse, R. M. E. and Allison, A. C. Nat. New Biol., 235:220 (1972).
24. Lin, P. and Wallach, D. F. H. Science, 184:1300 (1974).
25. Parr, E. L. and Oel, J. S. J. Cell Biol., 59:537 (1973).

VERTEBRATE IMMUNOLOGY

Specific Immunoregulation and Histocompatibility Systems

PHYLOGENY OF FUNCTIONAL HUMORAL TRANSPLANTATION IMMUNITY: COMPARATIVE STUDIES IN AMPHIBIANS AND RODENTS

Nicholas Cohen, William M. Baldwin III and V. Manickavel

Division of Immunology, Department of Microbiology, University of Rochester School of Medicine and Dentistry, Rochester, New York 14642

Mammalian transplantation alloantigens elicit complex immuno-protective and immunodestructive reactivities which can be demonstrated in vitro by cytotoxicity and blocking assays (1). The impact of these functionally disparate responses on the in vivo fate of transplants has been strongly evidenced by the dramatically prolonged (enhanced) survival or by the significantly accelerated rejection of test skin grafts on mice adoptively immunized with immune lymphoid cells or sera (2-4). In marked contrast to our emerging awareness that for mammals, the survival of allografts reflects a net immune response equal to the outcome of a dynamic balance between functionally opposing immune reactivities (5), has been our relative ignorance of whether humoral immunity plays a comparable role in regulating graft survival in ectothermic (cold-blooded) vertebrates. Indeed, we are cognizant of only a limited number of reports that transplants do evoke detectable alloantibodies in fish (6), salamanders (7) and frogs (8).

In this paper we will first review some of our early observations in amphibians and extrapolations from mammalian systems that led us to formulate the rather simple hypothesis that humoral alloimmunity is as important to the eventual survival of allografts in amphibians as it is in rodents. We shall then present new data from passive transfer studies with two amphibian species that directly substantiate this hypothesis.

EXTRAPOLATIONS FROM MAMMALIAN SYSTEMS

That humoral alloimmunity in amphibians plays a pivotal role in graft survival was suggested by the impressive biological constancy

411

and similarity of transplantation reactions among all vertebrates
(9). Specifically, the typically chronic rejection reaction of
outbred urodele amphibians (10) is similar in many ways to the
chronic rejection of skin allografts exchanged between mice histoincompatible only at the species' "minor" histocompatibility
(H) loci (11,12). Regardless of species, survival times of chronically rejected transplants frequently fail to fall into that
normal distribution pattern which describes rejection across a
major H-barrier. Rather, they are characterized by multiple rejection episodes (Fig. 1). This similarity, plus direct experimentation (13-15), suggested that only gene products from comparable minor H-loci elicit rejection in salamanders. In other words,
urodele amphibians behave as if they lack (totally or partially) a
major histocompatibility complex (16,17).

Data from murine studies indicate that phenomena, proven or
suspected to be causally associated with enhancement, are relatively easy to visualize and analyze across weak H-barriers (18). This
suggests that identical phenomena in the weakly histoincompatible
salamander system might also be manifestations of enhancement. One

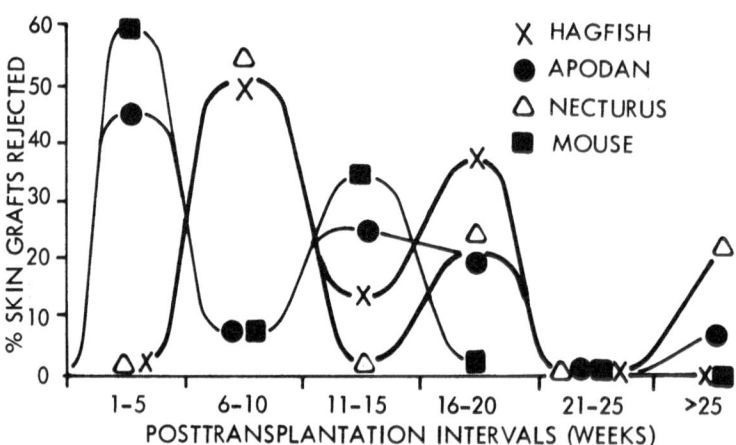

Fig. 1. Non-cumulative plot of chronic first-set skin allograft
rejection in four phylogenetically disparate species: Hagfish
(Hildemann, W., Thoenes, G., Transplantation 7:506 (1969); Apodan
(Cooper, E. & Garcia-Herrera, F., Copeia 2:224 (1968); Necturus
(10); and mice (3). Rejection in each species is characterized by
cycles of obvious graft destruction that alternate with periods of
quiescence (active immunoprotection?).

such phenomenon "proven" to be enhancement-associated in rats is the prolonged survival of renal allografts relative to skin allografts transplanted across the same weak H-barrier (19). This implies, but far from proves, that long-term survival of heart and other heterotopic organ grafts (relative to skin) in urodeles (20) might also be the end result of active enhancing antibody responses. Another finding suggesting that immunity elicited by urodele allo-antigens might be immunoprotective as well as immunodestructive is our repeated but unpredictable observation that second-set skin allografts sometimes survive as long as or significantly longer than first-set grafts from the same donor (3,10,13,20,21). That par-allel observations are also made in rodent systems when rejection is similarly chronic (22,23) lends credence to the application of the concept of positive and negative memory to amphibians (9).

IMPLANT-INDUCED IMMUNOMANIPULATION IN SALAMANDERS AND MICE

Many early researchers developed models in which alloantigenic pretreatment of recipients of weakly histoincompatible grafts (or such treatment plus nonspecific immunosuppression), predictably extended median survival times of test skin grafts (24-27; for dis-cussion, see ref. 3). Yet, there were no attempts to similarly manipulate transplantation immunity in phylogenetically primitive species. Thus, we designed a parallel model system in salamanders and mice in which hosts are initially exposed to antigen borne by tissue fragments that are implanted either subcutaneously (newt or mouse) or suprarenally (sr.) on the kidney cortex (mouse). Whether the preponderance of urodele or murine test grafts ex-hibited prolonged, first-set type, or curtailed survival can be controlled by the tissue origin and site of the implant, the inter-val between implantation and test grafting, the antigenic disparity between donor and host, and the administration of minimally immuno-suppressive amounts of antithymocyte sera (27). An example of im-plant-induced immunomanipulation in salamanders and across the H-3 + H-13 barrier in mice is presented in Fig. 2.

PASSIVE TRANSFER STUDIES IN MICE

These observations that under controlled conditions of allo-antigenic pretreatment, specific host immunoprotective responses can be exaggerated do not of course discriminate between humoral (enhancement) or cellular (classic tolerance, suppressor cells) reactivity as the preeminent effector of prolonged test graft sur-vival. Any argument, however, that long-term test skin graft sur-vival on normal or treated hosts in this system results from classic tolerance is weakened by numerous examples of cytotoxic activity of the hosts toward the test grafts. These include transient

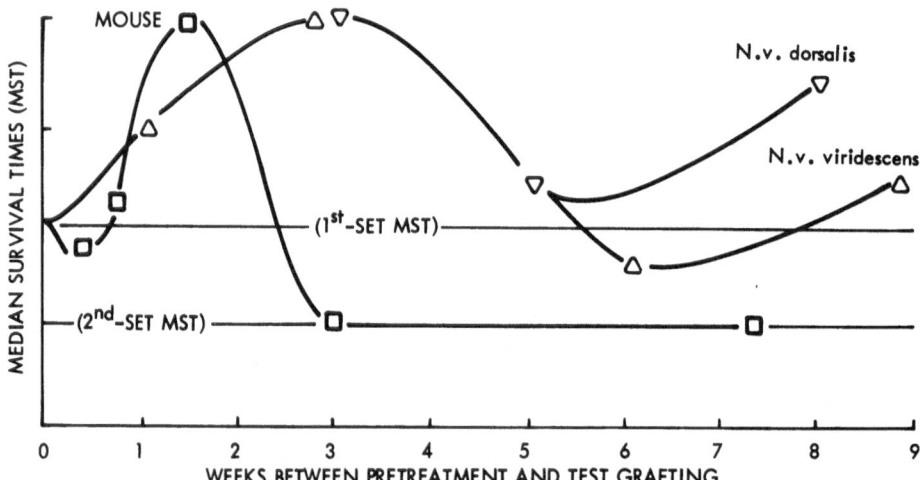

Fig. 2. Effects of alloantigenic pretreatment with liver implants from weakly histoincompatible donors on the survival of subsequent test skin grafts in mice and in two subspecies of salamanders as a function of the interval between pretreatment and test grafting.

rejection crises; destruction of long surviving test grafts following their removal and re-transplantation to the original hosts; and rejection of second test grafts by hosts carrying fully viable initial skin test grafts. More cogent is the additional fact that either lymphoid cells or sera harvested 5-12 days after sr. implantation (i.e., a situation favoring prolonged test graft survival) resulted in accelerated second-set type rejection of skin grafts on adoptively immunized mice (2,3). Opposing these immunodestructive responses in skin grafted or alloimplanted hosts were immunoprotective reactivities. Indeed, both splenocytes and sera from mice sensitized with a single orthotopic skin graft or sr. implant can passively transfer implant-induced immunosuppression to normal hosts (2,3). The type of functional immunity that is transferred is dependent on when after sensitization sera or cells are harvested and when they are transferred relative to the time of test grafting (Fig. 3). In addition, the strain combination used, the size of the sensitizing graft, the route by which the inoculum is injected, and the time of day when the harvest and transfers are performed all influence the transferred immune state (Chrispens and Cohen, unpublished data).

PASSIVE TRANSFER STUDIES IN AMPHIBIANS

The aforementioned studies in mice strongly support the

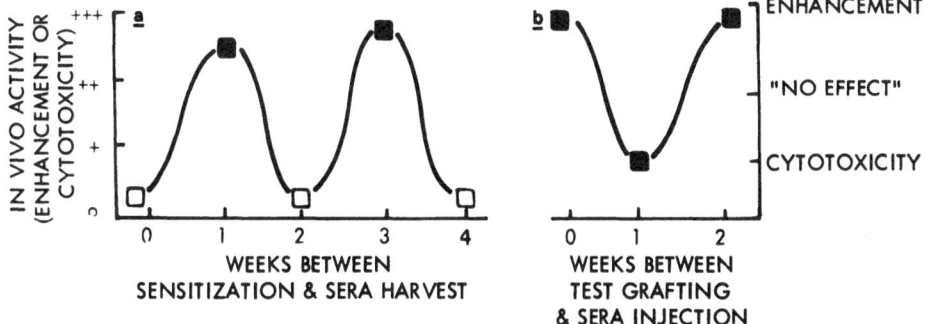

Fig. 3. Cyclical appearance of functional humoral immunity in mice
(2). a. Appearance of antibody after sensitization with a skin
graft; b. Net effect of this antibody in the serum recipient as a
function of time of injection. For example, sera harvested one
week after sensitization (in a.) enhance test graft survival when
given at the time of or two weeks after test grafting (in b.) but
accelerate graft rejection when given one week after test grafting.
Sera harvested two weeks after sensitization (in a.) have no effect
regardless of when they are transferred (in b.).

original hypothesis that normal tissue allografts routinely stimulate production of protective as well as destructive immune vectors.
The following passive transfer study reveals for the first time the
validity of this hypothesis for ectothermic as well as endothermic
vertebrates. Salamanders (Notophthalmus v. viridescens) and laboratory reared 8-10 month old clawed frogs (Xenopus laevis) were immunized with a single skin graft. Putatively immune sera were
harvested from salamanders at weekly intervals from 1-5 weeks post-
grafting (i.e., from 6 weeks before to 1 week after total rejection
of control grafts). Sera were collected from frogs one week
after grafting (from 5-10 days before total rejection was expected).
Each prospective serum donor was paired with a prospective serum
recipient so that both received their skin graft (immunizing or
test) from the same animal. In some instances, frogs received serum
from a donor that had been immunized with skin from a third party
(i.e., the donors of the test and immunizing graft were different).
Control animals received either normal sera or nothing.

Unpooled normal or putatively immune sera (0.02-0.05 cc) were
transferred i.p. or s.c. 1 or 2 weeks after test grafting. Other
serum aliquots were transferred to the freshly prepared graft bed
at the time of test grafting.

The rejection of skin allografts on control salamanders that
received normal sera was typically chronic and was morphologically
indistinguishable from that of grafts on untreated animals (Table 1).

TABLE 1. Curtailed and prolonged skin allograft survival in salamanders following adoptive immunization with alloimmune sera

Test graft survival time	Weeks sera harvested post-grafting	Route of serum (0.01 ml) transfer	Cumulative per cent (fraction[*]) test skin grafts rejected by (in weeks post-transplantation)				
			3	4	5	6	7
1st set type	none	none	3(3/93)	24(19/80)	40(26/65)	64(32/50)	71(35/49)
1st set type	non-immune	g.b.[**]	0(0/10)	30(3/10)	50(5/10)	80(8/10)	80(8/10)
1st set type	non-immune	s.c.[†]	0(0/8)	29(2/7)	57(4/7)	71(5/7)	86(6/7)
curtailed	3	g.b.[**]	22(2/9)	67(6/9)	78(2/9)	78(7/9)	78(7/9)
curtailed	5	g.b.[**]	0(0/8)	63(5/8)	71(5/7)	100(6/6)	100(6/6)
prolonged	2	i.p.[‡]	0(0/4)	0(0/3)	0(0/3)	33(1/3)	67(2/3)
prolonged	3	i.p.[‡]	0(0/6)	0(0/6)	0(0/6)	20(1/5)	60(3/5)

[*] Change in denominator reflects death of host
[**] Graft bed site at time of test grafting
[†] Subcutaneous site at the time of test grafting
[‡] Intraperitoneal transfers 2 weeks post-test grafting.

TABLE 2. Prolonged skin allograft survival in frogs (Xenopus) following adoptive immunization

Test graft survival time	Source of serum (route transferred)	Per cent (fraction) grafts rejected between: (in days post-transplantation)			
		0-11	12-17	18-21	22-30
1st-set type	none control (-)	0(0/6)	100(6/6)	0(0/6)	0(0/6)
1st-set type	non-immune (g.b.)	0(0/6)	83(5/6)	17(1/6)	0(0/6)
COMBINED		0(0/12)	92(11/12)	8(1/12)	0(0/12)
prolonged	1-week specific (s.c.)	0(0/3)	33(1/3)	67(2/3)	0(0/3)
	1-week "specific" (g.b.)	8(1/12)	58(7/12)	8(1/12)	25(3/12)[b]
	1-week "non-specific" (g.b.)	0(0/4)	25(1/4)	50(2/4)	25(1/4)
COMBINED		5(1/19)	47(9/19)	26(5/19)	21(4/19)

[a] All sera transferred at the time of test grafting

[b] 1 rejected at day 64

However, the transfer of 3 or 5 week sera (sera from salamanders that carried grafts for 3 or 5 weeks) to the graft bed at the time of test grafting effected curtailed test graft survival. Sixty five per cent of these grafts were totally destroyed by 4 weeks post-transplantation compared with only 25% of the control grafts (Table 1). The fact that 4 week sera did not appear to

affect test graft survival again points out a parallel between
amphibians and mammals in that such cyclical expression of humoral
immune reactivity has also been reported in endotherms (2,28-30).

In contrast to the cytotoxicity transferred by the previous
protocols, 2 and 3 week sera (but not 4 and 5 week sera) that were
transferred i.p. into salamanders that had already been grafted for
2 weeks were clearly associated with significantly prolonged test
graft survival. Whereas nearly half of the control grafts were
destroyed by week 5, none of the 10 test grafts on animals in these
two protocol groups were completely rejected by this time (Table 1).
Indeed, the incidence of rejection at 6 weeks was still well below
that of the controls. The fact that none of the 5 other transfer
protocols tested (not tabulated in Table 1) were associated with
marked change in test graft survival reveals that the differential
in vivo effectiveness of alloimmune salamander serum resembles that
of alloimmune murine sera in its dependency on the time of test
grafting relative to the time of transfer, the interval between
immunization and serum collection, and the route by which the sera
are transferred.

Data from a preliminary study have also associated enhancing
activity with transferred sera from skin grafted Xenopus. Control
skin allografts exchanged between siblings were vascularized by day
3-5, showed signs of incipient rejection by day 6-10, and were
totally destroyed (pigment cell death) between 12 and 17 days post-
grafting. Nonimmune sera placed on graft beds failed to alter this
temporal pattern. Neither did the i.p. injection of putatively
immune 1 week sera into 3 frogs that bore 1-week-old grafts. However, immune "antigenically specific" sera (raised against skin
grafts from the test graft donor (n=15)) or "antigenically non-
specific" sera from frogs immunized with third-party skin (n=4)
were associated with moderately prolonged test graft survival times
(Table 2). Whether the inability to demonstrate more dramatic prolongation relates to the stronger histoincompatibilities in Xenopus
vis a vis salamanders (20) or is a function of the transfer protocols used, remains to be determined.

In the first analysis, the apparent lack of specificity of enhancement in these amphibian studies is disconcerting in that this
phenomenon has been described as being as immunologically specific
as other immune reactions (4,31). However, it should be borne in
mind that the population of newts used in this study as well as in
others (13), displays a moderate degree of antigen sharing (revealed
by third party grafting). This, plus our purposeful use of Xenopus
siblings speaks to the cross reactivity of the transferred putative
antibodies. Moreover, recent data and mechanistic models presented
by Fabre and Morris (32) argue that passive enhancement of rat
renal allografts can readily occur with only "partial cover" of the
incompatible Ag-B specificities. Nevertheless, the specificity

question should be pursued directly rather than by extrapolation
by making use of inbred strains of Pleurodeles (6), axolotls (14)
and recently developed histocompatible clones of Xenopus (33).

CHRONIC REJECTION IN SALAMANDERS AND MICE
IS A FUNCTION OF ACTIVE ENHANCEMENT

The previous data support the hypothesis that regardless of
species, transplantation alloantigens elicit complex immunologic
reactivities. They also strongly imply that the very survival of
any first-set graft is dependent on the timing, sequence of appearance, and relative intensities of several functionally antagonistic
responses. Since transfer studies involving murine recipients of
weakly histoincompatible grafts revealed the early appearance of
enhancing serum, we have recently proposed that the very chronicity
of rejection across such weak barriers in salamanders as well as
mice is, in fact, the visible consequence of the tempering action
of early active immunologic enhancement of cytotoxic cellular and
humoral responses (34). We have supported this hypothesis by
selectively interfering with putative B-cell responses so as to
functionally eliminate or temporally delay humoral alloimmunity
and actually accelerate normally chronic rejection. To do this we
made use of the observation that in other in vivo systems cytosine
arabinoside (ara-C) preferentially eliminates serum blocking factors
to tumor-associated transplantation antigen (35). Indeed, the s.c.
administration of 5 daily injections of this antimetabolite accelerated the rejection of skin grafts across the H-Y barrier in mice
and multiple weak barriers in salamanders to a statistically significant extent (Table 3). Our most recent studies in mice further
point out that sera from ara-C treated skin grafted mice are

TABLE 3. Cytosine arabinoside (ara-C) curtails normally chronic
          rejection of skin grafted across weak H-barriers.

Animal[*]	Median survival times (95% confidence limits) of skin grafted on animals injected with:			
	Saline	Number	Ara-C	Number
Mice	32.0 (27.5-37.1)	12	12.5 (6.8-23.1)	18
Salamanders	28.5 (25.4-32.0)	13	18.0 (15.4-21.1)	15

[*]Mice and salamanders received daily s.c. injections of 20 mg/kg
and 18 mg/kg, respectively for 5 consecutive days. For mice, the
first injection was on the day of grafting; for salamanders, it
was 24 hours later.

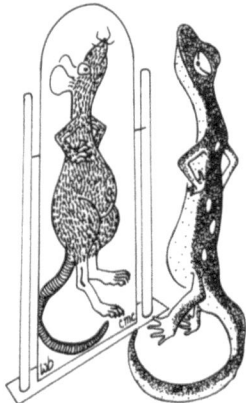

Fig. 4. Immunoprotective and immunodestructive transplantation
responses of salamanders reflect those seen in mice.

deficient in transferring prolonged survival when compared with sera
from the appropriate saline-injected skin grafted controls (36).
Experiments involving comparable serum-transfer from grafted ara-C
and control salamanders are in progress.

SUMMARY

Remarkably comparable observations from parallel experiments
in salamanders and mice utilizing three related model systems (im-
plant-induced immunomanipulation; passive transfer; and putative B
cell suppression) argue directly that functional humoral transplantation immunity is highly developed at the phylogenetic level of
Amphibia and that it plays a major role in regulating graft survival
in these species (Fig. 4). Although it is still conjectural whether
such humoral immunity and weak H-antigens evolved concurrently, the
argument that enhancing antibodies evolved exclusively in viviparous
species to protect the fetus from potential rejection by the maternal immune system no longer seems tenable (1).

ACKNOWLEDGEMENTS

The research cited has been supported by grants AI-08784 and
HD-07901 from the U.S. Public Health Service, grants from the Monroe
County Cancer and Leukemia Association, and grant IN-18 from the
American Cancer Society to the University of Rochester. N.C. is a
recipient of USPHS Research Career Development Award AI-70736;
W.M.B. is a clinical investigator trainee supported by USPHS Train-
ing Grant AI-AM-1004; and V.M. is a postdoctoral fellow supported
by USPHS grants CA-1198 and HD-07901.

REFERENCES

1. Hellström, K-E. and Hellström, I., Adv. Immunol. 18:209 (1974).
2. Baldwin, W. M. and Cohen, N., Transplantation 15:663 (1973).
3. Baldwin, W. M. and Cohen, N., Immunogenetics 1:33 (1974).
4. Jeekel, J. J., McKenzie, I. F. and Winn, H. J., J. Immunol. 108:1017 (1972).
5. Voisin, G. A., Transplant. Proc. 7:361 (1975).
6. Hildemann, W. H., Immunology 1:46 (1958).
7. Badet, M-T., Chateaureynaud-Duprat, P. and Voisin, G. A., C.R. Acad. Sc. Paris 278:1297 (1974).
8. Du Pasquier, L., Chardonnen, X. and Miggiano, V. C., Immunogenetics 1:482 (1975).
9. Hildemann, W. H. in Transplantation Antigens, B. D. Kahan and R. A. Reisfeld, eds., Academic Press, N. Y. (1972), p. 3.
10. Cohen, N., J. Exp. Zool. 167:37 (1968).
11. Hildemann, W. H., Transplant. Rev. 3:5 (1970).
12. Graff, R. J. and Bailey, D. W., Transplant. Rev. 15:26 (1973).
13. Cohen, N. and Hildemann, W. H., Transplantation 6:208 (1968).
14. DeLanney, L. E. and Blackler, K., in Biology of Amphibian Tumors M. Mizell, ed., Springer-Verlag, N. Y. (1969), p. 399.
15. Charlemagne, J. and Tournefier, A., J. Immunogen. 1:125 (1974).
16. Klein, J., Biology of the Mouse Histocompatibility-2 Complex (1975), 624 pp. Springer-Verlag, N. Y.
17. Collins, N., Manickavel, V. and Cohen, N., Advances in Exp. Med. and Biol. (this volume) (1975).
18. Hildemann, W. H. and Cohen, N., in Histocompatibility Testing, Curtoni, E. S. et al., eds., Williams and Wilkins Co., Baltimore, Md. (1967), p. 13.
19. Hildemann, W. H. and Mullen, Y., Transplantation 15:231 (1973).
20. Cohen, N., Amer. Zool. 11:193 (1971).
21. Cohen, N., Transplantation 10:382 (1970).
22. Graff, R. J., Hildemann, W. H. and Snell, G. D., Transplantation 4:425 (1966).
23. Hildemann, W. H. and Walford, R., Ann. N.Y. Acad. Sci. 87:56 (1960).
24. Baldwin, W. M. and Cohen, N., Transplantation 10:530 (1970).
25. Baldwin, W. M. and Cohen, N., Transplant. Proc. 3:217 (1971).
26. Baldwin, W. M. and Cohen, N., Folia Biol. (Praha) 18:181 (1972).
27. Cohen, N. and Latorre, J. A., Folia Biol. (Praha) 21:33 (1975).
28. Fitch, F. W. and St. Sinclair, N. R., Prog. Immunol. 2:358 (1974).
29. Gillespie, G. Y. and Barth, R. F., Cell. Immunol. 13:472 (1974).
30. Weston, B. J., Int. J. Canc. 9:66 (1972).
31. Miller, G., J. Nat. Cancer Inst. 30:1205 (1963).
32. Fabre, J. W. and Morris, P. J., Transplantation 18:436 (1974).
33. Kobel, H. R. and Du Pasquier, L., Immunogenetics 2:87 (1975).
34. Manickavel, V. and Cohen, N. Transplant. Proc. 7:451 (1975).
35. Heppner, G. H. and Calabresi, P. J., J. Nat. Cancer Inst. 48:116 (1972).
36. Manickavel, V. and Cohen, N., Fed. Proc. 34:1034 (1975).

GENETIC CONTROL OF IMMUNE RESPONSES IN CHICKENS

Albert A. Benedict and Leonard W. Pollard

Dept. of Microbiology, University of Hawaii

Honolulu, Hawaii 96822

INTRODUCTION

Those of us who are fond of dinosaurs were happy to learn that "dinosaurs are not extinct" (1), and those of us who are fond of birds had new meaning given to our work when Bakker (1) reported that "the colorful and successful diversity of living birds is a continuing expression of basic dinosaur biology". Based on bioenergetic and anatomical evidence Bakker proposes that mammals inherited their "warm-bloodedness" (endothermy) from therapsids and that birds inherited their endothermy from dinosaurs. This new classification of the class Aves makes it especially interesting to know the extent to which the structural and biological properties of the immunoglobulins, and the immune response (Ir) control mechanisms, have been conserved and have diverged in the mammalian and avian evolutionary branches.

Functionally, the humoral immune responses of birds, at least some gallinaceous species, resemble the mammalian responses (2). Unlike many lower vertebrates (3), but like mammals, many birds are brisk antibody responders to a variety of immunogens. Also, the affinity constants of chicken antibodies increase with time and approach the high values found in mammals (4). In many lower vertebrates antibodies have relatively lower binding constants; and "maturity" of affinity is a rather slow process. To extend this comparison we present evidence here and in the following paper by Wakeland that the immune responses and the expression of immunoglobulin allotypes in chickens are under genetic control mechanisms similar to those found in mammals.

Many of the immune responses in mammals are controlled by an-
tigen-specific, autosomal genes which are closely linked with genes
controlling expression of the major histocompatibility specificities (5). Recently, the chicken major histocompatibility complex
(MHC) was shown to be associated with Ir genes to the multideter-
minant synthetic branched polypeptide poly-L(tyr, glu)-poly-DL-ala--
poly-L-lys [(T,G)-A--L] (6), to tuberculin (7), and to the linear
random copolymers poly (L-glu^{60}-L-ala^{30}L-tyr^{10})n (GAT^{10}) and poly
(L-glu^{60}L-ala^{40})n (GA) (8). The B blood group locus in the chicken
represents the avian counterpart of the MHC in mammals. Incompatibility for the B locus leads to allograft rejection (9), the graft-
versus-host reaction (10,11), and the mixed leukocyte reaction (12).

RESPONSE OF INBRED CHICKEN LINES TO GAT^{10} AND GA

Several related random polymers, kindly supplied by Dr. Paul
Maurer, were used as immunogens. Inbred chickens used were mainly
lines 2, 3, and 7 which are homozygous for 10 blood group loci and
had inbreeding coefficients at the time of use of 0.979, 0.981, and
0.965, respectively (8). They were bred and supplied by Dr. Hans
Abplanalp, University of California, Davis. Both he and Mr. Phillip
Morrow collaborated in some phases of these studies. In response
to immunization with GAT^{10} and GA, line 7 gave no or very low responses to 2 injections of the polymers, 1 mg each, in Freund's complete adjuvant (FCA) as detected by radioelectrocomplexing (REC)
(13), and radioimmunoelectrophoresis (RIE) Table 1). Lines 2, 3,
and 7 have different genotypes at the B locus; namely, $\underline{B}^6\underline{B}^6$, $\underline{B}^2\underline{B}^2$,
and $\underline{B}^4\underline{B}^4$, respectively. The F$_1$ hybrids obtained by mating line 7
birds with either line 2 or 3 were high responders; thus, respon-
siveness was inherited as a completely dominant trait. The segregation of the progeny from inter se mating of the F$_1$ hybrids should
yield about 25% low responders and 75% responders to conform to

Table 1. Twenty-day secondary immune responses of inbred lines to
GAT^{10} and GA as determined by REC.

Line	GAT	GA
2	232[a]	42
3	158	48
7	1	1
22	90	64
11	(-)	54
13	(-)	220

[a]Median of 8 birds/group expressed as reciprocal of serum dilution which bound 50% of homologous antigen.

Mendelian expectations. Indeed, the non- and low-responder F_2 birds had the B genotype of line 7 ($\underline{B^4B^4}$). The mean $\log_{10}$ responses of birds with genotype $\underline{B^4B^4}$ were 0.69±0.14 and 0.3±0.15 for the (2x7)F_2 and (3x7)F_2 hybrids, respectively; whereas, the mean responses of birds heterozygous and homozygous for the responder lines at the B locus were 2.18±0.6 and 1.98±0.14, respectively. A higher percentage (35%) of low responders than expected resulted from the occurrence of only 5% of the homozygous genotypes of the responder lines. The other blood group loci segregated as expected. Nevertheless, there was a close association between immune responsiveness to GAT^{10} and the MHC, and no association with other blood group loci and H chain allotypes (Table 2).

GAT^{10}-nonresponder mice have the $H-2^{\underline{p}}$, $\underline{q}$ and $\underline{s}$ alleles (14,15) but they differ in their responses to related polymers. Mice with $H-2^{\underline{s}}$ allele respond to GA and to GAT^{10} when the mole percent of tyrosine is reduced to 4 (GAT^4) (16). Line 7 chickens were low responders to GA and GAT^4; thus, line 7 birds seem to be analogous to mice with the $H-2^{\underline{p}}$ and $\underline{q}$ alleles, and strain 13 guinea pigs at least in respect to lack of the GA gene.

Table 2. The relationship between responsiveness to GAT^{10} and blood group and allotype genotypes in (2x7)F_2 hybrids.

Locus	Genotype	No. Birds	Responders Low[a]	High	χ^2	p[b]
B	4/4	8	8(3.0)[c]	0(5.0)		
	4/6	12	0(4.6)	12(7.4)	21.5	<.005
	6/6	1	0(0.4)	1(0.6)		
D	1/1	5	2(1.9)	3(3.1)		
	1/3	10	3(3.8)	7(6.2)	0.62	.979
	3/3	6	3(2.3)	3(3.7)		
E	7/7	4	1(1.5)	3(2.5)		
	1/7	11	5(4.2)	6(6.8)	0.49	.993
	1/1	6	2(2.3)	4(3.7)		
P	3/3	3	2(1.2)	1(1.8)		
	3/10	10	2(4.0)	8(6.0)	3.41	.610
	10/10	7	4(2.8)	3(4.2)		
CS allotype	c/c	3	1(1.1)	2(1.9)		
	c/a	13	6(5.0)	7(8.0)	1.18	.948
	a/a	5	1(2.0)	4(3.0)		

[a]Dilutions of 1:20 or less of antiserum which bound 50% of GAT^{10}.
[b]Probability of a greater value of χ^2 assuming 5 d.f. No significant deviation from the expected results is apparent.
[c]Numbers in parenthesis are the expected values if responsiveness is segregating independently.

There are quantitative differences between the responses of responder lines, and there is considerable variability in the responses of individual birds. Although responsiveness is clearly related to the B alleles, perhaps factors not associated with MHC influence the level of the responses as seems to be the case of the response of mice (17). Whereas in GAT-responder mice, the genes controlling the quantity of antibody may be linked to the immunoglobulin heavy chain allotype linkage group (18), there was no such correlation between low responders and a heavy chain linkage group (CS) (19) in F_2 chicken hybrids (Table 2). Whether other modifying genes are involved remains to be determined.

Thus, mice (20), rats (21,22), guinea pigs (23), Rhesus monkeys (24), and chickens have histocompatibility-linked Ir genes controlling the responses to GAT[10] and to (T,G)-A--L. In mice the response to (T,G)-A--L is considered to be quantitative as low responding mice elicit primary IgM responses, but only high responders have secondary IgG antibody responses (25). Low responder chicken lines also synthesize anti-(T,G)-A--L, but the class of antibody has not been reported. In mice no IgM anti-GAT antibody has been detected and it has been suggested (26) that the all-or-none character of this response resembles the all-or-none character of the IgG response to (T,G)-A--L. The chicken anti-GAT response has different characteristics. Some of the "non-responders" are very low responders and make small amounts of 7S as well as 17S antibody. Responder birds produce 17S antibody but there is a rapid switch to 7S synthesis. Among rat strains it is difficult to make the separation between high and low responders to GAT[10], although a more clearcut division could be made in response to GT and GA (27). Similar difficulty is encountered in separating low and high responder chicken lines in response to DNP, although separation was attempted on the basis of differences of a mean titer value of a single doubling dilution using passive hemagglutination for detection of anti-DNP antibody which favors detection of IgM antibody (28). In this connection, the fact that low responder chickens make small amounts of antibody to GAT[10] probably reflects the ability of chickens to make antibody to the homopolymer, poly(glu)n (G); and thus small amounts of anti-G are synthesized to the G determinant of GAT[10]. This is described below.

                            RESPONSE TO OTHER POLYMERS

Distinctive Ir patterns in chickens are emerging to other copolymers. All inbred lines immunized with poly(glu[90]tyr[10])n (GT) respond poorly in contrast to their responses to GAT[10] and GA. Furthermore, even after booster inoculations 17S responses are still evident. Under the conditions employed we have not been able to make a quantitative division between high and low responders.

Nevertheless, results by RIE indicate that line 3 chickens respond less well than other inbred chickens. Maurer and Merryman (16) did not find significant responses to GT in most inbred mouse strains tested; whereas, division of nonresponder and responder strains to GT has been made in rats (27) and in the classic case of strains 2 and 13 guinea pigs (23).

A surprising finding was the cross-reactivity between anti-GA and anti-GT responses in chickens. No such cross-reaction was detected in guinea pigs (29). This cross-reactivity is explicable on the basis of chickens being able to make antibody to the glutamyl residues. Chickens respond to poly(glu)n (G) and their responses are chiefly 17S even after repeated boosters. The responses to GT are of a similar nature in quantity and quality of antibody. Thus, chickens respond to this homopolymer and this response apparently is responsible for cross-reactions between polymers containing the G determinants. The nature of the polymer seems to have an influence on the amount of anti-G produced, and this could mean that the other determinants might have varying abilities to serve as carriers or that the physical-chemical characteristics of the polymers are important for anti-G responses. No DHS has been detected to G either in animals immunized with G or with other polymers (GAT^{10}, GT, GA) and skin tested with G. The persistent 17S response and failure to develop DHS might be indicative of a T-cell independent response to G.

Line 3 chickens consistently make less anti-G antibodies to G, GA, GT and poly $(glu^{60}lys^{40})n$ (GL) than other inbred chickens as shown in Table 3 and Fig. 1. Whether the G response is linked to the B locus is being determined.

Table 3. Antibody response to GA assayed with G^a.

Chicken Line	Dilution of serum	
	0	1:2
2	62 ± 10^b (85,83,78,55,48,22)	57 ± 12 (77,69,60,43,11,10)
3	27 ± 13 (87,27,22,10,8,7)	19 ± 13 (83,8,6,6,5,5)

[a] Tyrosylated (2%) and radioiodinated.
[b] Mean % of G bound ± S.E.; responses determined by REC.

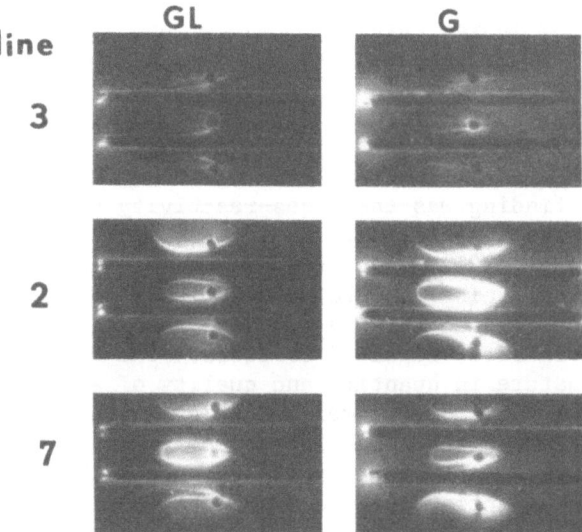

Figure 1. The radioimmunoelectrophoretic patterns of
secondary responses to GL and G as determined with
^{125}I-GAT. Each well represents an individual chicken.
The 17S Ig is the major antibody binding antigen.

RELATION OF Ir AND T-CELL FUNCTION

        In mammals several criteria are used to implicate T-lymphocytes
in immune responses regulated by the Ir genes (5). These include
development of delayed-type hypersensitivity (DHS), recognition of
carrier function, and the ability of responder T cells to be stimulated with antigen. The question whether histocompatibility-linked
non-responder chickens lack these functions has been partially
answered by the finding that line 7 birds synthesize anti-GAT
antibodies at greatly increased levels following immunization with
GAT[10] which had been complexed to immunogenic methylated BSA
(MBSA), and that the antibody is predominantly 7S (Fig. 2). Presumably BSA helper T cells are able to function; however, we have
no direct evidence for this. A surprising result was the reduced
anti-GAT responses in line 3 birds immunized with MBSA-GAT[10].
Nevertheless, a switch from 17S to 7S antibody occurred in the
primary response as did responses of line 3 to GAT (and line 7 to
MBSA-GAT[10]); thus, the 7S response was depressed (Fig. 2). Since
MBSA apparently is a poor carrier for the anti-GAT response in
line 3 birds, perhaps these birds will prove to be low responders
to BSA, or the coupling of GAT[10] to BSA suppresses 7S antibody
synthesis for other reasons. Studies are in progress to determine

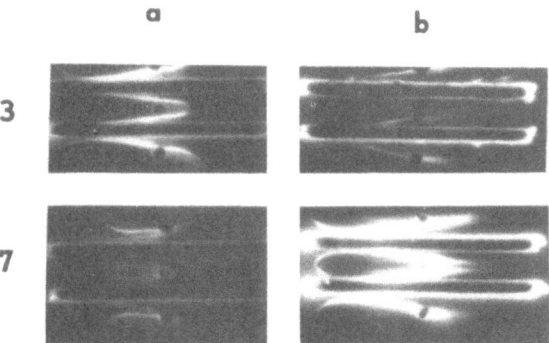

Figure 2. The radioimmunoelectrophoretic patterns of
primary response anti-GAT^{10} sera from chicken lines 3
and 7 after immunization with (a) GAT^{10}, and (b)
methylated bovine serum albumin-GAT^{10}. The major arc
binding ^{125}I-GAT^{10} is the 17S Ig for line 7 birds (a)
and 7S Ig for the others.

whether the suppressed response is associated with the MHC.

GAT-nonresponders fail to elicit DHS by wattle test, whereas
responders generally do. We do not know whether nonresponder T
cells fail to respond to specific antigen stimulation; nevertheless, these data are compatible with the functional expression of
the Ir genes as being related to T cells. However, the variation
in responses in highly inbred lines might indicate a multigenic
control which may prove to involve B cell functions. Attesting to
the possibility of multigene differences is the observation that
some high antibody responders to GAT give weak DHS reactions.
Zelko in our laboratory observed DHS-nonresponders in outbred
chickens, which had been boosted repeatedly with GAT in FCA, yet
they were good antibody producers. These findings are similar to
those made with rats (27). In fact, rats with identical haplo-
types at the major histocompatibility locus were similar in antibody response to GA and to GT but different in DHS to GA.

SUMMARY

In view of the delineation of the T and B lymphoid systems in
birds by virtue of the thymus and bursa of Fabricius, these animals
will be useful for obtaining further information on the roles of
the T and B lymphocytes in the genetic control of immune responses.

The parallel finding in birds and mammals that immune responsiveness and histocompatibility are genetically associated suggests a
basic functional interrelationship between these two phenomena. It
is not known whether histocompatibility and immune responsiveness
in birds depend on different, but linked loci, as is found in mammals, or involves a less evolved genetic complex. Nevertheless,
the finding that the genes controlling immune responsiveness, graft
rejection, the graft-versus-host reaction, and the mixed leukocyte
reaction are closely associated in the MHC in the mammalian and
avian species and the finding of a MHC in the toad (30) favors the
view that "this region has remained relatively unchanged over millions of years" (31).

Wolfe (32) pointed out a number of years ago that chickens
were excellent antibody producers. The finding that anti-G responses were elicited to the G homopolymer attests to the ability
of chickens to synthesize antibodies specific to a large number of
antigenic determinants, not unlike mammals. It will be interesting
to determine whether a single gene ("G gene"?) will permit T cell
responses to cross-reactive antigens, such as the PLL gene in guinea
pigs (33).

ACKNOWLEDGMENTS

This work was supported by United States Public Health Service
Grant AI 05660. We are grateful to Dr. Hans Abplanalp and Mr.
Phillip Morrow for their generous cooperation, to Dr. Paul Maurer
for the generous supplies of polymers, to Dr. W. E. Briles for determining the blood group antigens, to Edward Wakeland for determining allotypes, and to the following students without whose help
hundreds of radioimmunoassays would still be undone--Ellen Buena-
ventura, Lean Kuan Ch'ng, Les Chong, Joe Elm, Bruce Keswick, John
Zelko.

REFERENCES

1. Bakker, R. T., Scientific American, 232: 58 (1975).

2. Benedict, A. A. and Yamaga, K., in Comparative Immunology (J.
    J. Marchalonis, Ed.) (Blackwell Press, in press).

3. Kubo, R. T., Zimmerman, B. and Grey, H. M., in Phylogeny of
    Immunoglobulins (M. Sela, Ed.) (Academic Press, New York,
    1973).

4. Yamaga, K. and Benedict, A. A., J. Immunol., in press.

5. Benacerraf, B., Ann. Immunol. (Inst. Pasteur), 125: 143 (1974).

6. Günther, E., Balcarova, J., Hala, K., Rude, E. and Hraba, T.,
    Europ. J. Immunol., 4: 548 (1974).

7. Karakoz, J., Krejcí, J., Hala, K., Blaszczyk, B., Hraba, T. and
    Pekárek, J., Eur. J. Immunol., 4: 545 (1974).

8. Benedict, A. A., Pollard, L. W., Morrow, P. R., Abplanalp, H.
    A., Maurer, P. H. and Briles, W. E., Immunogenetics (in press).

9. Schierman, L. W. and Nordskog, A. W., Science, 134: 1008 (1961).

10. Jaffe, W. P. and McDermid, E. M., Science, 137: 984 (1962).

11. Schierman, L. W. and Nordskog, A. W., Nature, 197: 511 (1963).

12. Miggiano, V., Birgen, I. and Pink, J. R. L., Europ. J. Immu-
    nol., 4: 397 (1974).

13. Simons, M. J. and Benedict, A. A. in Contemporary Topics in
    Molecular Immunology (G. L. Ada, Ed.), 3: 205 (1974).

14. Martin, W. J., Maurer, P. H. and Benacerraf, B., J. Immunol.,
    107: 715 (1972).

15. Merryman, C. F. and Maurer, P. H., J. Immunol. 108: 135 (1972).

16. Maurer, P. H. and Merryman, C. F., Ann. Immunol. (Inst.
    Pasteur), 125: 189 (1974).

17. Maurer, P. H., Merryman, C. F. and Jones, J., Immunogenetics,
    1: 398 (1974).

18. Dorf, M. E., Dunham, E. K., Johnson, J. P. and Benacerraf, B.,
    J. Immunol., 112: 1329 (1974).

19. Wakeland, E. and Benedict, A. A., this Conference.

20. Benacerraf, B., in Genetic Control of Immune Responsiveness:
    Relationship to Disease Susceptibility (Academic Press, New
    York, 1972).

21. Günther, E., Rude, E. and Stark, O., Eur. J. Immunol., 2: 151
    (1972).

22. Armerding, D., Katz, D. H. and Benacerraf, B., Immunogenetics,
    1: 340 (1974).

23. Bluestein, H. G., Ellman, L., Green, I. and Benacerraf, B.,
    J. Exp. Med., 134: 1529 (1971).

24. Dorf, M. E., Balner, H., de Groot, M. L., and Benacerraf, B.,
     Transplant. Proc., 6: 119 (1974).

25. Grumet, F. C., J. Exp. Med., 135: 110 (1972).

26. Kapp, J. A., Pierce, C. W. and Benacerraf, B., J. Exp. Med.,
     138: 1107 (1973).

27. Armerding, D., Katz, D. H. and Benacerraf, B., Immunogenetics,
     1: 329 (1974).

28. Balcarova, J., Derka, J., Hala, K. and Hraba, T., Folia Bio-
     logica, 20: 346 (1974).

29. Bluestein, H. G., Green, I., Maurer, P. H. and Benacerraf, B.,
     J. Exp. Med., 135: 98 (1972).

30. Du Pasquier, L., Chardonnens, X. and Miggiano, V. C., Immu-
     nogenetics, 1: 482 (1975).

31. Ceppellini, R. in Progress in Immunology (B. Amos, Ed.) (Aca-
     demic Press, New York, 1971).

32. Wolfe, H. R., J. Immunol., 44: 135 (1942).

33. Green, K., Paul, W. E., and Benacerraf, B., Proc. Nat. Acad.
     Sci. (USA), 64: 1095 (1969).

THE GENETICS OF CHICKEN 7S IMMUNOGLOBULIN ALLOTYPES

Edward K. Wakeland and Albert A. Benedict

Dept. of Microbiology, University of Hawaii

Honolulu, Hawaii 96822

INTRODUCTION

Studies on the phylogeny of immunoglobulins (Ig) focus on the structural similarities and differences between the Ig of various vertebrate species. Such structural comparisons, particularly those utilizing amino acid sequencing data, have been used to reveal the theoretical evolution of Ig structural genes. Evolutionary genetic mechanisms, such as complete gene duplication, partial gene duplication, and gene fusion are common postulates of phylogenetic theory (1). Yet, there is a paucity of information on the genetic organization of the Ig structural genes in non-mammals. With hopes of obtaining this kind of information in avian species, we have begun studies on the genetic organization of chicken 7S Ig structural genes.

Although several investigators have reported the detection of allotypes on chicken serum proteins, the criteria used for associating the specificities with chicken Ig (2-6) of either the 7S (2-4) or 17S (3,5) Ig classes have not been always rigorous. For examples, some workers (2,3) reported the detection of 7S Ig and 17S Ig allotypes on the basis of the electrophoretic mobility of the specificities in whole serum. It has been assumed that the use of washed bacterial agglutinates as allotype antigen preparations (alloantigen) for the production of allotype antisera (alloantisera) results in the detection of only Ig allotypes. However, we have found that alloantisera prepared in this manner may occasionally detect the allotypes of other serum proteins. Also, Ivanyi (personal communication) has detected an allotype on a lipoprotein with alloantisera prepared against bacterial agglutinates.

Thus, we suggest that the Ig allotypic specificities should be demonstrated on isolated 7S or 17S Ig before they are considered to be Ig-specific allotypes.

To date, chicken Ig allotypes have not been demonstrated on isolated heavy (H) or light (L) polypeptide chains. Nevertheless, if a specificity is only detected on one class of immunoglobulin, it is probably located on the class specific H chain. Therefore, we concur with others (5) in assigning class specific allotypes to the H chain until the analysis of isolated H and L chains has been completed.

STRUCTURAL STUDIES ON CHICKEN ALLOTYPES

David (7) reported a specificity (b_1) on isolated 7S Ig which was destroyed by reduction and alkylation and by papain digestion. Also, Ivanyi (personal communication) produced alloantisera against specificities associated with 7S and 17S Ig found in fractions separated by electrophoresis and sucrose density ultracentrifugation. We have confirmed these results using isolated 7S and 17S Ig (8).

In our studies, we used inbred chicken lines 2, 3, and 7 which were described previously (9). Alloantisera were produced by immunization of recipients with washed bovine serum albumin (BSA)-anti-BSA precipitates containing about 5 mg of donor antibody in slight antibody excess. Immunizations between the 3 inbred lines produced alloantisera which detected 2 distinct specificities, termed CS-1 and CS-2. These specificities were located on the 7S Ig papain-produced Fab fragment. Anti-CS-1 and CS-2 antisera had weak precipitating ability, but bound 90% of the homologous ^{125}I-Fab when assayed by a double antibody radioimmunoassay (RIA) in which rabbit anti-chicken Fc antiserum was used to precipitate intact chicken antibody (Table 1).

As determined by RIA inhibition, CS-1 and CS-2 were not found on 17S Ig; therefore, these genetic variations probably occur in the Fd fragments of the 7S Ig H chains. In this connection, reduction and alkylation altered the binding of CS-1 with antiserum. There was reduced inhibition of binding and the slope of the inhibition curve was sufficiently altered to indicate modification of the determinants.

Specificities CS-3, CS-4 and CS-5 were demonstrated on intact 7S Ig by immunodiffusion. They were recognized by multi-specific alloantisera produced in line 2 birds (anti-CS-3 and anti-CS-5), or by alloantisera supplied by Dr. J. Ivanyi (anti-CS-3) and Dr. C. David (anti-CS-4). As shown in Table 2, these specificities were not detected by RIA on papain-produced fragments of 7S Ig. Also,

Table 1. Allotypic specificities on 7S Ig Fab fragments.

Antiserum[a]	$\%^{125}$I-Fab bound[b] Derived from line			Precipitation of 7S Ig from line		
	2	3	7	2	3	7
Anti-CS-1 (line 7 anti-2)	94.2	88.7	0	+	+	-
Anti-CS-2 (Line 2 anti-7)	0	0	90.3	-	-	-

[a]Antisera did not bind ^{125}I-Fc from any line.
[b]Values were corrected for non-specific binding of 2%.
Each alloantiserum was diluted 1:10 in borate buffer.

CS-3 and CS-5 were partially dependent on intact disulfide bonds, since reduction with 0.2 M mercaptoethanol and alkylation yielded products which did not precipitate with alloantisera. These specificities were not detected on 17S Ig and probably are located in a region of the 7S Ig H chain which is either directly digested by papain or is conformationally dependent on intact H chains.

Table 2. Allotypic Specificities on 7S Ig which are destroyed by papain digestion.

Antiserum	Precipitation of 7S Ig from line		Binding of[a]	
	3	2	Fab	Fc
Anti-CS-3[b]	+	-	-	-
Anti-CS-4[c]	-	+	-	-
Anti-CS-5[d]	-	-	-	-

[a]Binding of ^{125}I labelled papain fragments derived from homologous 7S Ig was assayed by RIA.
[b]The CS-3 specificity is detected by line 2 anti-outbred (1955) antiserum and by antisera AA11 and AA32 prepared by Ivanyi.
[c]The CS-4 specificity is detected by anti-b_1(David, 1969).
[d]The CS-5 specificity is detected by line 2 anti-outbred (1827) antiserum. CS-5 was not found among the inbred lines, but was detected in 21 of 77 outbred white leghorn chickens tested.

In summary, genetic variation in the structure of chicken 7S Ig was detected in 2 regions of the molecule: 1) within the Fab and probably associated with the Fd fragment of the H chain; and 2) within a region of the H chain which is sensitive to papain digestion. To date, no specificities shared by the 7S and 17S Ig or localized on the Fc fragment have been found.

GENETIC ANALYSIS

When analyzed with these alloantisera, each inbred line had a distinct allotypic phenotype as shown in Table 3. The CS-1 specificity was associated with CS-4 in line 2, and with CS-3 in line 3. All parental specificities were expressed in F_1 hybrids of either sex (Table 3). Thus, these specificities are codominant traits not associated with the sex chromosomes.

Analysis of sera from F_2 progeny produced by _inter se_ matings between the inbred lines is shown in Table 4. Only the phenotypes characteristic of parental homozygotes or F_1 heterozygotes were observed. Specificity CS-1 segregated in association with either CS-3 or CS-4, depending on the parental lines, and thus lines 2 and 3 expressed the phenogroups (10) CS-1,4 and CS-1,3, respectively. Based on the observed segregation ratios, these specificities define 3 alleles at a single "Mendelian" locus which we have designated "CS".

These results are consistent with the structural data which demonstrated that the specificities probably were genetic variation in 2 separate regions of the 7S Ig H chain. Thus, the line

Table 3. Allotypic phenotypes of inbred chicken lines and their F_1 hybrids.

Line	Phenotype	Specificities detected[a]				
		CS-1	CS-2	CS-3	CS-4	CS-5
2	CS-1,4	+	−	−	+	−
3	CS-1,3	+	−	+	−	−
7	CS-2	−	+	−	−	−
(2x3)F_1	CS-1,3,4	+	−	+	+	−
(2x7)F_1	CS-1,2,4	+	+	−	+	−
(3x7)F_1	CS-1,2,3	+	+	+	−	−

[a]Specificities CS-1 and CS-2 were detected by RIA inhibition; sera inhibiting >88% of binding were positive and those inhibiting <5.0% were negative. Specificities CS-3, CS-4, and CS-5 were demonstrated by immunodiffusion.

Table 4. Segregation analysis of CS specificities among F_2 hybrids.

Hybrid	Phenotype observed				No. birds with phenotype		χ^2	p[a]
	CS-1	CS-2	CS-3	CS-4	(observed)	(expected)		
(2x3)(2x3)	+	−	+		3	5.75[b]		
	+	+	−		7	5.75		
	+	+	+		13	11.5		
				Total	23	23	1.8	.33
(2x7)(2x7)	+	−		+	7	6.5[c]		
	−	+		−	6	6.5		
	+	+		+	13	13.0		
				Total	26	26	0.8	.965
(3x7)(3x7)	+	−	+		5	6.5[d]		
	−	+	−		5	6.5		
	+	+	+		16	13		
				Total	26	26	1.4	.500

[a]Probability of a greater value of χ^2 assuming 2 d. f. The observed values do not deviate significantly from the expected values.
[b]Assuming that CS-3 and CS-4 characterize alternative alleles at a single locus and that CS-1 is present on both alleles.
[c]Assuming that CS-1 and CS-4 are closely associated specificities characterizing one allele and that CS-2 specifies the alternative allele at a single locus.
[d]Assuming that CS-1 and CS-3 are closely associated specificities characterizing one allele and that CS-2 specifies the alternative allele at a single locus.

2 CS allele contained the CS-1 specificity in the "Fd" region, and the CS-4 specificity in the "papain sensitive" region. The line 3 CS allele differed from line 2 by having the CS-3 specificity in the "papain sensitive" region. Such an arrangement would result in two stable phenogroups -- CS-1,4 and CS-1,3.

The CS locus was not associated with the B locus or with four other chicken blood group loci as determined by statistical analysis of F_2 progeny. The B locus has been shown to be associated with the major histocompatibility complex (11), the mixed leucocyte reaction (12), and loci controlling the humoral immune response of these inbred lines to synthetic polypeptide antigens (13). Also, allotypes found on chicken 17S Ig and 7S Ig segregated in association among F_2 progeny (Ivanyi and Pink, personal communication) and thus the chicken may contain an H chain linkage group similar to that described in mammals (14).

SUMMARY

Four allotypic specificities on the 7S Ig characterized 3 codominant alleles segregating at a single locus. This locus has been designated CS (chicken 7S) and probably represents the position of the structural gene which produces the 7S Ig H chain constant region. The term "CS" was preferred over "CG" to emphasize the fact that chicken 7S Ig is structurally unique and not necessarily homologous to mammalian IgG (15). Nevertheless, in these initial studies the genetics of chicken Ig allotypes did not differ from the mammalian systems.

The specificities described may represent fixed, neutral mutations in the structure of the chicken 7S Ig H chain. In support of this we have found that CS-2, CS-3, and CS-5 are detected in some, but not all, jungle fowl sera (Foppoli, unpublished results). This suggests that these allotypic specificities may have been in the common ancestor of the primitive jungle fowl and the domestic chicken. In this connection, CS-3 was detected in 66 of 74 outbred white leghorns in Hawaii and in approximately 178 of 317 birds from various strains in England (Ivanyi, personal communication). More extensive population studies would be of interest to determine the stability of the phenogroups (i.e., CS-1,3 or CS-1,4) formed by associations of "Fd" and "papain sensitive" specificities.

Clearly, many interesting questions concerning the genetics of chicken Ig structural genes remain to be answered. For instance, no information is available on either the nature or location of the genes responsible for the L chain or for the H chain variable regions. An understanding of the genetic organization of chicken Ig structural genes, may result in a better understanding of the evolution of the humoral immune response as a complex genetic system.

ACKNOWLEDGMENTS

We wish to thank Dr. Hans Abplanalp for providing the inbred chicken lines and sera from the F_1 and F_2 hybrids, Dr. W. E. Briles for determination of blood group genotypes, and Drs. C. David and J. Ivanyi for generously supplying some of the alloantisera used. This study was supported by Research Grant AI-05660 from the National Institute of Allergy and Infectious Disease, National Institutes of Health.

REFERENCES

1. Hood, L. and Prahl, J., in Advances in Immunology, Vol. 14, pp 291-352 (Academic Press, New York, 1971).

2. Skalba, D., Nature, 204: 894 (1964).

3. McDermid, E. M., Petrosky, E. and Yamazaki, H., Immunology, 17: 413 (1969).

4. David, C. S., Kaeberle, M. L., and Nordskog, A. W., Biochemical Genetics, 3: 197 (1969).

5. Pink, J. R. L., Eur. J. Immunol., 4: 679 (1974).

6. Derka, J., in Proceedings of the VIIth International Symposium on Laboratory Animals, p. 107 (Hruba´ Skala, 1971).

7. David, C. S., Genetics, 71: 649 (1972).

8. Wakeland, E. K., and Benedict, A. A., submitted for publication.

9. Benedict, A. A. and Pollard, L. W., in this conference.

10. Stormant, C., Amer. Naturalist, 89: 105 (1955).

11. Schierman, L. W. and Nordskog, A. W., Science, 134: 1008 (1961).

12. Miggiano, V. C. and Pink, J. R. L., Eur. J. Immunol., 4: 397 (1974).

13. Benedict, A. A., Pollard, L. W., Morrow, P., Abplanalp, H. A., Maurer, P. H. and Briles, W. E., Immunogenetics, in press.

14. Mage, R., Lieberman, R., Potter, M. and Terry, W. O., in The Antigens, Vol. 1, pp 300-376 (Academic Press, New York, 1973).

15. Hersh, R. T., Kubo, R. T., Leslie, G. A. and Benedict, A. A., Immunochemistry, 6: 762 (1969).

USE OF THE GVH REACTION TO INVESTIGATE THE REGULATION OF THE

HUMORAL IMMUNE RESPONSE

R. Elie and W.S. Lapp

Department of Physiology, McGill University

Montreal, Quebec, Canada

Comparative studies in various vertebrate species have shown that the systems responsible for the recognition and elimination of foreign bodies have undergone increasingly complex evolutionary adaptations (1-11). This evolutionary process has led to the appearance in mammals of a sophisticated immune system involving different well organized lymphoid organs, highly specialized cell populations and various classes of immunoglobulins. The function of such a system implies complex cellular interrelations and control mechanisms.

An example of such complex cellular interactions has been identified using the graft-versus-host (GVH) induced immunosuppression phenomenon as an experimental model to study nonspecific immune regulatory mechanisms. Both in vivo (12-13) and in vitro (13-14) studies have shown that the GVH induced suppression of the plaque forming cell (PFC) response of the mouse to heterologous erythrocytes is due, at least in part, to the deficiency of a T cell derived mediator which plays a critical role in the activation of the B lymphocytes into antibody forming cells. Our recent work reported here suggests that the suppression of the T cell helper function is mediated by a feedback mechanism exerted by an adherent (A) cell which we presume to be a macrophage.

MATERIALS AND METHODS

GVH reactions were induced in 8 to 12 week old C57BL/6 X A F_1 (B6AF$_1$) mice by an intravenous injection into each recipient of 75 X 10^6 spleen and lymph node cells obtained from adult A strain mice. Four to five days later one half of the group was used as

439

spleen cell donors for in vitro studies, the other half received
5 X 10^8 sheep red blood cells (SRBC) in order to confirm that immunosuppression was induced.   Single cell suspensions were prepared from various lymphoid organs by gently tamping them through
a 50 mesh stainless steel screen (14, 15).

Restoration experiments were performed using a modified Marbrook culture chamber (MMCC) (14).   The modification consisted of
two concentric culture compartments separated by a 0.45 µm cell
impermeable Millipore filter.   The experimental protocol consisted
of culturing 10 X 10^6 responding spleen cells from 4-5 day GVH
animals (GVH-SC) plus 5 X 10^6 SRBC in the outer compartment (OC)
of the MMCC and 3 X 10^6 restoring cells of different origin in the
inner compartment (IC).   CMRL 1066 medium supplemented with 10-15%
fetal calf serum (FCS) was used.   The cell cultures were incubated
at 37°C in a 5% CO_2 humidified atmosphere for 4 days.   The number
of direct PFC per culture vessel was determined by a modification
of the Cunningham and Szenberg technique (16,17).   Thymus derived
cells were killed with an AKR anti-theta C3H serum plus complement
as described previously (13).

In vitro experiments designed to investigate the immunosuppres-
sive action of A cells on the PFC response to SRBC were performed
using the following protocol.   A cells and non-adherent (NA) cells
were prepared from spleens obtained from normal and GVH mice.   The
spleen cells were suspended in Eagle's medium supplemented with
10% FCS at a concentration of 10 X 10^6 cells per ml.   The cells
were incubated in Falcon plastic Petri dishes for 1.5 hours at 37°C
after which the NA cells were removed by washing 2X.   The A cells
were scraped from the plastic Petri dishes with a rubber policeman.
Both NA and A cell populations were washed once and suspended in
CMRL 1066 medium supplemented with 15% FCS.   Increasing numbers of
A cells were added to 5 X 10^6 normal NA cells and 2.5 X 10^6 SRBC
and cultured in a standard Marbrook chamber (18) under the conditions described above.

                              RESULTS

Restoration of the In Vitro PFC Response to SRBC of GVH-SC by
Different Lymphoid Cell Populations Across a Cell Impermeable Membrane.

In order to investigate if normal lymphoid cells release a
soluble factor which could restore the PFC response of GVH-SC,
10 X 10^6 GVH-SC were cultured with 5 X 10^6 SRBC in the OC of the
MMCC while 3 X 10^6 thymus cells (TC), lymph node cells (LNC), spleen
cells (SC) or bone marrow cells (BMC) taken from normal B6AF$_1$ mice
were placed in the IC.   The 0.45 µm Millipore filter separating
the IC and the OC prevented cell movement between the two culture

compartments without interfering with the transfer of soluble factors.
Fig. 1 shows that normal TC, LNC and SC cultured in the IC significantly restored the PFC response of the GVH-SC whereas BMC failed to
do so. However, TC, LNC and SC treated with an anti-theta C3H serum
plus complement failed to restore. These results confirm earlier
work (12-15) suggesting that GVH induced immunosuppression is due, at
least in part, to the suppression of T cell helper function.

The next series of experiments were performed to study the time
post GVH induction that suppression of the T cell helper function
could be observed in the different lymphoid organs. The results in
Fig. 2 show that SC obtained from B6AF$_1$ mice on the day of GVH induction greatly restored the <u>in vitro</u> PFC response of 5 day GVH-SC.
However, within a few days after the parental cell TC and LNC taken
from GVH B6AF$_1$ mice even as late as 17 and 25 days post GVH induction
were able to restore the PFC response as well as TC and LNC taken
from normal animals (Fig. 2). These results, therefore, suggest that
GVH induced suppression of the T cell helper function is a local
rather than a systemic phenomenon.

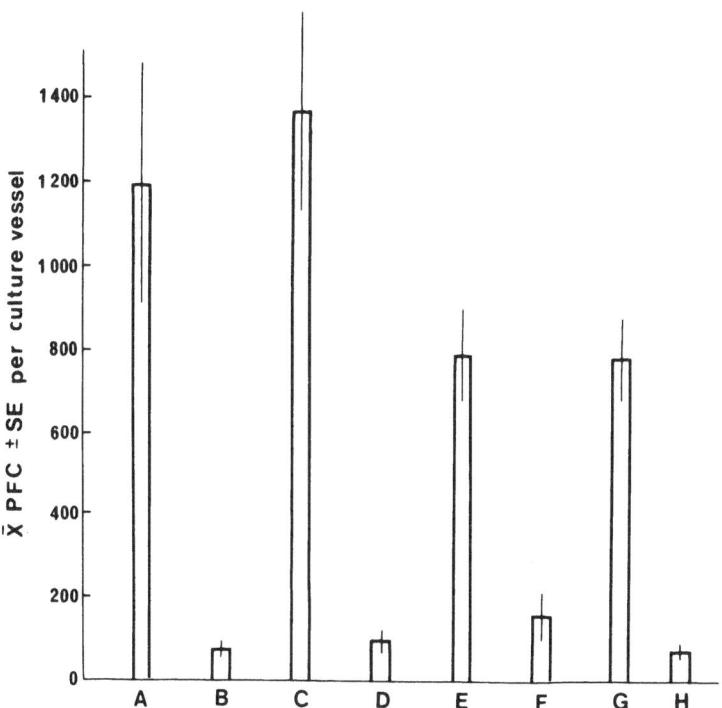

Fig. 1. <u>In vitro</u> PFC response to SRBC of 5 day GVH-SC restored across
a cell impermeable membrane by normal TC (C), LNC (E), SC (G) and BMC
(H) and by anti-theta serum treated TC (D) and LNC (F). Bars A and B
represent the PFC response of normal SC and 5 day GVH-SC respectively.

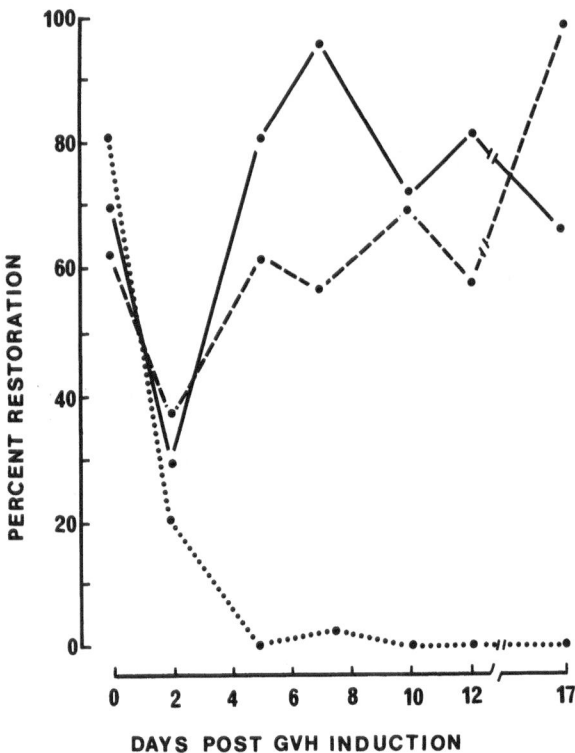

Fig. 2. In vitro PFC response of 5 day GVH-SC restored across a cell
impermeable membrane by TC ●—●, LNC●--● and SC●···● taken from B6AF$_1$
mice at different days post GVH induction. The results of 3 experiments were pooled and are presented as percent restoration calculated
as follows:

$$\frac{\bar{x} \text{ PFC restored GVH-SC} - \bar{x} \text{ PFC non-restored GVH-SC}}{\bar{x} \text{ PFC normal SC} - \bar{x} \text{ PFC non-restored GVH-SC}} \times 100.$$

Study of the Role of A cells in the GVH Induced Immunosuppression

        Earlier work reported by Sjöberg (19) suggested that the immuno-
suppression observed in GVH-SC was caused by the adherent cells.
Experiments were therefore carried out to test the ability of A cell
deprived GVH-SC to restore the PFC response of GVH-SC. The results
shown in Fig. 3 demonstrate that day 5 GVH-SC depleted of their A
cell fraction and placed in the IC of the MMCC were able to restore
the in vitro PFC response of GVH-SC as well as normal SC. Fig. 3
further demonstrates that treatment with anti-theta serum plus complement abrogated the restoring ability of day 5 GVH-NA cells.

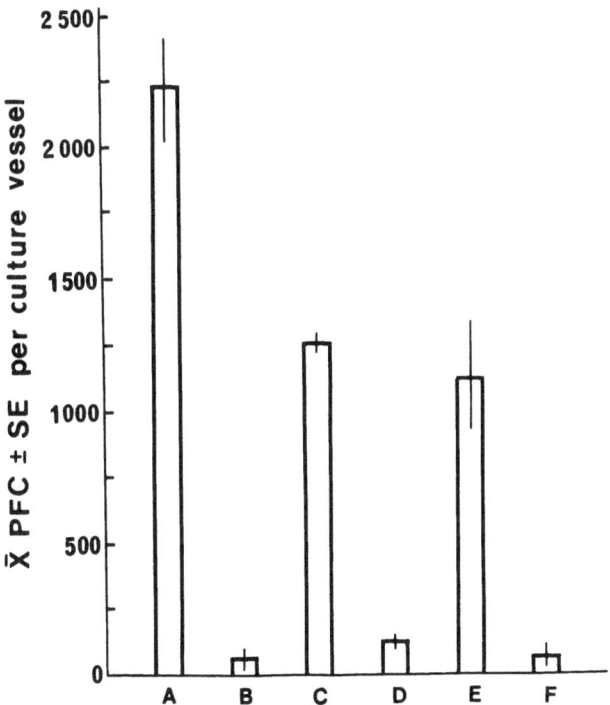

Fig. 3. <u>In vitro</u> PFC response to SRBC of 5 day GVH-SC restored across
a cell impermeable membrane by normal SC (C), GVH-SC (D), GVH-NA cells
(E) and anti-theta treated GVH-NA cells (F). Bars A and B represent
the PFC response of normal SC and non-restored GVH-SC respectively.
5 day GVH spleens were used as a source of restoring cells.

The results reported thus far suggest that A cells in the spleens
of GVH mice exert a suppressive effect on T cell helper function.
Experiments were therefore designed to determine whether or not the
suppressive effect was due to qualitative or quantitative changes in
the A cell population or to both. The first series of experiments
tested for a correlation between the number of A cells and the <u>in vivo</u>
PFC response in the spleens of GVH mice. At different times post GVH
induction a minimum of three mice were sacrificed to determine the
proportion of A cells in the spleen. At the same time a minimum of
two mice were injected with SRBC and the number of PFC determined
four days later. Similar determinations were performed on normal
animals. Fig. 4 shows that the proportion of A cells in the spleen
increased with time and reached a maximum value at day 10-11 post

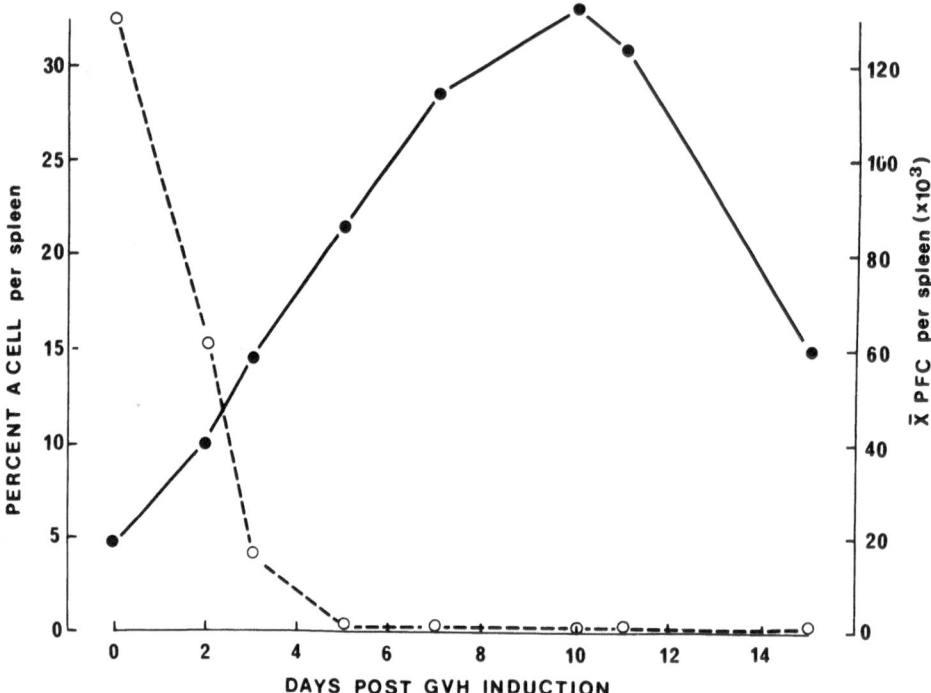

Fig. 4. Relationship between the proportion of A cells •—• and the number of PFC o--o in the spleens of GVH mice at different times post GVH induction. The total number of viable cells increased linearly from 53×10^6 at day 0 to a maximum of 136×10^6 at day 10 and remained nearly constant until day 15 post GVH induction.

GVH induction followed by a decrease at day 15. In contrast to the increase in the number of A cells there was a sharp decline in the total number of PFC per spleen (Fig. 4).

Experiments were then designed to determine whether a qualitative change had also occurred in the A cell population of GVH spleens. The results in Fig. 5 show that A cells from GVH-SC could

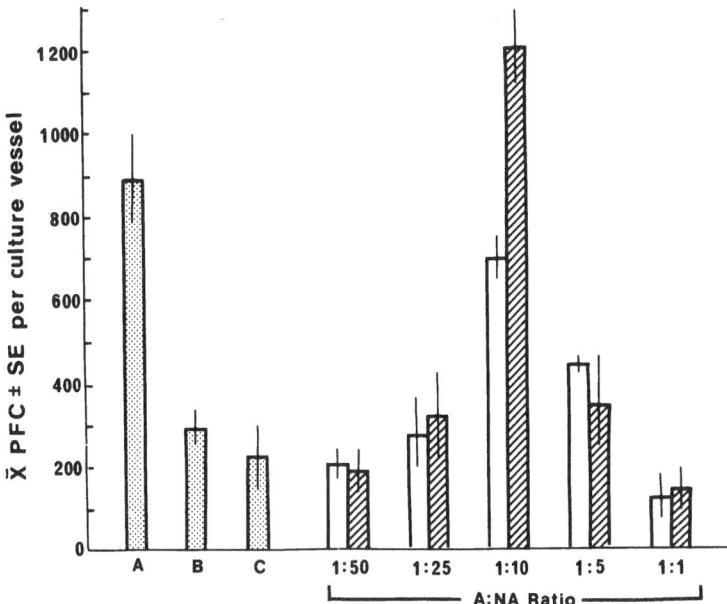

Fig. 5. Effect of increasing numbers of GVH ☐ or normal ▨ A
cells on the in vitro PFC response to SRBC of non-adherent spleen
cells. Bars A, B and C represent the PFC response of normal SC,
GVH-SC and GVH-NAC respectively.

substitute for normal cells and cooperate with normal NA cells
in the initiation of the in vitro PFC response to SRBC. The results
also show that regardless of the source of A cells (normal SC or
GVH-SC), the in vitro PFC response was related to the ratio of A to
NA cells in culture (Table IV). The maximum PFC response was obtained when the mixture contained 1 A to 10 NA cells. When the
ratio of A to NA cells exceeded that level the PFC response was
inhibited. These results suggest that the suppressive effect
exerted by A cells on T cell helper function in GVH spleens is
due mostly to a quantitative rather than a qualitative change in
the A cell population.

DISCUSSION

Previous reports on in vivo (12, 13) and in vitro (14, 15)
restoration of the PFC response have shown that the GVH induced
immunosuppression is due, at least in part, to the deficiency of a
non-specific T cell factor which is essential for the T cell helper
function. It has been demonstrated that the in vitro PFC response
of 5 day GVH-SC can be restored by a soluble factor released by
normal thymus, spleen and lymph node T cells in the absence of
antigenic stimulation.

The results shown in Fig. 2 demonstrate that within a short
period of time post GVH induction, splenic T cells lose their ability to restore. In contrast TC and LNC taken from GVH mice as
late as 17 days post GVH induction restored the PFC response of
5 day GVH-SC as well as normal TC and LNC. These results suggest
that the GVH reaction induces a local rather than a systemic depression of the T cell helper function. However, suppression of
T cell helper function in GVH-SC was not irreversible since removal
of A cells permitted the GVH-NA cells to restore the PFC response.
These results suggest that T cells in GVH spleens still possess
their ability to perform helper function for the induction of antibody synthesis, but that their helper function is suppressed by the
action of the A cell population.

An inverse correlation was demonstrated between the in vivo
PFC response and the number of AC in the spleen of GVH mice. The
total number of PFC per spleen decreased with time post GVH induction, while the number of A cells showed a marked increase. However, the A cells in GVH spleens did not appear to be solely suppressor cells but rather served to regulate the inductive phase of
the immune response. GVH-A cells were able to reconstitute the
anti-SRBC PFC response of normal NA cells (Fig. 5). The maximum
PFC response was obtained at the ratio of one A cell to ten NA
cells for both GVH and normal A cells. When the ratio of A to NA
cells exceeded that level the PFC response was markedly suppressed.
These results seem to indicate that the excessive number of A cells
was responsible for the depressed humoral immune response observed
in GVH animals. Similar results have been reported by others. It
has been shown by Hoffmann and Dutton (20) that an excessive concentration of A cell product suppressed the immune response of
mouse spleen cells. Waldman and Gottlieb (21) have recently reported that high numbers of macrophages inhibited PHA transformation
of rat T lymphocytes. They suggested that the suppressive effect
was elicited by a low molecular weight, heat stable factor released
into the culture fluid only by viable macrophages. Therefore it
appears that small numbers of A cells have a stimulatory effect on
the antibody response whereas large numbers have an inhibitory

effect by depressing T cell function.

Although the present results suggest that suppression is due to a feedback effect exerted on T cell helper function by an increase in the A cell population, a qualitative change of the A cells cannot be ruled out. Two sets of evidence reported here support the hypothesis that the GVH reaction induces functional changes in the A cell population with an increased number of suppressor cells. Firstly, GVH-A cells were not as efficient as normal A cells in reconstituting the PFC response of the normal NA cell population (Fig. 5). Secondly, spleens from day 3 and day 15 GVH mice contained the same percentage of A cells, however day 15 GVH mice were fully immunosuppressed, whereas day 3 GVH mice produced a significant PFC response (Fig. 4). Experiments by others have shown that splenic and peritoneal A cells taken from GVH mice 7 or more days post GVH induction released an inhibitory factor which suppressed the immune response and normal T cell function (19,22,23). Scott has obtained similar results with A cells taken from mice injected with Corynebacterium parvum (23).

In summary, these results suggest that at least one type of A cell in the spleen of GVH immunosuppressed mice is not simply an inhibitory cell but rather a regulatory cell and most likely functions to regulate normal T cell helper function. It seems highly probable that this regulatory effect is exerted via a feedback control mechanism similar to most biological control systems, in which the same A cell and/or its product may both stimulate and suppress T cell function.

ACKNOWLEDGMENTS

This investigation was supported by the Medical Research Council of Canada and the National Cancer Institute of Canada. R.E. was a MRC of Canada Fellow. Present address is: Departement des Sciences Biologiques, Universite du Quebec a Montreal, P.O. Box 8888, Montreal, P.Q., Canada W.S.L. is a MRC of Canada Scholar.

We thank Mrs. H.C. Lee, Mrs. A. Lee Foon, and Miss R. Siegrist for their careful technical assistance.

REFERENCES

1. Good, R.A., and Papermaster, B.W., Adv. Immunol. 4, 1 (1974).
2. Good, R.A., Finstad, J., Pollara, B. and Gabrielsen, A.E., in Phylogeny of Immunity, ed. R.T. Smith, P.A. Miescher and R.A Good, 145, (1966).

3. Finstad, J., Papermaster, B.W and Good, R.A., Lab. Invest 13, 490, (1964)
4. Grey, H., J Immunol. 91, 819, (1963)
5. Clem, L.W. and Small, P.A , J. Exp. 125, 893, (1967).
6. Clem, L.W., De Boutaud, F., and Sigel, M.M., J. Immunol. 99, 1226, (1967).
7. Shuster, J. and Goodman, J.W., Nature 219, 298, (1968)
8. Lopez, D.M., Sigel, M.M., Cell. Immunol. 10, 287, (1974).
9. Miller, J.F.A.P. and Mitchell, G.F., Transplant. Rev. 1, 3, (1969)
10. Claman, M.N. and Chaperon, E.A., Transplant. Rev. 1, 92, (1969).
11. Unanue, E.R., Adv. Immunol. 15, 95, (1972).
12. Grushka, M. and Lapp, W.S., Transplantation 14, 157, (1974).
13. Lapp, W.S., Wechsler, A., and Kongshavn, P.A.L., Cell. Immunol. 11, 419, (1974).
14. Elie, R., Abrahams, R., Parthenais, E. and Lapp, W.S., Proc. 8th Leuc. Cult. Conf. Acad. Press. 175 (1974).
15. Parthenais, E., Elie, R., and Lapp, W.S., Cell. Immunol. 13, 164, (1974)
16. Cunningham, A.S. and Szenberg, A., Immunology 14, 599, (1968).
17. Kongshavn, P.A.L. and Lapp, W.S., Immunology 22, 227, (1972).
18. Marbrook, J., Lancet 2, 1279, (1967).
19. Sjöberg, O., Clin. Expl. Immunol. 12, 365 (1972).
20. Hoffmann, M., and Dutton, R.W., Science 172, 1047, (1971)
21. Waldman, S.R., and Gottlieb, A.A., Cell Immunol. 9, 142, (1973).
22. Nelson, D.S., Nature 246, 306, (1973).
23. Scott, M.T., Cell. Immunol. 5, 469, (1972).

IMMUNE FACILITATION OF ALLOGRAFT SURVIVAL ACROSS RESTRICTED DIFFERENCES AT THE H-2 COMPLEX

William C. Davis[*] and Gregory J. Ferebee

Washington State University

Pullman, Washington

Numerous studies have now documented that a number of parallels exist between the overt immune response of lower and higher vertebrates to allografts.[1,2] In both, the immune response is influenced by a number of factors the most prominent of which are the genetic disparity between the donor and host and the type of tissue employed as an allograft. Whether across weak or strong histocompatibility barriers, skin grafts elicit the most vigorous response. This is manifested as chronic rejection across weak barriers and acute rejection across major barriers. Heart and kidney grafts, however, elicit a varied response.[3,4,5] In the urodels,[6] and certain semi-inbred strains of fish,[7] heart grafts persist indefinitely or are rejected over a long time course. In inbred strains of rats[3,4,5] and mice,[8,9] kidney and in some instances, whole heart grafts are either rejected as rapidly as skin grafts or exhibit a prolonged survival time. In each group of animals, a correlation has been found between the strength of the genetic incompatibility and the duration of graft survival.[10] A similar correlation has been found between the immunogenetic strength of histocompatibility antigens and the capacity of alloantibody to enhance graft survival.[11] That is, it has been shown that it is easier to enhance the survival of grafts across weak barriers than strong barriers.

One of the hopes of many investigators interested in analyzing the mechanisms of immunological enhancement, has been that the development of animal models at all levels of phylogeny would provide a means of characterizing the individual components of enhancement in a setting where the immunological machinery is less complex, and then, trace the evolution of this phenomenon into its more complex form in higher vertebrates. I should like to direct my comments to the development of such models in higher vertebrates with emphasis on recent findings with congenic strains of mice.

Enhancement of normal tissue grafts in outbred animals.
Currently, efforts to demonstrate enhancement, or as some prefer immunoblocking, in outbred animals has proven difficult.[1,3] Although ample evidence has shown that pretreatment with preparations of antigens, such as whole blood, bone marrow, lymph node cells and crude semisoluble preparations of cell extracts can prolong graft survival, administration of alloantibody has lead to acute rejection.[3] Only on occasion, such as in the rabbit and baboon, has there been reports that some preparations of whole alloantiserum and native or pepsin digested IgG prolong graft survival. In addition, it has been difficult to identify donor-recipient combinations where genetic compatibility is such that the differential susceptibility of organ grafts to rejection can be identified.[1,3]

Enhancement of allograft survival in the rat. Striking results have been obtained with inbred strains of rats.[1,5] In these animals, a sharp difference has been noted between the host response to skin, kidney[3,5] and heart[4] allografts. Except across minor histocompatibility differences, skin, whether because of the site of grafting or inherent immunogenicity, has presented a formidable barrier. Regardless of the regimen of antibody administration employed, it has been impossible to increase the survival of skin grafts more than a few days across all but the weakest of incompatibilities. By contrast, a broad range of differences in immunogenetic strengths have been noted with kidney grafts.[11] Depending on the strain combination employed, first-set graft survival, across either the major H-1 locus or non-H-1 loci, is similar to that of skin grafts or prolonged. Hildemann and Mullen[11] have noted that across the major H-1 locus, graft survival time may vary from 8 to 50 days, across non-H-1 differences survival may vary from 76 to 197 days. In situations where the antigenic load has been reduced by employing F1 hybrids as donors the range of survival may be broadened even further, 7 to 321 days. Similar observations have been made by other investigators.[3] In both H-1 and non-H-1 combinations the passive transfer of antibody increases graft survival time to a considerable extent, with the most pronounced effect being evident across the weaker incompatibilities. In fact, instances have been reported where enhancement has lead to a permanent acceptance of grafts across non-H-1 differences.

A point of particular relevance brought out by these studies has been the observation that the regimen of antibody administration influences the survival time. Unlike studies with skin and tumor grafts, repeated injections of antibody have proven to be more effective than a single injection.[11] Additional information has been obtained on the immunological status of rats with long

surviving grafts. The important point here, however, is that these
animals have provided an excellent model for elucidating the
mechanisms of immunological enhancement of normal tissue grafts.

Enhancement of allograft survival in the mouse. Until recently,
it has not been possible to take full advantage of the immense
amount of knowledge acquired from the use of inbred mice to study
the mechanisms of enhancement except across minor histoincompatibilities. The size of the animals has made it difficult to
develop simple surgical techniques for grafting whole organs to
perform comparable studies to those done in rats.[8,9] In addition,
investigations with skin grafts across the major H-2 complex in
congenic resistant strains of mice have suggested that it is
exceedingly difficult to extend graft survival time by treatment
with alloantibody.[13] These studies have indicated that it is
only possible to enhance graft survival across restricted antigenic
differences at the K end of the H-2 complex.[13] Our studies,
however, have shown this applies only to skin grafts and also that
heart tissue is more suitable for distinguishing differences in
immunogenetic strength in the mouse. Although it has been known
since 1959 that it is possible to transplant neonatal heart tissue
and obtain pulsatile activity, few laboratories have used this
tissue in their studies. With the demonstration of a technique
for implanting heart tissue in the ear, however, interest has
increased.[14,15] The technique is simple and readily performed.

An incision is made at the base of the ear, a pocket formed
with a blunt probe and a piece of heart tissue from a neonatal
mouse (1- to 3-day-old hearts are best) inserted and positioned
toward the center of the ear. One half of a heart, comprised of
either or both auricular and ventricular tissue can be used as the
graft. Between 90 to 100% of the grafts vascularize and develop
electrical activity by 6 days. Survival can be followed by macroscopic inspection or by using microelectrodes (at 50 microvolts).[15]
Electrical activity persists in syngrafts and disappears rapidly
in allografts as rejection ensues.

In the strain combinations that we have examined, the mean
survival time of first-set heart grafts has been quite similar to
those of skin grafts. Across restricted differences at either the
D or K and of the H-2 complex, however, graft survival time of
heart grafts is slightly broader.

In contrast to the results with skin grafts, it has been
possible to enhance the survival of heart grafts across differences
involving the whole H-2 complex as well as differences at either the
K or D end. The main variables that have been encountered in
demonstrating enhancement of normal tissue grafts have been the
haplotype combination employed and the regimen of antibody
administration. As shown in the table, in the strains examined

Immune Facilitation of Heart Allograft Survival in Congenic Resistant Strains of Mice Differing
At the H-2 Complex

Group	Donor	H-2 haplotype	Recipient*	H-2 haplotype	Number of mice	Treatment	MST ± S.E.	Days prolongation
1	B10.A	a	B10.M	f	23	---	11.4 ± 1.0	
2	"	a	"	f	10	B10.M anti B10.A	13.3 ± 1.1	+ 1.9
3	B10.A(2R)	h2	B10.A(5R)/SJL	i + s	9	---	10.5 ± 0.0	
4	"	h2	"	i + s	19	B10.A(5R)/SJ anti B10.A(2R)	17.1 ± 0.6	+ 6.6
5	B10.S	s	B10.A	a	20	---	11.2 ± 0.5	
6	"	s	"	a	19	B10.A anti B10.S	18.6 ± 0.8	+ 7.4
7	B10.A	a	B10.D2	d	9	---	11.3 ± 0.8	
8	"	a	"	d	8	B10.M anti B10.A	21.0 ± 2.3	+ 9.7
9	B10.D2	d	B10.A/B10.F	a + f	17	---	13.8 ± 1.4	
10	"	d	"	a + f	18	B10.A/B10.F anti B10.D2	17.9 ± 0.4	+ 4.1
11	"	d	"	a + f	16	SJL/B10.A anti B10.D2	24.5 ± 2.5	+ 10.7
12	B10	b	B10.D2/B10.A(2R)	d + h2	18	---	15.5 ± 0.9	
13	"	b	"	d + h2	20	B10.D2/B10.A(2R) anti B10	36.7 ± 3.3	+ 21.2
14	B10.A	b	B10.A(2R)	h2	11	---	11.8 ± 0.9	
15	"	b	"	h2	12	B10.M anti B10.A	16.3 ± 0.8	+ 4.5
16	"	a	B10.AKM	m	12	---	16.3 ± 3.4	
17	"	a	"	m	22	B10.M anti B10.A	48.6 ± 10.3	+ 32.3
18	B10.A	a	B10.AKM/B10.A(2R)	m + h2	138	---	15.3 ± 0.8	
19	"	a	"	m + h2	41	B10.M anti B10.A	43.6 ± 4.8**	+ 28.6
20	"	a	"	m + h2	9	B10.M anti B10.M(11R)	61.8 ± 13.9	+ 46.3

*Recipients received serial injections (0.2 ml i.p.) biweekly of ammonium sulfate (50% saturated) precipitated immune ascites (10 mg/ml).
**Grafts still persisting at 140 days.

thus far, the mean survival time (MST) has been increased from
1.9 to 7.4 days in combinations differing at the whole H-2 complex
(compare groups 1 through 6), 4.1 to 21.2 days in combinations
differing only at the K end (compare groups 7 through 13) and 4.5
to 46.3 days in combinations differing at the D end.

The regimen of antibody administration is of critical
importance in prolonging graft survival. In the experiments that
we have completed thus far, large increases in graft survival time
have been achieved only by giving mice serial injections of antibody over an eight to twelve week time course. No absolute
schedule of injections has been established as being most effective
at this juncture. Depending on the strain combination employed,
injection of antibody (whole or ammonium sulfate precipitated
immune ascites is the source of antibody in our studies[15]) on a
2- or 3-day or biweekly schedule has yielded similar results. In
one strain combination that we have examined extensively, B10.A
to B10.AKM/B10.A(2R), the serial injection of antibody on a
biweekly regimen increased the mean survival time of heart grafts
from 15.3 to 43.6 days (compare groups 18 and 19) with individual
survival times ranging from one month to over a year. By contrast,
a single injection or multiple injections of antibody given over a
short time course, i.e. 5 to 10 days has had minimal effect in
prolonging survival.

Another point brought out in these studies is that the extent
of prolonged graft survival is also influenced by the immune
reagent employed. As noted in the data presented here, the MST of
graft survival may be altered by 6.6 days, as in B10.D2
to B10.A/B10.F (compare groups 10 and 11), or as much as 18.2 days
as in B10.A to B10.AKM/B10.A(2R) (compare groups 19 and 20). At
this juncture, no adequate explanation is available for this
observation. However, two possibilities can be considered: One
is that the differences in activity are associated with the titer
of the antibody directed towards the antigens present in the donor
tissue. The other is that the differences are associated with the
interaction of antibodies directed towards antigens shared by both
the donor and host as well as those unique to the donor. Further
studies are needed to distinguish between these possibilities.

In summary, a number of significant observations have emerged
from phylogenetic studies of immune responsiveness which are of
importance to the study of immunological enhancement. First, the
studies have shown that the type of tissue graft employed is of
paramount importance. Because of their greater immunogenicity,
skin grafts tend to obscure differences in the immunogenetic
strength of histocompatibility antigens determined by both the
major and minor histocompatibility loci. Though the reason is not
totally clear, heart and kidney grafts tend to reveal such differences. Second, the investigations have revealed that it is

easier to enhance the survival of kidney and heart allografts, as emphasized in our studies, with inbred rats and mice. Third, evidence has been obtained which indicates that repeated injections of antibody can be more effective than single injections in maximizing the survival of allografts. Fourth, the studies with heart and kidney grafts in inbred mice and rats, have demonstrated that it is possible to enhance the survival of normal tissue grafts across both major and minor histocompatibility differences. These findings should lead to some exciting investigations in the near future.

References

1. Hildeman, W.H., in Transplantation Antigens: Markers of Biological Individuality, 3 pp. (Academic Press, New York and London, 1972).

2. Cohen, N., Am. Zool., 2: 193 (1971).

3. Stuart, E.P., McKearn, T.J., and Fitch, Transplant Proc., 6: 53 (1974).

4. Barker, C.F. and Billingham, R.E., Transplant. Proc., 3: 172 (1971).

5. White, E., Hildemann, W.H., and Mullen, Y., Transplantation, 8: 602 (1969).

6. Cohen, N. and Rich, L.C., Am. Zool., 10: 536 (1970).

7. Kallman, K.D., Transplant. Proc., 2: 263 (1970).

8. Corry, R.J., Winn, H.J., and Russell, P.S., Transplant. Proc., 5: 733 (1973).

9. Skoskiewicz, M., Chase, C., Winn, H.J., and Russell, P.S., Transplant. Proc., 5: 721 (1973).

10. Hildemann, W.H., Transplant. Rev., 3: 5 (1970).

11. Hildemann, W.H. and Mullen, Y., Transplantation, 15: 231 (1973).

12. Feldman, J.D., Adv. Immunol., 15: 167 (1972).

13. McKenzie, I.F.C. and Snell, G.D., J. Exp. Med., 138: 259 (1973).

14. Huber, B., Demant, P., and Festenstein, H., Transplant. Proc., 5: 1377 (1973).

15. Davis, W.C., Transplant. Proc., 5: 625 (1973).

16. Klein, J., Biology of the Mouse Histocompatibility-2 Complex.
     Principles of Immunogenetics Applied to a Single System.
     620 pp. (New York, Springer-Verlag, 1975).

*This research is supported by grants from the NIH AI-10290,
GM-00691, and FR5465 and the Washington State Heart Association.

INDUCTION OF UNRESPONSIVENESS TO ORGAN TRANSPLANTS IN CONGENIC

STRAINS OF RATS AND OTHER MAMMALS

Gunther H.THOENES

Immunbiologisches Labor,1.Medizinische Klinik,Universi-

tät München,Ziemssenstr.1,8 München 2,Germany

It is beyond doubt that the phylogeny of species has not only
led to the relatively simple process of immune elimination,but also to a complicated mechanism which limits the immune response.It
seems that by such an immune regulation the organism has become
able to coexist with certain foreign agents without overt problems.
This unresponsiveness can be called "enhancement" and a heated de-
bate rages between protagonists and antagonists as to whether "tolerance" is the most extreme form of this immune regulation.In any
case,the immunological unresponsiveness in face of a fully developed machinary seems to be the greatest achievement which phylogeny
of species has accomplished in this field.This is especially evident with regard to the tolerance of the self,allowing autoagres-
sion only as a state of disease.Inasmuch as true autoimmune diseases are manifested only in mammals (-so far as I know-) the need
for immunological unresponsiveness might also be the greatest in the
mammalian species.Despite the general validity which enhancement
could very well have in cases like autoimmunity and tumorigenesis,
I have elected to limit my presentation to the field of transplan-
tation.Regardless whether we speak of tolerance or of enhancement,
any specific unresponsiveness depends on antigenicity.With reference again to the phylogenetical context,the transplantation antigens
appear to be the most fundamental expression of the divergent development of species.The problem of "antigenic strength" is an inherent question of interest in immunologic phylogeny.The polymorphism in cell surface antigens might be required to maintain the integrity of the individual.However,the capability to produce specific unresponsiveness counteracts in principle the incompatibility
between normal outbred individuals.But transplantation antigens
and the induction of specific unresponsiveness toward them appear
to play a major role for a life-sustaining heterozygosity by inhibi-

ting the maternal graft-versus-host-reaction against her offspring,
histoincompatible from the paternal line (1).All these examples indicate the importance which the ability for specific immunological
unresponsiveness constitutes on the phylogenetical vertebrate level.

TRANSPLANTATION IN MAMMALS

Most experimental immunologists have long been occupied with
transplantation of cells and skin.But it has been experimental organ transplantation which created fruitful unrest to further unra-
vel the significance and mechanism of unresponsiveness through immunological enhancement.Skin transplantation has been practiced in mice as well as in hagfish,but in order to establish the practical
usefulness of enhancement and to recognize the overall participation
of it in most,if not all,forms of transplantation immunity,kidney
grafting in rats produced the breakthrough.Skin grafting seems to
be a rigid test of rejection,but much too stringend for protection.
The question why this is so,is intimately related to the understanding of the mechanism itself.As long as the investigation of molecular processes in vivo and in vitro remains a difficult task often inconsistent with the actual relationships which exist,it appears reasonable to proceed in a deductive manner as well.Many researchers have thus collected valuable knowledge on the natural history of specific unresponsiveness in organ transplantation.This
concerns the obvious differences in susceptibility for the enhancement of skin versus kidney,heart versus liver etc. It also includes
the differences between the several species accessible for organ
transplantation.Histoincompatibility and immunosuppression has been
considered primarily in terms of rejection.During the past few years,
however,it has become apparent that even in untreated recipients,
probably every rejection process in accompanied by immunological en-
hancement.The balance between both processes is very delicate and
the predominance of either one depends on such factors as histoincompatibility,immunosuppression as practiced clinically and possibly
on the immuneresponsiveness of the recipient as well as the quality
of its immune response.We need to analyse this multifactorial system
which eventually leads to unresponsiveness.

ALLOGRAFT ENHANCEMENT IN RATS

The rat seems to be the animal with the least relevance nowa-
days for the clinical practice of human transplantation,but its significance for recognizing the chances which biology allows for
irregular allograft survival is greater than any large mammal closer
to humans can provide.In learning with the aid of this easy-going
model we might proceed to immunological engineering in more complex
situations.Just as every species is not equally susceptable to enhancement,a remarkable dissociation between skin and kidney graft

survival after autoenhancement in rats was first observed by WHITE
and HILDEMANN (2) and was confirmed by others (3,4,5,6).Other
authors,however,have been able to show a definite unresponsiveness
for skin grafts as well after an organ graft had been accepted for
long periods of time (7,8,9).This brings me to the first two statements:

1.Specific unresponsiveness to a graft must depend on certain peripheral factors like greater or lesser vulnerability to the rejection mechanism.
2.A continuous stimulation of enhancing factors balancing rejection
   gradually diminishes or exhausts the specifically directed rejection capacity.

The longer an organ graft has remained in a recipient,the more
successful a subsequent skin graft will survive.A difference in the
susceptibility of grafted tissues with respect to enhancement therefore does not really exist,but rather reflects the degree of sensitivity to the remaining rejection processes.

This rejection can be controlled more easily,the smaller the
antigenic differences are.On the basis of their results with passive enhancement,HILDEMANN and MULLEN (10) presented evidence for
a new rule of transplantation immunology.(+) It seems very appropriate to link enhancement to histocompatibility factors too,there-
by eliminating the exclusive dependence of rejection on histoin-
compatibility.This seems especially important because it is likely
that every rejection process concurs with enhancement.In terms of
immunogenicity in either of these cases,one should assume that semiallogeneic grafts across strong H-barriers are not different
than fully allogeneic ones.The fact that we nevertheless found semiallogeneic grafts generally be predestined for a long survival
through autoenhancement (Fig.1) is still in accordance with HILDE-
MANN's rule:The term "weak" (+) could suggest a lower immunogenic
quality of certain H-antigens.But it has been shown (11) that the
enhancement effect does not necessarily depend on the antibody titer of the applied serum.Thus,I believe that immunogenic quality
will not prove to be the major issue,but rather the frequency distribution of antigenic sites on the cell surface.According to
WIGZELL (12),Fl-hybrid (semiallogeneic) cells contain half the
amount of antigenic specificities present on parental cells.If enhancement is determined by "antigenic strength",this can mean first
of all,a differential distribution of antigenic sites.

This is supported by results obtained with congenic rats.In
addition to using grafts from hybrid donors,we have been able to
use kidneys from H-1 congenic donors.These grafts lack the so-
called "weak" non-H-1-antigenic differences.It is shown unequivocally in Fig.2 that such "weak" antigens contribute significantly

---

(+) "The weaker the histoincompatibility,the greater the effecti-
    veness of specific immunoblocking antibodies".

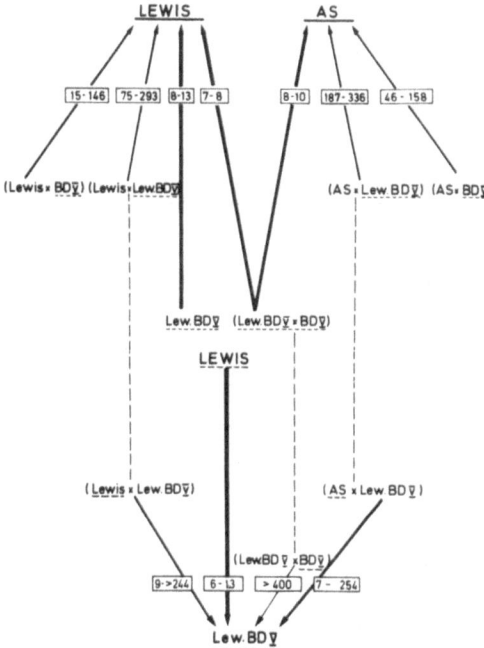

Fig.1.The survival ranges of kidney grafts,semiallogeneic to the graft recipient (⟶) are shown in comparison to the survival ranges of fully allogeneic transplants (➡). The recipients are Lewis and AS (both H-1^l) and Lew.BDv (H-1^d).The semiallogeneic grafts show in general longer survivals,possibly due to a lesser representation of alloantigens and a more effective enhancement.

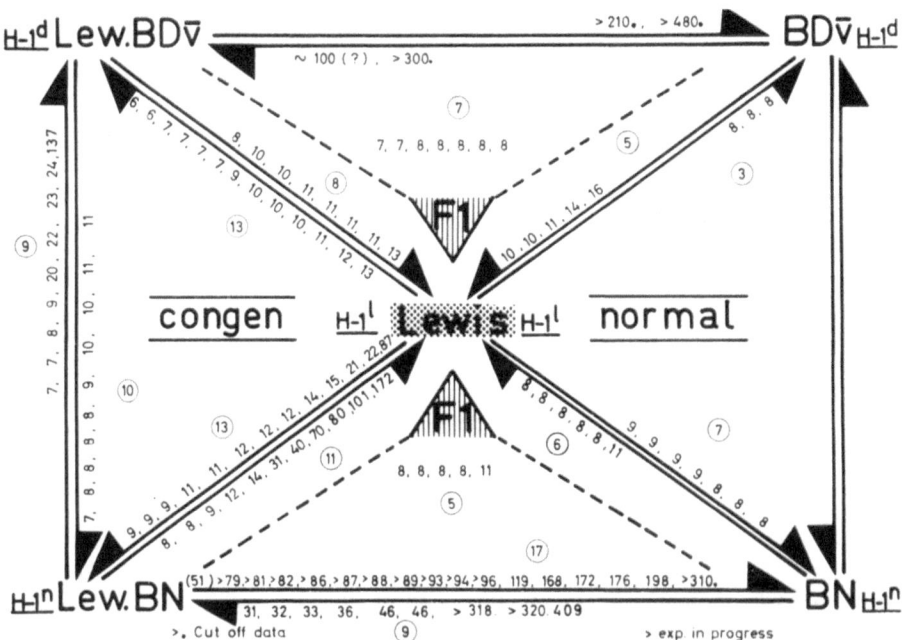

Fig.2.Individual survival times after kidney transplantation in congenic (H-1),normal (H-1 + non-H-1) and "weak" (non-H-1) combinations are shown.The additive effects of weak alloantigens in Fl-kidneys from a cross between congenic and background strain is seen.

to curtail graft survival: Fl hybrids between the "congenic line"
(Lew.BN) and the "donor strain" (BN) provide grafts which are rejected very consistently at a higher rate than are the transplants
exchanged between the "congenic line" and the "inbred partner"
strain (Lewis).The survival times of the latter grafts across the
isolated H-1 difference (given as the day of death) show a broader
range and a more favorable delay which is especially pronounced in
the congenic pair Lew.BN   Lewis.The data in Fig.2 are presented
in an uncomputed manner in order to give a more detailed,natural
view.This concerns,for example,the H-1 different combination Lew.BN
◄──►Lew.BDv,where the kind of interallelic donor-recipient combination clearly influences additionally graft survival,Lew.BDv ──►
Lew.BN being rejected more rapidly than in the reverse direction.
As has been shown for mice by Mc KENZIE and SNELL (11), the several
private H-specificities provide different immunogenicities and the
more immunogenic graft seems to be enhanced more easily.We do not
have comparable investigations as yet for rats but the differential
immunogenicity of private specifities can certainly influence the
interallelic dissimilarity in graft survivals of untreated rats as
well.The contradiction between HILDEMANN's (10) and Mc KENZIE's (11)
findings with regard to the lesser enhanceability across "weaker"
incompatibility is difficult to reconcile.In addition to the possibility that unfavorable immune response genes could be involved,
one has to take the different graft-types investigated (kidney versus skin) into account.In persuing the original concept of (active)
autoenhancement across non-H-1 differences (13),we have continued
to investigate active enhancement in other weak and strong combi-
nations.It was shown that life-long survival through enhancement
can be achieved regardless of whether additive non-H-1 differences
are present or not.The quality of survival in terms of kidney function and morphology,however,was definitely better when enhancement
across isolated H-1 took place (14).This section may then be concluded with the third statement:
3.As more antigenic sites are involved in a transplant combination,
   the more rejection predominates enhancement.

(AUTO-) ENHANCEMENT ACROSS NON-H-1 BARRIERS

When we started transplanting H-1-identical,non-H-1 different
Lewis and AS rats of the H-1^1 allele   several years ago, we happen-
ed to find almost indefinite survival times with only low grade
signs of cell infiltrations in the kidney grafts.No signs of immune
complex deposition were observed in these very compatible combina-
tions.We considered the fact that anti-donor antibodies could be
shown for long periods of time after transplantation to be suggestive evidence for autoenhancement (15).When we recently turned to an
other non-H-1 combination Lew.BN and BN, shown in Fig.2, a very unexpected observation was made.In spite of long survival of BN recipients with Lew.BN kidneys,moderate to heavy proteinuria deve-

loped during the first three months.The results were highly repro-
ducible.A typical immunecomplex glomerular disease of extra- and
endomembranous patterns (Fig.3) with positive intertubular capillaries (Fig.4) was found in the transplant by immunofluorescence.Al-
though it has been reported that immune deposits can be found in
transplants of human origin (16),this often is ·complicated by the
problem of recurrent disease and it rarely has been as pronounced
as in these rats.To the best of my knowledge a comparable immune
complex glomerulopathy for allografted rats has not yet been reported (17).It must be mentioned from other experiments in our laboratory that the same BN strain is resistant to the induction of
an autoimmune complex nephritis (STENGLEIN,THOENES,GÜNTHER,submit-
ted for publication).Therefore,it could be possible in principle
that the immune complexes found after kidney allografting in BN recipients constitute alloantigen immune complexes.The permanent confrontation of the recipient with a vital graft seems to be the prerequisite,since simple and continual presensitization with lymphoid
cell extracts does not produce the disease.Renal lesions in form of
immune deposits as sequela during a chronic graft-versus-host reaction have been shown in mice (18) and for a host-versus-graft syn-
drome as well (19).Very similarly,in this non-H-1 weakly incompatible combination Lew.BN → BN,kidney transplantation is obviously accompanied by the formation of (allo-?)antigen-antibody complexes.
The BN-immunoglobulin,acid-eluted from glomeruli,indeed showed a
positive reaction with Lew.BN (donor) lymphocytes but at the same
time with its own (BN,recipient's) lymphoid cells as well.This would
basicly mean that we are dealing with an autoimmune response against
cellular membrane antigens possibly of the nature of transplantation
antigens.This brings to mind the nuclear antigens in erythematodes
or the tubular cell antigen,all three being cellular substances and
the latter two clearly functioning as autoantigens leading to immune
complex glomerulonephritis.It is very likely that every type of au-
toantigen requires special conditions for autoimmunization.In the
postulated case of autoimmunization against transplantation antigens,it can be assumed that the continuing autoenhancement process
would be the right prerequisite in order to convert the strictly
alloantibody production into a general autoantibody response.Again
we should be reminded that this immune complex glomerulonephritis
depends on chronic transplantation reactions either of the GvH/
HvG-type as cited above or on the enhanced survival of kidneys
across non-H-1 differences. Regardless of whether or not autoimmunity is involved in addition to autoenhancement,it is difficult in
general to provide direct evidence for circulating immune complexes.
Therefore I regard this observation as valuable,"almost-direct" evidence for the immune complex mechanism involved in enhancement and
autoenhancement.
    The formation of transplantation antigen-immune complexes pro-
bably occurred in this case under unfavorable ag/ab-ratio conditions as far as the glomerular function is concerned.Glomerular
immune complex disease usually occurs with complexes formed in anti-

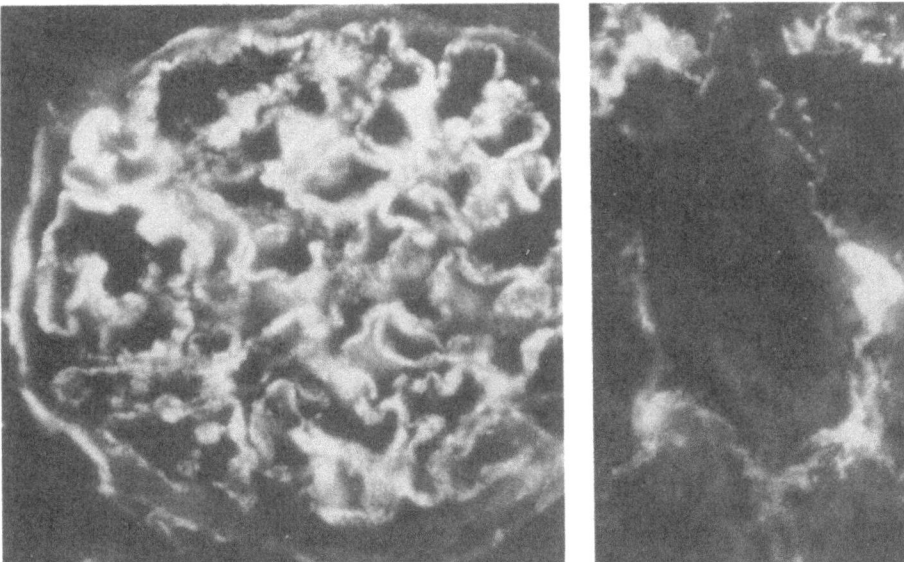

Fig.3.Transplant-Immunecomplex-Nephritis. Fig.4.Intertub.Capillaries
Positive immunofluorescence,Rat-IgG,Lew.BN → BN.

gen excess.Since complex deposition has not been observed in other
enhancement situations,it must be assumed that the regular enhancing immune complex is non-nephritogenic and possibly formed in antibody excess.Besides the fact that this observation has important
implications for using enhancement as a therapeutical mean in organ
transplantation,it has proved the occurrence of immune complexes in
long-surviving graft recipients whose survival is believed to be
due to autoenhancement.The following statements are:
4.There are indications that enhancement is caused by circulating
  immune complexes,at least,in part.
5.Under unfavorable conditions enhancement can lead to organ disease.

HAMSTER XENOGRAFTS IN RATS

     It may be of interest in this context of comparing "antigenic
strength" and enhanceability to ask whether the rat would also enhance the survival of a cross-species organ graft as closely related as possible.STEINMULLER (20) has shown that hamster skin on
newborn rats survived the longest compared with other xenogeneic
donors.And LANCE et al.(21) showed that "tolerant" mice retained
rat skin grafts in the continual presence of antirat antibodies.
This seems encouraging and indeed we found that rats survive with
hamster kidneys almost as long as with allografts (Fig.5).The
operation technique is somewhat complicated and bladder-to-bladder

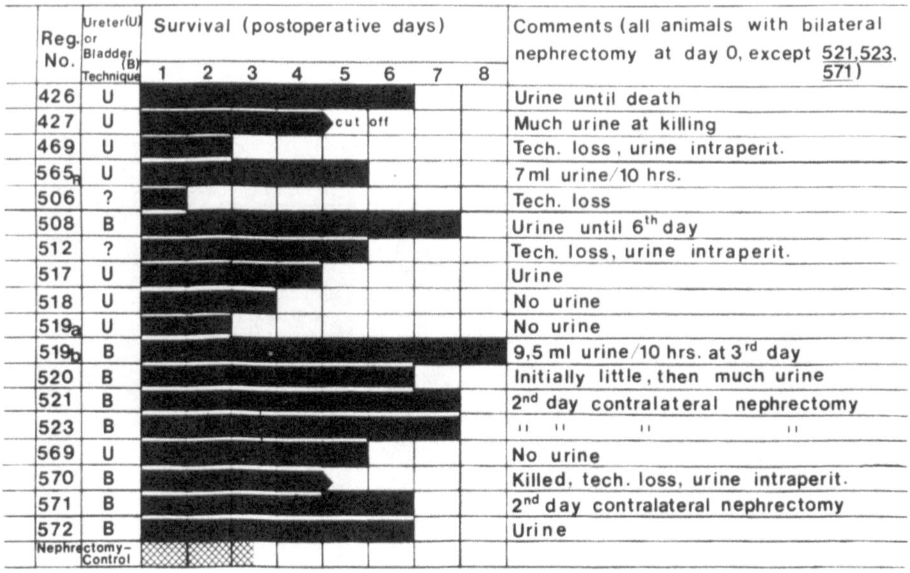

Reg. No.	Ureter(U) or Bladder(B) Technique	Survival (postoperative days) 1 2 3 4 5 6 7 8	Comments (all animals with bilateral nephrectomy at day 0, except 521,523, 571)
426	U		Urine until death
427	U	cut off	Much urine at killing
469	U		Tech. loss, urine intraperit.
565a	U		7 ml urine/10 hrs.
506	?		Tech. loss
508	B		Urine until 6th day
512	?		Tech. loss, urine intraperit.
517	U		Urine
518	U		No urine
519a	U		No urine
519b	B		9.5 ml urine/10 hrs. at 3rd day
520	B		Initially little, then much urine
521	B		2nd day contralateral nephrectomy
523	B		" " " "
569	U		No urine
570	B		Killed, tech. loss, urine intraperit.
571	B		2nd day contralateral nephrectomy
572	B		Urine
Nephrectomy-Control			

Fig.5.Hamster kidneys in rats,functioning up to 8 days post op.

anastomosis must be used sometimes.However,we have not as yet been successful in achieving prolonged survival by passive or active sensitization.No efforts have been made so far to use purified blocking antibodies.In the case of active sensibilization with a crude hamster lymphoid cell extract two weeks before transplantation, no urine production began and the vessels showed an intensive staining with anti-IgM and C3.In future experiments this model may be useful in finding out what the difference is between presensitization leading to accelerated rejection on the one hand and to graft enhancement on the other.

ALLOGRAFT ENHANCEMENT IN OTHER MAMMALIAN SPECIES

The intention of giving a survey of what enhancement can do in mammalia larger than rat and mouse has to take into account the fact that the prerequisites are very different from case to case with regard to operational details,kind,dosage and route of application of antigen and/or antibody,immunosuppression used additionally (ALG or drugs),evaluation of survival data and -last but not least- genetic heterogeneity of the animals.Nothing reliable is known about the role which a genetically determined responsiveness of the recipient might play in rejection and enhancement.Therefore a survey of selected data available up to now can only be of limited value.A very approximate measure is appropriate under those conditions in order to depict selected data from several authors (Fig.6).Three findings

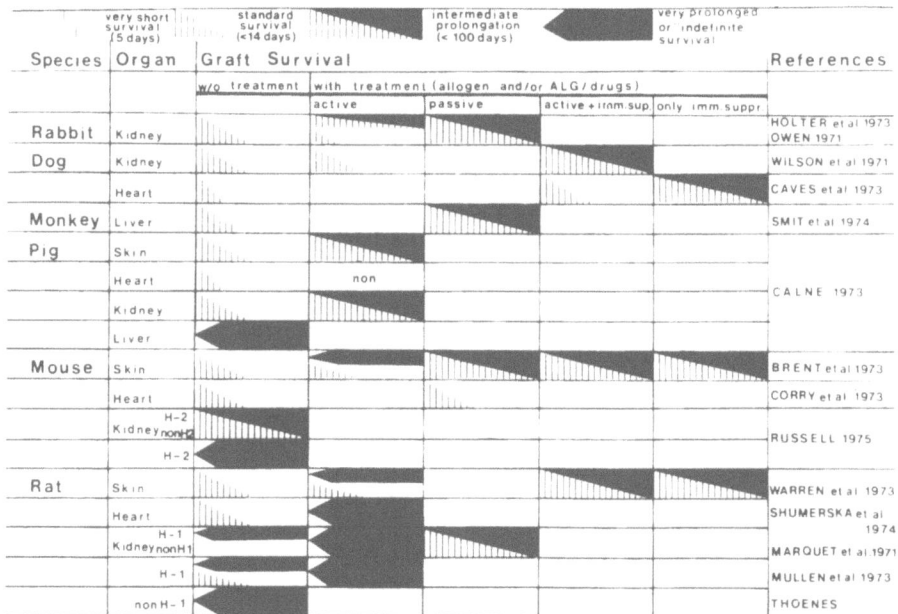

Fig.6.A rough information is given regarding enhancement success
       in other mammals,compared to rats.

may be deducted from these facts:
1.Although a significant prolongation of survival in larger grafted
animals can be achieved by active or passive enhancement or added
immunosuppression,"indefinite" survival has not been reached in ge-
neral.An exeption seems to be the liver in pigs which curiously
survives without any treatment.
2."Indefinite" or very prolonged survival is achieved mainly in
small inbred animals,rarely without,but in most cases with enhancement induction which is probably due to greater genetical homogeneity and better matched histocompatibilities.
3.In order to achieve better results with enhancement in larger
animals,we probably should investigate more systematically whether
best matched animals actually produce long survival times when
treated actively or passively with polyspecific antigens or antibodies,including immunosuppression,as has already been done in part
for pigs and monkeys (22,23).

    With respect to the phylogeny of the immunological system of
alloantigens and antibodies,the major issues seem to be "antigenic
strength" and"immune responsiveness".On the vertebrate level,
mammals and birds have developed the most divergent antigenic dis-
similarities.The concurrent development of enhancement capability,
being most effective against "weaker" antigenic differences,might
have caused a selective pressure for the expression of more or

"stronger" cellular determinants in order to maintain individuality. The differential state of immuneresponsiveness of individuals may also have to be interpreted in terms of survival advantage or disadvantage during the phylogeny of species.

1. Palm,J.,Transplantation Proc.,2:162(1970).
2. White,E.and Hildemann,W.H.,Transplantation Proc.,1:395(1969).
3. Fabre,J.W.and Morris,P.J.,Transplantation,14:634(1972).
4. Jenkins,A.McL.and Woodruff,M.F.,Transplantation,12:57(1971).
5. Kim,J.P.,Shaipanich,T.and al.,Transplantation,13:322(1972).
6. Ockner,S.A.,Guttmann,R.D.and al.,Transplantation,9:39(1970).
7. Marquet,R.L.,Heystek,G.A.and al.,Transplantation Proc.,3:708(1971).
8. Bitter-Suermann,H.,Transplantation,17:75(1974).
9. Salaman,J.R.,Elves,M.W.and al.,Transplantation Proc.,3:577(1971).
10. Hildemann,W.H.and Mullen,Y.,Transplantation,15:231(1973).
11. McKenzie,I.F.C.and Snell,G.D.,J.Exp.Med.,138:259(1973).
12. Wigzell,H.,Transplant.Rev.,3:86(1970).
13. Thoenes,G.H.,White,E.and al.,J.Immunol.,104:1447(1970).
14. Thoenes,G.H.,Urban,G.and al.,Immunogenetics,1:239(1974).
15. Thoenes,G.H.,White,E.,Transplantation,15:308(1973).
16. Hume,D.M.,Sterling,W.A.and al.,Transplantation Proc.,2:361(1970).
17. Mahabir,R.N.,Guttmann,R.D.and al.,Transplantation,8:369(1969).
18. Gleichmann,H.,Gleichmann,E.and al.,J.Exp.Med.,135:516(1972).
19. Hard,R.C.,Moncure,C.W.and al.,Lab.Invest.,28:468(1973).
20. Steinmuller,D.,Transplantation Proc.,2:438(1970).
21. Lance,E.M.,Levey,R.H.and al.,Proc.Nat.Ac.Sci.,64:1356(1969).
22. Calne,R.Y.,in:Immunological aspects of transplantation surgery, ed.by R.Calne,MTP,Lancaster,England,1973,p.296.
23. Smit,J.A.,Myburgh,J.A.,Transplantation,18:63(1974).
24. Wilson,R.E.,Maggs,P.R.and al.,Transplantation Proc.,3:705(1971).
25. Caves,P.K.,Dong,E.and al.,Transplantation,16:252(1973).
26. Warren,R.P.,Lofgreen,J.S.and al.,Transplantation,16:458(1973).
27. Brent,L.,Hansen,J.A.and al.,Transplantation,15:160(1973).
28. Holter,A.R.,Neu,M.R. and al.,Transplantation Proc.,5:593(1973).
29. Corry,R.J.,Winn,H.J.and al.,Transplantation Proc.,5:733(1973).
30. Russell,P.S.,Chase,C.M.and al.,Transplantation Proc.,7:345(1975).
31. Owen,E.R.,Transplantation Proc.,3:562(1971).
32. Shumerska,T.,Betel,I.and al.,Transplantation Proc.,3:708(1971).

Acknowledgements.I am grateful for the active cooperation and the kind support of Drs.H.Bazin,E.Günther,G.Hübner,K.Pielsticker, R.Roeßler, as well as of I.Döring,H.Gaitzsch,G.Schubert and G.Urban.The neat secretarial work of R.Hauser is especially acknowledged.
Supported by Deutsche Forschungsgemeinschaft,SFB 37,C 5.

MANY QUESTIONS (AND ALMOST NO ANSWERS) ABOUT THE

PHYLOGENETIC ORIGIN OF THE MAJOR HISTOCOMPATIBILITY COMPLEX

Jan Klein

Department of Microbiology, The University of Texas

Southwestern Medical School, Dallas, Texas 75235

WHAT IS MHC?

The major histocompatibility complex, MHC, (HL-A in man, H-2 in the mouse, RtH-1 in the rat, B in the chicken, etc.) can be defined on the basis of its involvement in four phenomena: allograft reaction in vivo, allograft reaction in vitro, genetic control of immune response, and genetic control of complement activity.

Allograft Reaction in vivo

In the mouse, there is a whole series (perhaps several hundreds) of histocompatibility (H) loci (1), and a difference between the donor and the recipient at any of these loci can lead to skin graft rejection, and presumably also to rejection of other tissue grafts. The cluster of loci forming the MHC leads to rapid rejection of skin grafts (usually within the first two weeks after transplantation), whereas a difference at any of the non-MHC (so-called minor) loci leads to delayed and often protracted rejection (usually not earlier than three weeks after grafting). However, this criterion for distinguishing major from minor H loci is not absolute. Recently, several H-2 mutations have been described which often allow prolonged survival of skin grafts exchanged between mice differing at the affected locus (2,3). For example, the mean survival time of skin grafts transplanted from $H-2^{bg1}$ donors to $H-2^b$ recipients, in a coisogenic situation, is 31 days and the range is from 14 to 59 days (3). This survival is actually longer than the survival of skin grafts transplanted across some minor H loci. For example, in the congenic combination C57BL/10 → B10.BY which represents an

H-1^C difference, the median survival time is 15 days with 95% confidence limits between 14 and 16 days (4). It thus appears that
the strength of the MHC is at least partially caused by its genetic
and immunological complexity, i.e., by the fact that the complex is
composed of several H loci, each of which controls antigens with
multiple determinants, and by the fact that these loci and these
determinants display a cumulative effect (5). However, the cumulative effect is clearly not the full explanation of MHC strength;
some qualitative difference between the MHC and non-MHC loci must
also exist.

Allograft Reaction in vitro

Cell-mediated lymphocytotoxicity (CML). So far, CML has been
demonstrated only across differences in the MHC; differences at
minor H loci, singular or multiple, do not lead to killing in the
CML assay. In this respect, CML might be the best test-system for
the detection of MHC differences. However, here too a word of
caution is appropriate for two reasons. First, no systematic
attempt has been made so far to explore the role of non-MHC differences in CML; it is possible that involvement of some minor H loci
in CML might still be discovered. Second, the CML assay, as
presently used, has been designed to detect MHC differences; it is
possible that different experimental conditions (e.g., different
length of stimulation, different target cells, etc.) might be required to detect CML against non-MHC antigens. After all, CML is
believed to be an in vitro form of the allograft reaction, and
allograft reaction is the test by which all H loci, major and minor,
are detected.

Lymphocyte activation can be achieved in vitro in the form of
mixed lymphocyte reaction (MLR) and in vivo in the form of graft-vs-
host reaction (GVHR). There is no doubt that in most cases differences at the MHC lead to strong lymphocyte activation, both in vitro
and in vivo. However, there is also no doubt that, in the mouse, at
least one non-MHC locus (Mls, cf. ref. 6) also leads to strong MLR.
Furthermore, in the mouse, significant involvement in MLR (7,8) and
GVHR (9) has been reported for several other non-MHC loci. Finally,
as in the case of CML, the optimal conditions for minor loci MLR or
GVHR might be different from those currently employed for the detection of MHC lymphocyte activation. Hence, clearly, lymphocyte
activation is not the prerogative of the MHC, although the MHC does
play a major role in it.

Genetic Control of Immune Response

There have been enough reports in different species of verte-

brates of the genetic control of the immune response by the MHC to
justify the use of this trait as a criterion for the definition of
the MHC. However, the genetic control of the immune response is by
no means solely the property of the MHC. A number of non-MHC linked
Ir genes have been described (for a review cf. ref. 10), and it is
clear that the immune response is a polygenically controlled trait.

Genetic Control of Complement Activity

It has been known for some time (11) that the H-2 complex is
closely linked to a serum protein gene (Ss), but this fact has
generally been considered as an evolutionary accident, unrelated to
the function of the complex. However, recently it has become known,
first, that the S region containing the Ss gene is somehow involved
in regulation of complement activity (12); and second, that the subunit structure of the Ss protein shows a certain similarity to the
structure of the H-2 molecule (13). Furthermore, most recent studies
in man (14) and rhesus monkey (15) suggest that genes regulating
complement activity are also associated with MHC's of these species.
Obviously, more comparative studies are needed before any generalizations can be made on the involvement of the MHC in complement-
associated functions, but the three documented cases at hand suggest
that such an involvement might eventually become another criterion
for the definition of the MHC. The possible MHC-complement connection
is the more attractive as it may also tie the MHC to the immunoglobulin system. Recent amino acid sequence data on the human C3a
component (16) indicate homology between this complement component
and immunoglobulin variable regions (D. J. Capra, personal communication) and thus suggest a common origin of at least some of comple-
ment-component-genes with immunoglobulin genes. Such homology can
then be extended also to the H loci of the MHC (see below).

Conclusion

It is apparent from the above discussion that no single criterion
adequately defines the MHC since each criterion alone can also be
applied to some non-MHC loci. However, taken together, the aforementioned criteria provide a reasonable basis for identification of
the MHC.

WHEN DID MHC EMERGE DURING EVOLUTION?

I shall attempt to answer this question by considering one by
one the phenomena defining the MHC.

Allograft Reaction in vivo

Tissue incompatibility reactions in the broadest sense probably
exist in all phyla of Metazoa. On the other hand, true allograft
reactions, i.e., reactions mediated by immunocytes capable of specific
recognition and development of immunological memory, can exist only
in species in which such immunocytes are present. The capacity to
mount an allograft reaction is probably developed in all classes of
Chordata, as well as in some of the higher invertebrates, particularly
Annelida and Echinodermata. However, the allograft reaction of invertebrates is relatively weak and of the chronic type. Strong acute
type of allograft reaction is a characteristic of all mammals and
birds, and some (but not others) amphibians, reptiles, and fishes.
Thus, among fishes, Teleostei reject skin grafts in acute fashion,
whereas Chondrostei reject grafts in a chronic fashion; among amphibians acute graft rejection is frequently observed in Anura and
chronic rejection in Urodela and Apoda (for a review see ref. 17).

To what extent the incompatibility reactions developing in the
absence of typical immunocytes can be considered predecessors of
allograft reactions is not known. However, as discussed below, some
of these reactions possess many features remarkably similar to those
characterizing allograft reactions (they were termed by Burnet "para-
immunological" reactions, see ref. 18).

In vitro Allograft Reactions

Of the two in vitro tests for allograft reactivity, CML, to my
knowledge, has not been demonstrated outside the class Mammalia; but
this is probably because of technical difficulties in setting up non-
mammalian CML assay. Such an assay should provide very useful data
on the evolution of the MHC. My prediction is that the presence or
absence of CML reactivity in different classes of vertebrates will
correlate closely with the strength of the allograft reaction in vivo,
i.e., species that can acutely reject grafts will also be able to
mount CML response in vitro.

The second of the in vitro tests, the MLR (and its in vivo
homologue, GVHR), should, by definition, be restricted to the animal
phyla with typical lymphocytes. I can foresee that, as the work on
lower vertebrates and invertebrates will progress, there undoubtedly
will be claims of in vitro lymphocyte stimulation in a great variety
of species. There will be problems regarding what to call a lymphocyte and what to call an MLR. I would expect, however, that like in
the case of the CML, the occurrence of classical MLR in different
species will again parallel the presence of acute graft rejection
in vivo. Preliminary studies (19) support this prediction.

Genetic Control of Immune Response

The MHC associated control of immune response can be studied at
two levels, humoral (by means of quantitating antibodies in the serum)
and cellular (by means of measuring delayed hypersensitivity reactions).
It is generally assumed, but not proven, that the genetic system controlling the two levels is the same. Measuring differences in the
antibody response is a more common way of asserting the presence of
Ir genes. By this assay, MHC-linked Ir genes have been demonstrated
in guinea pigs (20), mice (21), rats (22), chickens (23), monkeys (24),
and possibly man (25). My prediction is that they will be demonstrated
in all species with acute graft rejection, CML, and strong MLR. By
definition, they cannot be demonstrated in any of the species that do
not possess the immunoglobulin system, i.e., below the level of
vertebrates.

MHC Associated Complement Activities

Although the complement system is usually thought to have
developed in parallel with the immunoglobulin system, it is possible
that at least some of the complement components, particularly those
of the alternate pathway, are phylogenetically much older than immunoglobulins. Indeed, there is, for instance, evidence for the presence
of C3 proactivator in starfish hemolymph (26), in which typical
immunoglobulins have not been detected. The original function of
complement components might have been regulatory, and the lytic
function could have been acquired much later. Unfortunately, except
for the mouse (12), man (14), and the rhesus monkey (15), we know
nothing about the association of complement genes with MHC. Further
studies may well prove that these genes are among the oldest components of the major histocompatibility system.

Conclusion

The MHC seems to be present in all mammals and birds; it appears
to be absent in <u>Agnatha</u>; and apparently is present in some but absent
in other species of fishes, amphibia, and probably reptiles. Thus,
it appears to be of polyphyletic origin, developing simultaneously
in different classes of vertebrates. It can be expected, therefore,
that substantial differences will be found in the genetic organization of the MHC in different classes of animals.

WHAT MIGHT BE THE NATURAL FUNCTION OF THE MHC?

A discussion of a possible function of the MHC is beyond the
scope of this paper; I shall limit myself to a statement that at this
moment, of the many theoretical possibilities, a regulatory function

of the MHC seems to me the most appealing. According to this hypothesis, the MHC codes for a series of cell surface molecules which
regulate certain steps in cell differentiation. This differentiation
may involve transformation of a bone-marrow-derived (B) lymphocyte
into an antibody-producing plasma cell and transformation of a thymus-
derived (T) lymphocyte into an effector ("killer") cell. A detailed
description of this function will be presented elsewhere (27).

IS MHC RELATED TO ANY OTHER GENETIC SYSTEMS?

In the mouse, two systems recently have come under scrutiny as
possible genetic relatives of the MHC, namely, the immunoglobulin
system and the T/t complex.

The Immunoglobulin (Ig) System

Although there is no direct evidence for the evolutionary homology of the MHC and Ig systems, such homology is favored by many.
The circumstantial evidence suggesting genetic relationship between
the two systems is fourfold. First, on the cell surface the MHC
antigens are associated with β^2-microglobulin molecules (28), and
β^2-microglobulin is believed to represent a free domain of the Ig
molecule (29). Second, the MHC is functionally tied to the Ig
system via its control of antibody production by the Ir genes.
Third, Staphylococcus aureus protein A, known to bind exclusively
to the Fc region of immunoglobulin G, interacts in a similar way
with H-2 antigens (30). And fourth, there are claims of certain
similarities in the subunit structure of MHC and Ig molecules. Thus,
according to Peterson et al. (30), the H-2 and HL-A molecules are
tetramers with molecular weight of about 130,000 daltons, composed
of two light chains (β^2-microglobulin) and two heavy chains. The
heavy chains are held together by disulfide bridges and each chain
consists of three domains, each domain containing one disulfide
bridge.

The hypothesis that the MHC and the Ig systems are evolutionary
homologues is certainly attractive in many respects. But it must be
emphasized that the above cited evidence for the purported homology
is not unquestionable. The β^2-microglobulin is also known to be
associated with a series of other cell surface molecules (28), and
at present, one cannot rule out the possibility that the β^2-micro-
globulin molecules are merely some kind of nonspecific stabilizing
factor of most membrane proteins. With regard to the linkage of the
Ir genes to the MHC, one must keep in mind that the mechanism of the
Ir gene action is not known; once the mechanism becomes known, we all
might be surprised how little it has to do with the Ig genes themselves. As for the biochemical evidence, we have heard so many
claims about MHC biochemistry that many of us have learned to take up

a "wait and see" position to any new claims. However, if one is an
optimist, one may want to speculate that the two systems, MHC and Ig,
indeed have a common evolutionary origin, and that a considerable
degree of homology between the systems has still been preserved.
One can go even one step further and hypothesize when the separation
of the MHC and Ig systems might have occurred. According to Ohno (31),
the vertebrate ancestors underwent at least one round of tetraploidi-
zation resulting in the doubling of their genomes. One can still
observe direct consequences of this event in contemporary fishes and
amphibians. One of the genetic complexes doubled during the tetra-
ploidization process might have been the MHC ancestor, and after the
doubling, one set of genes on one pair of chromosomes might have
evolved into the Ig system, and the other set on another pair of
chromosomes into the MHC. Most likely, even before the doubling,
the MHC ancestor was already a complex rather than a single gene.
Further divergence of the doubled complexes might have occurred by
intrachromosomal duplication. If one wants to carry this <u>Glasperlen-
spiel</u> still further, one can postulate an evolutionary homology
between the Mls locus (6) and the MHC, and the origin of Mls from
the archetypal MHC gene by detached gene duplication. The sequence
of events can then be visualized as shown in Fig. 1.

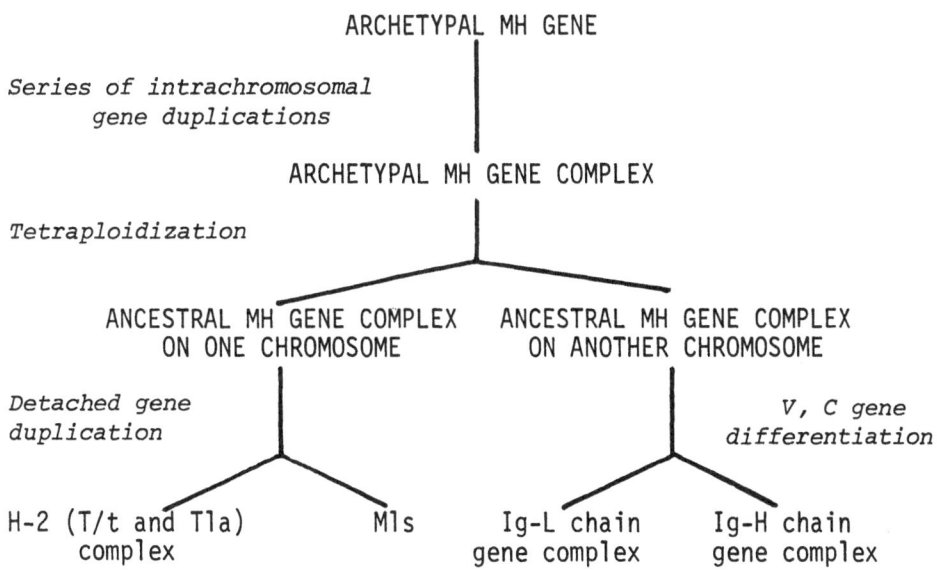

Fig. 1 *Highly speculative interpretation of presumed homologies
between H-2, Mls, and Ig systems.*

The T/t System

Although an evolutionary homology between T/t and H-2 systems
was postulated 5 years ago (32), the postulate has been taken more
seriously only very recently, primarily because of three new developments that point out a definite relationship between the two systems.
First, Bennett and her coworkers demonstrated (33) that, like H-2,
the T/t genes are also expressed on the cell surface. Second,
Vitetta and her coworkers showed (34) that the product of at least
one of the t genes is amazingly similar in its subunit structure
and molecular weight to the products of the H-2 loci. Third,
Hammerberg and Klein (35) provided evidence for a relationship
between the H-2 and t systems at the population level.

If indeed there is homology between the H-2 and T/t systems,
one would expect that it dates very far back on the evolutionary
scale, almost certainly prior to the emergence of <u>Chordates</u>. One
can fit the relationship between the two systems into the scheme
in Fig. 1 by postulating that the archetypal MH gene underwent a
series of intrachromosomal duplications producing a long stretch
of homologous genes. A functional differentiation then occurred
along this string of duplicated genes and resulted in specialization
and diversification into several gene clusters, one of them being
the MHC (H-2).

WHAT MIGHT HAVE BEEN THE FUNCTION OF THE MH ARCHETYPAL GENE?

Ohno (31) postulated that vertebrates carry only very few (if
any) genes whose ancestors did not exist among lower animal species.
And indeed, some of the vertebrate genes can be traced back to the
most primitive forms of life. Thus, for instance, genetic homologues of hemoglobin genes were found in plants (36), suggesting
that a common ancestor of these genes existed before the separation
of the animal and plant kingdoms. The evolution of hemoglobin genes
through the animal kingdom is well documented (37).

It seems, therefore, reasonable to postulate that archetypal MH
genes existed long before the actual emergence of the MHC in vertebrates. What might have been the function of these genes? Since we
do not know the true function of the MHC, an attempt to answer this
question is unlikely to succeed. However, one is tempted to speculate that there might be more than superficial resemblance between
the vertebrate MHC and invertebrate incompatibility systems, as has
been first suggested by Burnet (38). Incompatibility systems have
been demonstrated in a great number of species, both animal and
plant (for a review, see ref. 39). I find particularly striking
the resemblance to the MHC of the incompatibility system in a fungus

Schizophyllum commune, a representative of the Basidiomycetes.
The haploid spore of this fungus germinates to produce a mold-like
mycelium made up of filaments of uninucleate cells (homokaryon).
When two homokaryotic filaments grow together, their cells can fuse
and form a dikaryon with each cell carrying two nuclei. The dikaryon constitutes a prerequisite to sexual reproduction of the
fungus. However, the fusion between two filaments can occur only
if the corresponding mycelia belong to different mating types with
the recognition of the proper mate being controlled by two sets of
incompatibility factors, A and B (for a review, see ref. 40). The
A set of incompatibility factors is controlled by two closely linked
loci, α and β, which are expressed on the cell surface. Each gene
has a pleiomorphic effect, affecting not only cell-compatibility but
also further differentiation and morphogenesis of the dikaryon (if
fusion occurs). The α and β loci are extremely polymorphic: at
least 9 alleles have been identified at the α locus, and 32 alleles
at the β locus. Thus, approximately 9 x 32 = 288 different A factors
can exist in natural population. The α and β genes appear to have
been derived by gene duplication from a common ancestral gene.

The resemblance of the incompatibility system of S. commune to
the vertebrate MHC system is manifold. Both systems code for cell
surface structures involved in tissue (cell) compatibility reactions;
in both cases there are two closely linked genetic regions controlling the cell surface products; the two regions appear to be homologous in their origin and were most likely derived from one
ancestral gene; and finally both the fungi incompatibility system
and the vertebrate MH system are highly polymorphic.

I am fully aware of the danger of drawing evolutionary
homologies on the basis of superficial resemblances. Such resemblances might be coincidental or they might be the result of an
evolutionary convergence. Nevertheless, the temptation is almost
too great to be resisted. Somewhat safer would be to speculate
that the MHC precursor was a gene expressed on the cell surface
and somehow involved in differentiation, perhaps as a regulatory
gene providing "on" and "off" signals for cell growth and for
elimination of unwanted cells. If the gene was also a precursor
for the Ig system, then one might speculate further that its
product was a molecule with a molecular weight of some 12,000 daltons and consisted of some 100 amino acid residues (corresponding
to a gene for one Ig domain). These gene then repeatedly duplicated
and different sets of the duplicated genes either fused or were
placed under the control of a single regulating genetic element.
Three or four such genes might have been needed to produce what is
now known as the H-2K (or alternatively H-2D) locus in the H-2
system of the mouse.

WHAT MIGHT HAVE BEEN THE STIMULUS FOR THE DEVELOPMENT OF MHC?

If all invertebrates and primitive vertebrates can do without the MHC, why do the more advanced vertebrates need it? What changes in the life-style of higher vertebrates required development of such a complicated genetic system? Burnet (41) suggested two possible reasons for the development of the MHC. One reason was protection against parasitism on one's own kind. When free-swimming marine provertebrates ancestral to cyclostomes first appeared, they were exposed to a danger of parasitism by their own young or by related species. This danger provided an urgent demand for the development of a more sophisticated capacity to recognize the difference between self and non-self and thus led to the emergence of the MHC. The second reason, was a protection against parasitism by an embryo on its own mother. According to Burnet "when a living embryo is nourished in the tissues of the parent, the situation is barely distinguishable from parasitism, and oscillation between a controlled situation and uncontrolled parasitism must have occurred not infrequently" (36). Therefore, "the first evolutionary task of the free-swimming progenitors of the vertebrates was to devise a way of recognizing whether a group of living cells within its body was self or not-self" (36). However, it seems to me that, if anything, the opportunity of turning into intraspecies parasite was even greater in invertebrates than in vertebrates, and yet, the invertebrates apparently did not need the MHC to prevent this from happening. Similarly, the MHC is well developed in birds where the danger of an embryo becoming a parasite on its mother is minimal.

I would like to suggest, therefore, that there was a more prosaic reason for the emergence of the MHC. In comparison to invertebrates, the vertebrate body in general is bigger, far more complex, and its tissues and organs are far more specialized. In particular, the circulatory system achieved a degree of sophistication not known before. It rapidly disseminates its content throughout the body, to the very finest and most sensitive areas. All this complexity and elaborateness makes the vertebrate body extremely vulnerable to attacks by parasites, particularly microorganisms. The very efficient circulatory system can spread in a very short time invading organisms into the remotest corner of the body. Under these circumstances the inefficient non-specific defense mechanisms of the invertebrates became totally inadequate for vertebrates. There was a need for a dynamic, specific defense mechanism which would effectively cope with the new situation. The first step toward such a mechanism was the emergence of the primitive immunoglobulin system such as that known in contemporary primitive vertebrates. However, soon even this system was not enough and there was a need for amplifying and regulatory mechanism that would increase the effectiveness of the Ig system. This mechanism was provided by the MHC. At the same time, the Ig system itself was developing toward a higher degree of sophistication by improving its own molecules and by developing close ties with the complement system. The result of all these improvements was a very elaborate, but very efficient, supersystem of which the MHC is only one part.

ACKNOWLEDGEMENTS

The author's experimental work cited in this communication was supported by grants AI11879 and AI11650 from the National Institutes of Health. I thank Drs. James Forman and Donald J. Capra for critical reading of the manuscript and Ms. JoAnne Tuttle for her secretarial assistance.

REFERENCES

1. Snell, G. D., Immunogenetics, 1:1(1974).
2. Klein, J., Hauptfeld, V., and Hauptfeld, M., in L. Brent and J. Holborow (eds.) Progress in Immunology II, Vol. 3, p. 197. (North-Holland Publ. Co., Amsterdam, 1974).
3. Melief, C. J. M., Schwartz, R. S., Kohn, H. I., and Melvold, R. W., Immunogenetics, in press, 1975.
4. Graff, R. J., Hwldemann, W. H., and Snell, G. D., Transplantation, 4:425(1966).
5. Klein, J., Folia Biol. (Praha), 12:168(1966).
6. Festenstein, H., Transplantation, 18:555(1974).
7. Adler, W. H., Takiguchi, T., Marsh, B., and Smith, R. T., J. Immunol., 105:984(1970).
8. Mangi, R. J. and Mardiney, M. R., J. Immunol. 105:90(1970).
9. Cantrell, J. L. and Hildemann, W. H., Transplantation, 14:761 (1972).
10. Klein, J., Biology of the Mouse Hsstocompatibility-2 Complex. (Springer-Verlag, New York, 1975).
11. Shreffler, D. C., Genetics, 49:973(1964).
12. Hinzová, E., Démant, P., and Iványi, P., Folia Biol. (Praha), 18:237(1972).
13. Capra, D. J., Vitetta, E. S., and Klein, J., J. Exp. Med., submitted 1975.
14. Fu, S. M., Kunkel, H. G., Brusman, H. P., Allen, F. H. Jr. and Fotino, M., J. Exp. Med., 140:1108(1974).
15. Ziegler, J. B., Alper, C. A., and Balner, H., Nature 254:609 (1975).
16. Hugli, T. E., Vallota, E. H., and Müller-Eberhard, H. J., J. Biol. Chem., 250:1472(1975).
17. Cohen, N. and Borysenko, M., Transplant. Proc., 2:333(1970).
18. Burnet, F. M., Contemp. Topics Immunobiol., 4:13(1974).
19. Cooper, E. L. and DuPasquier, L., in L. Brent and J. Holborow, (eds.) Progress in Immunology II, Vol. 2, p. 301 (North-Holland Publ. Co., Amsterdam, 1974).

20. Ellman, L., Green, I., Martin, W. J., and Benacerraf, B.,
    Proc. Nat. Acad. Sci. USA, 66:322 (1970).
21. McDevitt, H. O. and Chinitz, A., Science, 163:1207(1969).
22. Günther, E., Rüde, E., and Stark, O., Eur. J. Immunol.,
    2:151(1972).
23. Günther, E., Balcarová, J., Hála, K., Rüde, E., and Hraba, T.,
    Eur. J. Immunol., 4:548(1974).
24. Dorf, M. E., Balner, H., deGroot, M. L., and Benacerraf, B.,
    Transplant. Proc. 6:119(1974).
25. Levine, B. B., Stember, R. H., and Fotino, M., Science,
    178:1201(1972).
26. Day, E. in L. Brent and J. Holborow (eds.): Progress in
    Immunology II, vol. 2, p. 288 (North-Holland Publ. Co.,
    Amsterdam, 1974).
27. Klein, J., Contemp. Topics Immunobiol., in press 1975.
28. Neauport-Sautes, C., Bismuth, A., Kourilsky, F. M., and
    Manuel, Y., J. Exp. Med., 139:957(1974).

29. Peterson, P. A., Cunningham, B. A., Berggard, I., and
    Edelman, G. M., Proc. Nat. Acad. Sci. USA, 69:1647(1972).
30. Peterson, P. A., Rask, L., Sege, K., Klareskog, L., Anundi,
    H., and Ostberg, L., Proc. Nat. Acad. Sci. USA 72:1612(1975).
31. Ohno, S., Evolution by Gene Duplication (Springer-Verlag,
    Heidelberg, 1970).
32. Gluecksohn-Waelsh, S. and Erickson, R. P., Cur. Topics.
    Devel. Biol., 5:281(1970).
33. Bennett, D., Boyse, E. A., and Old, L. J., in L. G. Silvestri
    (ed): Cell Interactions, p. 247 (North-Holland Publ. Co.,
    Amsterdam, 1972).
34. Vitetta, E. S., AVtzt, K., Bennett, D., Boyse, E. A., and
    Jacob, F., Proc. Nat. Acad. Sci. USA, in press 1975.
35. Hammerberg, C. and Klein, J. Nature, submitted 1975.
36. Ellfolk, N. and Sievers, G., Acta Chem. Scand., 25:3532(1971).
37. Goodman, M., Moore, G. W., and Matsuda, G., Nature, 253:603
    (1975).
38. Burnet, F. M., Nature, 232:230(1971).
39. Esser, K. and Blaich, R., Adv. Genetics, 17:107(1973).
40. Koltin, Y., Stamberg, J., and Lemke, P. A., Bacteriol. Rev.,
    36:156(1973).
41. Burnet, F. M., Acta Pathol., Microbiol. Scand., 76:1(1969).